Contents

The Effectiveness of Rehabilitation for Cognitive Deficits

Edited by
Peter W. Halligan
Department of Psychology
Cardiff University

and

Derick T. Wade
Oxford Centre for Enablement
University of Oxford

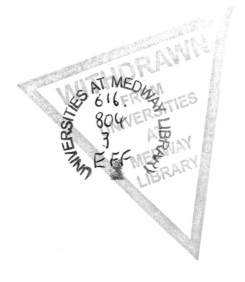

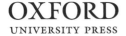

OXFORD
UNIVERSITY PRESS

OXFORD

UNIVERSITY PRESS

Great Clarendon Street, Oxford OX2 6DP

Oxford University Press is a department of the University of Oxford.
It furthers the University's objective of excellence in research, scholarship,
and education by publishing worldwide in

Oxford New York

Auckland Cape Town Dar es Salaam Hong Kong Karachi
Kuala Lumpur Madrid Melbourne Mexico City Nairobi
New Delhi Shanghai Taipei Toronto

With offices in

Argentina Austria Brazil Chile Czech Republic France Greece
Guatemala Hungary Italy Japan South Korea Poland Portugal
Singapore Switzerland Thailand Turkey Ukraine Vietnam

Oxford is a registered trade mark of Oxford University Press
in the UK and in certain other countries

Published in the United States
by Oxford University Press Inc., New York

© Oxford University Press, 2005

The moral rights of the author have been asserted

Database right Oxford University Press (maker)

First published 2005

Reprinted 2006

A catalogue record for this title is available from the British Library

Library of Congress Cataloging in Publication Data

(Data available)

ISBN 0-19-8526547
        978-019-852654-4

10 9 8 7 6 5 4 3 2

Typeset by Cepha Imaging (P) Ltd., Bangalore, India
Printed in Great Britain
on acid-free paper by Biddles Ltd., King's Lynn

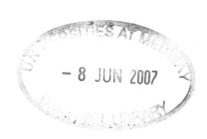

Acknowledgements

The editors would like to acknowledge the support offered by The Rivermead Development Fund, Departments of Medicine at Maastricht University, The Lewis Family Trust and Brain Injury Rehabilitation Trust for the conference that this book is based on.

We would also like to thank Hadyn Ellis, Udo Kischka, Mansel Aylward, Robert McCrum, Kath Little, Sue Dentten, Lorraine Woods, and Laura Morris for their advice and assistance all of which facilitated the conference and this subsequent book.

Finally we would also like to thank the staff at Oxford University Press.

The painting of the flowers in the cover illustration is taken from a painting by Peggy Palmer after her stroke in 1989.

List of contributors

Erica Barbuto — York University, Toronto ON, Canada.

Anna Basso — Department of Neurological Sciences, University of Milan, Milan, Italy.

Veronica Bradley — Hurstwood Park Neurological Centre, Haywards Heath, UK.

Ruth Brunsdon — Macquarie Centre for Cognitive Science, Macquarie University, Sydney, Australia.

Paul W. Burgess — Institute of Cognitive Neuroscience, UCL (University College, London), UK.

Nancy Carney — Div of Medical Informatics, Oregon Health and Science University, Portland OR, USA.

Keith D. Cicerone — JFK-Johnson Rehabilitation Institute, Edison NJ, USA.

Linda Clare — School of Psychology, University of Wales Bangor, Bangor, UK.

Max Coltheart — Macquarie Centre for Cognitive Science, Macquarie University, Sydney, Australia.

John R. Crawford — School of Psychology, King's College, University of Aberdeen, Aberdeen, UK.

Hugo du Coudray — Div of Medical Informatics, Oregon Health and Science University, Portland OR, USA.

Jonathan J. Evans — Dept of Psychological Medicine, University of Glasgow, Glasgow, UK.

Elizabeth L. Glisky — Dept of Psychology, University of Arizona, Tucson AZ, USA.

Peter W. Halligan — School of Psychology, Cardiff University, Cardiff, UK.

Julie D. Henry — School of Psychology, University of New South Wales, Sydney, Australia.

Argye E. Hillis — Dept of Neurology, Johns Hopkins Hospital, Baltimore MD, USA.

David Howard — School of Education, Communication and Language Sciences, University of Newcastle, Newcastle upon Tyne, UK.

Narinder Kapur — Dept of Neuropsychology, Addenbrooke's Hospital, Cambridge, UK.

Nadina Lincoln — School of Psychology, University of Nottingham, Nottingham, UK.

Hans J. Markowitsch — Dept of Psychology, University of Bielefeld, Bielefeld, Germany.

Jane Marshall — Department of Language and Communication Science, City University, London, UK.

Catherine A. Mateer — Dept of Psychology, University of Victoria, Victoria BC, Canada.

Lyndsey Nickels — Macquarie Centre for Cognitive Science, Macquarie University, Sydney, Australia.

Norman W. Park — York University, Toronto ON, Canada.

George Prigatano — Dept of Clinical Neuropsychology, Barrow Neurological Institute, Phoenix AZ, USA.

Ian H. Robertson	Dept of Psychology, Trinity College, Dublin, Ireland.
Jon S. Simons	Institute of Cognitive Neuroscience, UCL (University College, London), UK.
McKay Moore Sohlberg	Ph. D. Communication Disorders and Sciences, University of Oregon, Eugene OR, USA.
Joke M. Spikman	Neuropsychology Unit, University Hospital Groningen, Groningen, The Netherlands.
Elizabeth Styles	St Edmund Hall, Oxford University, Oxford, UK.
Adriaan H. van Zomeren	Neuropsychology Unit, University Hospital Groningen, Groningen, The Netherlands.
Derick T. Wade	Oxford Centre for Enablement, Oxford, UK.
Barbara A. Wilson	MRC- Cognition and Brain Sciences Unit, Cambridge, UK.
Andrew Worthington	Brain Injury Rehabilitation Trust, West Heath, Birmingham, UK.

Introduction

Is rehabilitation of cognitive deficits effective?

Thousands of rehabilitation professionals worldwide treat millions of people with acquired brain damage. Rehabilitation covers a wide range of interdisciplinary interventions and today extends beyond traditional medical care, but in this book we focus on one important and definable component of neurological rehabilitation, namely *cognitive rehabilitation*. Although neurological rehabilitation has long undertaken treatments aimed at physical deficits, it is generally recognized that many disabilities are not the sole consequence of the structural damage but reflect the interaction of the cognitive, psychosocial, emotional, and economic circumstances of the person.

In particular, cognitive deficits after brain damage often militate against full recovery to a greater extent than more obvious physical deficits. Recognition of this, and the growing developments in the cognitive neurosciences has led to an exponential growth of cognitive rehabilitation over the past 25 years, and to the assumption that there are now established cognitive-based therapies which are effective in treating or alleviating their functional consequences.

Unlike more observable neurological losses (e.g. hemiparesis), cognitive disorders do not always represent a naturally identifiable type of problem. The emergence of 'cognitivism' in the 1950s as the dominant approach in psychology, and later cognitive neuropsychology in the 1970s revitalized the diagnosis and rehabilitation of patients with acquired brain damage by providing a conceptual framework that helped explain the myriad of high level deficits that followed brain damage.

This advance was clinically useful in refining diagnosis and informed normal functional models. It was not long however before cognitive neuropsychology also began to influence treatments for rehabilitation. In 1989, Sohlberg and Mateer's now classic text helped locate cognitive rehabilitation alongside more established rehabilitation approaches. They reported an assembly of therapies that attempt to retrain, alleviate, or compensate for the deficits caused by selective cognitive impairments (e.g. Prigatano 1999; Basso, Cappa and Gainotti 2000; Wood and Fussey 1999; Ponsford, Sloan and Snow 1995; Fleminger and Powell 1999; Riddoch and Humphreys 1994; Ellis and Christensen 1989; Wilson 2003).

At the same time there have been several big advances in neurological rehabilitation over the last 25 years. The most important has been the development of a better model to analyse the genesis of disability (now termed activity limitation), the modified WHO ICF model (see chapter four, and Wade and Halligan 2004).

The conference that inspired this book was based on the modified WHO ICF model, a model that looks beyond impairment to the functional consequences of that impairment and the ways in which associated disability can be minimised for the individual. Hence we refer specifically and deliberately to rehabilitation for (patients with) cognitive deficits.

Many of the authors base their chapters on the model, distinguishing between impairment of cognitive functions (which typically implies little about consequence) and the resultant changes in behaviour, now called changes in activities but more normally referred to as disabilities. The model also emphasizes that there are not 'cognitive disabilities', but there are disabilities that are related to and caused by cognitive impairments.

A third big advance over the last 25 years has been in the quality and quantity of research into many aspects of rehabilitation, including the effectiveness of treatments aimed to reduce the problems arising from cognitive losses. Earlier studies were often hampered by a lack of appropriate control groups, inadequate assessment measures, failure to consider confounding variables such as pre-injury history and status, time since injury, ongoing treatments, the psychosocial environment, poor sampling techniques, inappropriate statistical analyses and so on (Robertson 1993; Winocur et al. 2000).

Now randomized, controlled studies are widely used in medical rehabilitation research, and are (despite all contrary comments) still the best method of evaluating interventions when they can be used. While the small number of randomized, controlled trials of cognitive rehabilitation have an important role in evaluating the effectiveness of cognitive rehabilitation, in reviewing the current evidence base this book draws primarily (but not exclusively) upon evaluations using single-subject designs, retrospective, controlled, and uncontrolled comparative group studies.

Fourthly, the enormous advances in computer technology have made it practical to undertake both systematic searches of the published literature and often meta-analysis of the published data. Consequently many (but by no means all) studies relating to a specific topic can be identified and firm conclusions can be drawn from the results, conclusions that are often not apparent when looking at all the studies individually. This book draws upon systematic reviews and meta-analyses.

Effectiveness

There were several reasons for focusing on the effectiveness of rehabilitation for cognitive deficits. First there is the growing increase in patients recognized as suffering from cognitive deficits. Rehabilitation professionals increasingly encounter such patients, and the consequences of these deficits are not trivial. Many therapists feel uncertain about the best way to help their patients. This is especially so because there has been an explosion of research into rehabilitation for people with cognitive problems, but busy clinical staff cannot hope to keep up-to-date with it. Evidence suggests that clinicians who recognise the need for information do not always access the most reliable and least biased sources (Smith 1996). Consequently they may consider that they are failing to help their patients, believing from optimistic publications that there are well-established and effective treatments.

Over the past decade, however, dissenting voices have been raised regarding the usefulness of the cognitive neuropsychological approach as a model for planning rehabilitation interventions. Despite a relatively better grounded theoretical basis than most other forms of rehabilitation, there is little agreement as to whether these theories work, and several large systematic reviews of cognitive rehabilitation have failed to confirm its effectiveness in treating and alleviating the functional consequences of cognitive disorders.

In 1997 (and later in 2002 and 2004) the Technology Evaluation Centre (TEC) Assessments (informing parts of the US's health insurance industry) concluded that there was inadequate data from the published peer-reviewed literature to validate the effectiveness of cognitive rehabilitation either as an isolated treatment, or even as a component of a multimodal rehabilitation program. It is also unclear whether the cognitive approach has actually changed therapeutic practice to any great extent. Even where cognitive interventions have been shown to work, it is not always clear how such 'therapies' might actually work.

Although evidence supports several forms of cognitive rehabilitation, some researchers have argued that cognitive neuropsychology lacks an adequate theory of rehabilitation capable of providing a general guide for effective and functionally relevant treatments (Caramazza 1989; Baddeley 1993; Basso 1989; Caramazza and Hillis 1993). Attempts to consider and develop this crucial link have recently begun (Caramazza and Hillis 1993; Baddeley 1993; Shallice 2000) and this book will facilitate this refocusing of cognitive neuropsychological efforts on the clinical relevant issues of remediation effectiveness.

The apparent gap between neuropsychological theory and effective clinical practice provides one of the driving forces behind this book. In appraising the merits or weaknesses of potential treatments, we also recognized the need to situate these questions within the wider context of the conceptual and theoretical models used, and the operational definitions used to define cognitive deficits; how do normal cognitive processing systems operate, how are they instantiated in the brain, and how are these matters are measured? Moreover, as Prigatano points out in chapter 1, 'we are not only asking how effective cognitive rehabilitation is, we are asking the worth of cognitive rehabilitation from the perspective of patients, families, and society'.

Consequently, we set out to collect and collate such information in this book. The principles adopted were simple. Contributions to the book should:

- Be based on systematically acquired evidence wherever possible
- Acknowledge uncertainty openly, not making dogmatic statements without supporting evidence
- Cover important, common clinical problems
- Review the basic science relating to unimpaired cognitive functioning, giving a theoretical basis based on anatomy, pharmacology and physiology as appropriate and known
- Review the detection and measurement of specific cognitive deficits
- Review treatments aimed at the level of impairment
- Review treatments aimed directly at behaviour (disability)

In order to achieve this we approached people who were excellent in their field, were capable of taking a critical point of view, and could review the evidence thoroughly.

The book is divided into 7 sections. The first part of the book provides the relevant context, both historical and theoretical. Without a context it is difficult to evaluate any information. Prigatano reviews how brain injuries sustained in war have provided great stimulus both to the theoretical foundations of neuropsychology, and to some of the early formulations of the process of rehabilitation. Coltheart draws attention to the conceptual and operational differences between cognitive-neuropsychological rehabilitation and cognitive rehabilitation. The former are characterized by their reliance on cognitive models of the impaired processing system for assessment and treatment, emphasis on restoration rather than compensation, and capacity to deal with acquired and developmental disorders. Mateer describes the major conceptual approaches for working with individuals with acquired cognitive impairments, and provides guidelines for selecting effective intervention strategies. Finally, Wade advocates the use of WHO ICF model when thinking about cognitive rehabilitation, and shows how research into effectiveness needs to consider careful study of both individual patients and group studies.

In considering the effectiveness of cognitive rehabilitation it was not possible or sensible to consider all cognitive domains and hence we targeted four well established and common cognitive deficits: attention, memory, language, and executive functions found after brain damage. We were well aware that these domains are not easily distinguished in clinical practice, and that they are interrelated and interdependent, but nonetheless they appeared sufficiently separate in the literature to warrant separate discussion.

If cognitive rehabilitation is to provide a basis for rehabilitation, then the first step is to clarify the nature of the normal cognitive process and where these processes take place in the brain. Consequently, each of the four common deficits have introductory chapters which hopefully provide useful reminders of the functional (i.e. cognitive neuropsychological) and anatomical (i.e. cognitive neuro-science) descriptive overview of the cognitive process involved.

For cognitive rehabilitation to be successful it must be based on knowledge of the individual patient's cognitive strengths and weaknesses as operationally defined in terms of task performance. Accordingly, we wished to review the available methods and tests used to detect deficits and quantify subsequent improvements. This is especially important because the interpretation of research is often dependent upon the nature of the data collection tools used. For example, apraxia in one specific study will be defined (usually) by the specific test used, which may not be measuring the same phe-nomenon as the apraxia investigated in a second specific study which uses a different specific test.

The conceptual and assessment reviews are followed by a comparison between two different approaches to treatment – interventions aimed at altering the cognitive impairment itself, and inter-ventions aimed more broadly at reducing the activity limitations seen in association with cognitive losses. Although somewhat artificial in terms of the WHO ICF model, it remains an important and realistic distinction given the historical and behavioural indices currently used and evidence available.

The reviews suggest that evidence exists describing the efficacy of some forms of cognitive rehabilita-tion. However, some researchers have argued that cognitive neuropsychology lacks an adequate theory of rehabilitation capable of providing a guide for effective and functionally relevant treatments.

Therefore, in the penultimate section, Robertson shows how progress in neuroscience provides us with an opportunity to place the rehabilitation of brain damage on a more scientific basis based upon experience-dependent plasticity of the adult brain. In a related chapter, Hillis suggests that a useful theory of cognitive rehabilitation will require several features including a model of the cognitive pro-cesses underlying the task; a proposal regarding the underlying neural mechanisms and how changes are effected; and finally an account of how neuroplasticity is influenced by pharmacological agents.

Many patients with brain damage present with multiple and no doubt interacting cognitive deficits depending on the nature and extent of the pathological insult, and hence we felt it necessary, and useful, in the last section of the book to consider the effectiveness of rehabilitation for patients with three common pathologies (diseases) – stroke, traumatic brain injury, and neurodegenerative dementia (Alzheimer's disease).

Although further research has been published since the conference in September 2002, the thrust of the conference and the book remain substantially unchanged. The underlying anatomy and neuro-physiological facts have seen new developments using imaging techniques such as fMRI and MEG, and new findings from cognitive neuroscience are making a significant contribution to the develop-ment of a scientific basis for the practise of neurorehabilition in general (Roberston 1999; Taub, Uswatte and Elbert 2002; Nadeau 2002). Evidence still supports the general conclusion that the prac-tice of tasks limited by cognitive deficits does improve activity performance, but there is less evidence to support the general use of specific training of underlying cognitive skill.

What is changing is the realization that cognitive rehabilitation comprises one part of a much larger rehabilitation exercise, where the effectiveness of any specific treatment is determined by the complex interaction of several factors including local service provision, and overcoming the psychosocial barriers that society and the patient bring to the rehabilitation process.

The challenge for cognitive neuropsychology remains whether it is capable of moving beyond the initial success of diagnostic specificity to developing an equally rich theory of rehabilitation that can inform and explain effective clinical treatments. Although much of this book is informed by the avail-ability of such research evidence, progress in cognitive rehabilitation must also be driven by identifying important clinically relevant questions and where necessary initiating the research lead.

Professor Peter W Halligan, Cardiff University
Professor Derick T Wade, Oxford University
April 2005

References

Baddeley, A. D. (1993). A theory of rehabilitation without a model of learning is a vehicle without an engine: A comment on Caramazza and Hillis. *Neuropsychological Rehabilitation*, **3**, 235–44.

Basso A, Cappa S, and Gainotti G. (eds) (2000). *Cognitive Neuropsychology and Language Rehabilitation.* Hove: Psychology Press.

Caramazza, A. (1989). Cognitive neuropsychology and rehabilitation: An unfulfilled promise? In *Cognitive approaches in neuropsychological rehabilitation* (eds X. Seron and G. Deloche), pp. 383–98. Hillsdale, NJ: Lawrence Erlbaum Associates.

Caramazza, A. and Hillis, A. E. (1993). For a theory of remediation of cognitive deficits. *Neuropsychological Rehabilitation*, **3**, 217–34.

Ellis, D. and Christensen, A-L. (1989). *Neuropsychological treatment after brain injury.* Boston: Kluwer Academic Publishers.

Fleminger, S. and Powell, J. (1999). Evaluation of Outcomes in Brain Injury Rehabilitation. *Neuropsychological Rehabilitation.* **9**(3-4). Special edition. Psychology Press.

Nadeau, S. E. (2002). A paradigm shift in neurorehabilitation. *Lancet Neurol.* **1**(2), 126–30.

Ponsford, J., Sloane, S. and Snow, P. (1995). *Traumatic Brain Injury: Rehabilitation for Everyday Adaptive Living.* Hove: Lawrence Erlbaum Associates.

Prigatano, G. P. (1999). *Principles of neuropsychological rehabilitation.* New York:Oxford University Press.

Riddoch, M. J. and Humphreys, G. W. (1994). *Cognitive Neuropsychology and Cognitive Rehabilitation.* Hove: Lawrence Erlbaum Associates.

Robertson, I. H. (1993). Cognitive rehabilitation in neurologic disease. *Curr Opin Neurol*, **6**(5), 756–60.

Robertson, I. H. (1999). The rehabilitation of attention. In *Cognitive Neurorehabilitation* (eds D. T. Stuss, G. Winocur and I. H. Robertson), chapter 19. Cambridge: Cambridge University Press.

Shallice, T. (2000). Cognitive Neuropsychology and rehabilitation: is pessimism justified? *Neuropsychological Rehabilitation*, **10**(3), 209–17.

Smith, R. (1996). What clinical information do doctors need? *BMJ*, **313**(7064), 1062–8.

Sohlberg, M. M. and Mateer, C. A. (1989). *Introduction to Cognitive Rehabilitation: Theory and Practice.* New York: The Guilford Press.

Taub, E., Uswatte, G. and Elbert, T. (2002). New treatments in neurorehabilitation founded on basic research. *Nat Rev Neuroscience*, **3**(3), 228–36.

Wilson, B. A. (2003). Neuropsychological Rehabilitation: Theory and Practice (Studies on Neuropsychology, Development, and Cognition). Lisse, Netherlands: Swets and Zeitlinger.

Winocur, G., Palmer, H., Stuss, D. T., Alexander, M. P., Craik, F. I., Levine, B., Moscovitch, M., Robertson, I. H. (2000) Cognitive rehabilitation in clinical neuropsychology. *Brain Cognition* **42**(1), 120–3.

Wood, R.L. and Fussey, I. (1999). *Cognitive rehabilitation in perspective.* London: Taylor & Francis.

Section 1

Historical and conceptual issues

1 A history of cognitive rehabilitation

George P. Prigatano

Abstract

Historical accounts are always shaded by the perspective of the historian who recounts past events: thus multiple perspectives are needed when attempting to obtain an accurate history of cognitive rehabilitation. The present attempt is simply one account that may be useful to the interested reader. Other accounts are referenced in this chapter.

Introduction

The history of cognitive rehabilitation must begin with a definition of cognitive rehabilitation. Wilson (2002) pointed out that the term 'cognitive rehabilitation' has been defined differently by various practitioners. This has to be taken into consideration and produces challenges to the historian.

Wilson (2002) presents a provisional model of cognitive rehabilitation that emphasizes the need to treat disabilities and handicaps, but she does not totally exclude the need to treat underlying neuropsychological impairment. From the perspective of this reviewer, cognitive rehabilitation refers to nonpharmacological and nonsurgical interventions by healthcare providers that aim to improve or restore problem-solving capabilities of brain function that have been disturbed by a known or suspected brain lesion(s). This broad definition includes many functions under problem-solving abilities such as memory, attention, language, impulse control, speed of information processing, etcetera. It builds on an earlier definition: 'the term cognition will be used to refer to the basic ability of the brain to process, store, retrieve, and manipulate information to solve problems' (Prigatano *et al.* 1986). Cognitive rehabilitation must also help patients to manage residual neuropsychological disturbances as they emerge into interpersonal situations (Prigatano 1999).

Zangwill (1947) described three activities that fall under cognitive rehabilitation: restoration, substitution, and compensation. The first includes 'direct retraining' or restitution efforts to restore impaired function. Teaching or training efforts intended to help patients use alternative problem-solving strategies when a given problem-solving approach has been disturbed by brain dysfunction are categorized as 'substitution' training. The third activity of cognitive rehabilitation is teaching patients to use compensatory methods to solve problems that cannot be addressed by direct retraining or substitution training. Typically, compensatory activities require an artificial approach to solving a problem. The approach can use both 'internal' and 'external' strategies to facilitate problem solving (see Dixon and Bäckman 1995) and frequently requires 'extra effort' and 'time' (Dixon, de Frias and Bäckman 2001; Prigatano and Kime 2003).

Clinicians can usually identify efforts that reflect direct retraining interventions or compensatory interventions. Substitution training falls between these two extremes, and therefore is not always easily defined. In fact, Luria (1948/1963) thought that substitution phenomena occurred naturally in many patients after the onset of brain injury. He explicitly stated that he had little to offer in terms of this type of retraining. His efforts were directed toward restoring problem-solving components of brain function by two methods. The first was reduction or removal of diaschises via pharmacological agents and 'methods of deblocking' (pp. 368–9). The second, 'restoration of function by reorganization of functional systems' (p. 380), often requires extensive and lengthy training efforts (Luria, Naydin, Tsvetkova and Vinarskaya 1969). Framed in this manner, what can be said about the history of cognitive rehabilitation?

Early efforts at cognitive rehabilitation

Efforts at cognitive rehabilitation can only exist if patients survive a brain insult. Thus, the history of cognitive rehabilitation is closely tied to the history of modern medicine, particularly neurosurgery. Finger's (1994) book on the origins of neuroscience provides references relevant to this review. He notes that the Egyptians were among the first, if not the first, to 'provide systematic medical records' (p. 6). Edwin Smith's Surgical Papyrus is frequently referenced in descriptions of how aphasia was first treated or managed. According to Finger's (1994) description, the Egyptians had a practical approach to classifying treatment. An ailment was either treated, contended with, or not treated – reportedly, aphasia fell in the last category. No treatment appeared to be effective (see Finger 1994, p. 371).

Today many still hold this common belief that no cognitive rehabilitation activity is effective for aphasia. Perceptions, however, partially changed at the end of the nineteenth and beginning of the twentieth century. At that time, the practice of neurosurgery greatly improved due to a variety of reasons discussed elsewhere (see Finger 1994). Finger (1994) notes that William Macewen's successful surgical removal of a brain tumor in 1879 ushered in a new era of surgical treatment for brain lesions. Finger (1994) refers to 'reeducation efforts' for aphasic patients dating to 1833, but the works of Broca (1865) and Charles Mills (1904) are frequently cited as the first efforts to retrain aphasic patients. Nonetheless, major efforts at cognitive rehabilitation appeared in Europe and America only after The First and Second World Wars. Most of the seminal work in this arena was propelled by the social responsibility of rehabilitating brain-injured soldiers given their significant personal sacrifices. A brief history of the methods of assessment and approaches to rehabilitation for patients with higher cerebral dysfunctions is found elsewhere (Prigatano 1986a, b). Although efforts at rehabilitating victims of war formed the basis of contemporary cognitive rehabilitation, there is one notable exception.

Sheppard Ivory Franz

Colotla and Bach-y-Rita (2002) recently documented the life and work of Sheppard Ivory Franz. Franz, who was trained in psychology and physiology, criticized von Monakow for not adequately considering the potential role of re-education (an early term for cognitive rehabilitation) in influencing recovery after a brain disorder (Franz 1924). Franz was especially interested in documenting the long-term changes associated with retraining activities to aid recovery from aphasia and hemiplegia. His patients typically had suffered stroke or the effects of syphilis on the central nervous system. Franz' early work shows the influence of his teachers, which included Wundt and James McKeen Cattell. Franz carefully recorded stimulus and response activities and plotted the findings over many treatment sessions. He worked with patients from the perspective of repetition or practice, but recognized the importance of altering the stimulus conditions and finding materials that would hold the patient's interest. He firmly believed that recovery was often a slow, arduous process and that attempts at stimulating recovery of higher brain functions should not be abandoned prematurely.

From 1912 to 1924, Franz was editor of *Psychological Bulletin* and served as President of the American Psychological Association in 1920. Ultimately, he migrated to the University of California, Los Angeles where he became Professor of Psychology. The building that houses the Department of Psychology is now called Franz Hall. He also became Chief, Psychological and Educational Clinic of Children's Hospital in Hollywood, California. Interestingly, the history of cognitive rehabilitation includes very little about the rehabilitation of brain-injured children. Most of the early work focused on adults or animals.

In this latter regard, Franz' student, Karl Lashley, was quite influential in providing models of how various brain lesions did or did not affect the learning process (Franz and Lashley 1917). Lashley's work influenced theories of brain organization and focused on the problem of recovery (Lashley 1938). His work influenced his student, Karl Pribram, who was both a neurosurgeon and soon to become a theoretical neuropsychologist. Of minor historical interest: Pribram was one of my mentors.

The tragedy of war and early efforts at cognitive rehabilitation

The First World War devastated the European population. The first contemporary efforts to work with cognitive deficits systematically occurred in Germany with brain-injured soldiers who had survived focal gunshot or shrapnel wounds to the brain. This early work was performed by two German clinician investigators: Walter Poppelreuter (1917) and Kurt Goldstein (1942). Poppelreuter's early work was published in 1917 but was translated by Zihl with the assistance of L. Weiskrantz (1990). Poppelreuter's work highlights the classic approach of applying experimental methods to the understanding of visual disturbances and how retraining activities might influence, or at least partially influence, the recovery process. Although his work was seminal, another German physician trained both in psychiatry and neurology disagreed with this approach. That physician was Kurt Goldstein. Goldstein argued that far more was needed to rehabilitate brain dysfunctional patients successfully. His early work is the basis of holistic approaches to neuropsychological rehabilitation (see Prigatano 2001).

The works of Poppelreuter and Goldstein are well known. Nonetheless, few historical accounts of neuropsychological rehabilitation are available in general and in cognitive rehabilitation in particular. Prigatano *et al.* (1986) documented the early influence of Oliver Zangwill (1947), Kurt Goldstein (1942), A. R. Luria (1948/63), and the more contemporary influences of Yehuda Ben-Yishay and Leonard Diller (1983).

Boake (1991) specifically reviewed the history of cognitive rehabilitation after traumatic brain injury. He cited the early work of Poppelreuter, Goldstein, Franz, Luria, and Zangwill. He also noted the contributions of Joseph Wepman and the more contemporary influences of Diller and Ben-Yishay. In 1996, the journal *Neuropsychological Rehabilitation* published an overview of historical contributions to different aspects of neuropsychological rehabilitation edited by Boake. One article in that special issue concentrated on the contributions of Luria. Another provided unique insights into the early work of Ben-Yishay in Israel. Prigatano (1999) also listed the influence of several earlier researchers and clinicians on holistic approaches to neuropsychological rehabilitation.

However, Freda Newcombe (2002) provided the most contemporary brief historical review. In her scholarly approach, she highlighted important aspects of 'the forgotten past' in neuropsychological rehabilitation. She describes cognitive rehabilitation activities that emanated from an interaction of many disciplines, including neuropsychology, experimental psychology, cognitive neuropsychology, and learning and behavioral modification theories. She cites the contributions of clinicians and researchers from the United Kingdom, America, Russia, Germany, France, and the Netherlands but refers to Kurt Goldstein as 'The Great Precursor' of cognitive and/or neuropsychological rehabilitation for many reasons.

Goldstein's contributions to neuropsychological rehabilitation

Newcombe (2002) cited several of Goldstein's contributions that make him the great precursor of our current activities:

1. Systematic and long-term follow-up of patients
2. Recognition of the individuality of patients and the variability of performance over time
3. The need for psychometric assessment and the recognition of their limitations (e.g., the standard IQ test)
4. The importance of working with the problem of fatigue in all of its manifestations throughout brain rehabilitation
5. The careful observation of patients' response to failures and their natural preferences for using one form of compensation or substitution over another, and
6. The need to connect cognitive rehabilitation to 'real world' activities (i.e., patients' ability to return to work).

Perhaps more than any other person, Goldstein emphasized the need to attend to patients' personal and social needs when attempting cognitive rehabilitation activities. He also (1942) emphasized the importance of patients' phenomenological state and active management of the catastrophic reaction. We have found this concept very useful in helping patients to return to work after brain injury (Prigatano *et al.* 1986; Prigatano 1999).

Goldstein also recognized two other important points. First was the importance of working with both cognitive and personality deficits simultaneously. He considered a strict cognitive rehabilitation approach as reflected in the early work of Poppelreuter as inadequate. Goldstein also emphasized the importance of distinguishing the direct and indirect symptoms of traumatic brain injury for both scientific analysis and rehabilitation. The direct effects of brain injury were those that emanated from damaged brain tissue. In John Hughlings-Jackson terms, these are the 'negative symptoms'. He also identified indirect symptoms as those that reflect the struggle to adapt to the effects of brain injury or the tendency to avoid the struggle. Practicing clinicians have recognized the importance of this conceptualization, which built on Hughlings-Jackson's early concepts. These observations, among others, set Goldstein apart as the prime influence on cognitive rehabilitation, at least as practiced in the United States and many other places in the world. For this reason, he justly deserves the title bestowed on him by Freda Newcombe.

Although many of Goldstein's observations were not published until 1942, his work developed from his efforts in working with soldiers from The First World War. At that time he had to leave Germany because of his Jewish heritage. While a student in New York City, Ben-Yishay was influenced by Goldstein's teachings as he documents in his reflections on the 'evolution of the therapeutic milieu concept' (Ben-Yishay 1996). The next great surge of interest in rehabilitation came from dealing with soldiers in the Second World War, primarily from Russia.

A. R. Luria and his contributions to neuropsychological rehabilitation

Goldstein (1942) was a psychiatrist and neurologist primarily interested in the rehabilitation of brain-injured patients. He also developed theoretical models concerning the nature of human behavior (Hall and Lindzey 1978). In contrast, Luria was a psychologist who also trained as a physician. He was especially interested in how culture and social milieu influence brain development, particularly the distribution of higher cortical functions (Luria 1966). He developed methods of assessment that reflected his understanding of how higher cerebral functions were organized and how they may become disorganized after brain lesions. As Christiansen and Caetano (1996) note, Luria's interest in rehabilitation appeared late in his career. Luria died in 1977 and his 1969 publication, which appeared eight years before his death, with Naydin, Tsvetkova, and Vinarskay, provided perhaps the most clear and concise statement of his thoughts on the restoration of higher cerebral functions after focal brain injuries.

Before reviewing his work, it is important to reflect on the title of his last paper on this topic – 'Restoration of higher cortical function following local brain damage'. As with Goldstein and Poppelreuter before him, many of Luria's patients (who underwent early forms of cognitive rehabilitation) had local brain lesions. These patients provided unique scientific data that clarified how the brain is organized and how different lesions disrupt that organization. As Goldberg (2001) noted, Luria was perhaps more interested in the insights that rehabilitation of brain-injured patients offered about brain organization than in dealing with the human suffering associated with brain injury. It is important to recall, however, that Luria *was* interested in this problem as reflected by his collaborative work, reported in a book entitled *A Man with a Shattered World*. That text, written by a patient with the help of Luria, reflected Luria's humane understanding of what brain-injured patients experience. He attempted to encourage such patients not to abandon their rehabilitation efforts. A careful reading of the book, however, reveals that Luria acknowledged that this patient never fully recovered and that he was a 'hero' in his efforts to deal with his own losses or tragedies. This topic is discussed in more detail elsewhere (Prigatano 1999). Let us pause, however, to identify Luria's contributions to cognitive rehabilitation.

Borrowing from von Monakow's concept of diaschisis, Luria emphasized that a focal brain lesion may produce physiological inactivity in normal brain regions. This was the process of diaschisis. He noted that this normal area of brain function may not return to its normal physiological activity without specific interventions. He referred to this process as 'restoration of synaptic conduction' (p. 368) or 'deblocking'. He believed that restoration was perhaps best accomplished through pharmacological methods, and he advocated the use of neostigmine (an anticholinesterase drug) to aid this process. His emphasis that neurons could temporarily be de-inhibited by anticholinesterase drugs was a revolutionary concept that has not yet been fully developed. Yet, as noted in the Introduction to his text, the use of pharmacological methods in and of itself does not constitute efforts at cognitive rehabilitation. What then were his specific contributions to cognitive rehabilitation?

First, Luria emphasized that the manifestations of cognitive deficit emerge from a disturbance of different functional overlapping brain systems. He used disturbances in writing as an example. He emphasized that a patient's cognitive deficit could not be retrained without obtaining a detailed neuropsychological analysis of the underlying disturbance. By identifying the primary deficit underlying a behavioral cognitive failure, a plan of cognitive rehabilitation could be outlined (Luria *et al.* 1969, p. 383).

Luria emphasized the importance of determining what area of the functional system remained 'intact'. That area became the focus of the rehabilitation process. That is, the therapist worked with what was unaffected to compensate for what was affected. Luria then emphasized the importance of 'complete, extended programming of the restorative activity' (Luria *et al.* 1969, p. 384). In other words, patients received numerous training experiences so they could use the 'intact link' to perform an impaired function and to reorganize an underlying functional system. This theory was extremely insightful, but it has been a difficult model to follow even though contemporary efforts at cognitive neuropsychological rehabilitation are based on Luria's approach.

The work of Christiansen and colleagues borrowed heavily from Luria's ideas. However, few papers, if any, specifically show how Luria's approach has been used to restore an impaired higher cerebral function. Thus, Luria's contributions have mainly pointed to retraining an underlying cognitive deficit, but have not led to specific methods of retraining that have proven to be of substantial help to patients. Given this reality, many moved away from the hope of restoring an impaired brain function to trying to help patients live and cope effectively with residual neuropsychological impairments. It is here that the evolution of a therapeutic milieu, or holistic approaches to neuropsychological rehabilitation, began.

The evolution of the therapeutic milieu concept in brain injury rehabilitation

Yehuda Ben-Yishay (1996) documented the circumstances that led to the development of holistic approaches in neuropsychological rehabilitation. Treating soldiers from the Yom Kippur war in the Middle East who sustained brain injuries was the basis for the third major movement in cognitive rehabilitation. Ben-Yishay, trained primarily in counseling and rehabilitation psychology, had the responsibility of attempting to improve the interpersonal and social interactive functioning of brain dysfunctional patients. His earlier work had focused on efforts at cognitive rehabilitation after stroke; he now applied these methods, coupled with other experiences, to establish a therapeutic milieu. For the first time, the power of the 'therapeutic community' in brain injury rehabilitation became obvious. Patients were given templates for how to approach various kinds of cognitive and interpersonal problems. They were trained systematically to try to improve their attention, visuospatial problem-solving skills, motor functions, and so on. The overall goal, however, was for patients to confront the effects of their brain injury and to develop adaptations or compensations that they could use to re-enter a social world (see Rattok, Ben-Yishay et al. 1992). This approach greatly influenced efforts at brain-injury rehabilitation in the United States in the late 1970s and early 1980s.

In 1980, Prigatano developed a neuropsychological rehabilitation program at the Presbyterian Hospital in Oklahoma City primarily based on Ben-Yishay's concepts. In fact, Ben-Yishay served as a consultant to that program during its first two years. In the context of that program, two additional difficulties emerged (Prigatano et al. 1986). One was the problem of impaired awareness. Progressively, it became clear that patients did not experience their deficits in the same way that those around them experienced those deficits. Many had diffuse rather than focal brain injuries. They seemed to minimize their disturbances when describing them, and this behavior was a roadblock to successful rehabilitation. At that time, only Edwin Weinstein's work was available in behavioral neurology and neuropsychiatry to better understand the phenomena of impaired awareness vs. denial of disability in brain dysfunctional patients (Weinstein and Kahn 1955). His contributions to neuropsychological rehabilitation have also been documented (Prigatano and Weinstein 1996).

The second problem that emerged was the need to manage the emotional and motivational disturbances that brain-injured patients experience. For the first time, a holistic approach formally incorporated individual and group psychotherapy as part of its rehabilitation efforts. Although this chapter is on the history of cognitive rehabilitation, it would be remiss if it did not point out that neuropsychological rehabilitation, at a minimum, should include both cognitive rehabilitation and psychotherapeutic interventions. Holistic approaches also incorporate other activities (Prigatano 1999). The legacy of Kurt Goldstein's approach, however, was to emphasize the need to work with the 'entire human being' as opposed to specific cognitive deficits.

Focused cognitive rehabilitation approaches

Not everyone, however, has shared this holistic perspective. Particularly in Europe and in some parts of the United States, efforts at focusing specifically on cognitive rehabilitation emerged in the mid- to early 1980s. The impetus for this work was not the treatment of brain-injured soldiers, but individuals who had survived automobile accidents, anoxic encephalopathy, cerebrovascular accidents, or the surgical removal of brain tumors. This approach to cognitive rehabilitation is represented most clearly in the writings of Wilson (1987), Sohlberg and Mateer (1989) and Robertson and Halligan (1999). This approach is often highlighted in published accounts such as the book by Stuss, Winocur and Robertson (1999) entitled *Cognitive Neurorehabilitation*.

These approaches borrow heavily from methods emanating from neuropsychology, cognitive neuropsychology, and experimental neuropsychology. They, too, are reflected in Newcombe's (2002) historical account. These approaches evolved in different fashions. Some evolved to help patients cope with their disability as opposed to their underlying impairment (Wilson 2002). Others have not abandoned the hope of treating the underlying impairment (Robertson and Halligan 1999).

The underlying assumption, however, of contemporary cognitive rehabilitation is that if the nature of the cognitive deficit and the principles of neuroplasticity are understood, the appropriate training might, in fact, substantially improve a cognitive deficit.

In retrospect: three great traditions

The history of cognitive rehabilitation reflects three great traditions that influence current practices. First is the tradition of scientific analysis of the recovery process after brain injury; second is the use of systematic methods of retraining or compensating for impaired cognitive function. These two traditions reflect the work of von Monakow, Franz, Hughlings-Jackson, Luria and Poppelreuter.

The third great tradition is that of Kurt Goldstein: Cognitive retraining activities must consider the entire organism or person. From this context holistic approaches to neuropsychological rehabilitation that include the therapeutic milieu, psychotherapeutic interventions, actively working with family members of brain dysfunctional patients, protected work trials, and working with rehabilitation staff who provide services to patients have emerged. Goldstein was also influenced by many of the theorists involved in the first two traditions.

In the context of these traditions, we have to deal with the 'practical present'. That is, clinically, we must treat a wide variety of patients and determine what types of cognitive retraining activities are most practical or helpful for them at different times during the rehabilitation process.

During the acute stages of brain injury, many patients do not need a holistic approach. They need specific efforts at intervention, which might include pharmacological treatments, surgical interventions, and focused methods of cognitive rehabilitation. These approaches must be based on adequate scientific analysis of the problem and adequate scientific assessment of the efficacy of the treatment being proposed.

For patients who will return to independent living and possibly gainful employment (or at least a productive lifestyle), more than focused cognitive rehabilitation is often needed. The entire fabric of these individual's lives has been disrupted. Interpersonal relationships are different as well as their own sense of self-value and worth. Helping these individuals to manage their cognitive deficits and to re-establish meaning in life becomes crucial, and the Goldstein tradition points the way toward accomplishing these goals (Prigatano 1999). Given these realities, what does the past reveal about what cognitive rehabilitation should provide today?

How does the past influence cognitive rehabilitation today?

Galaburda (1985) noted that Norman Geshwind's contribution flowed from his ability to combine classical thinking with contemporary scientific insights. He argued that knowing the 'useful past' helps achieve advances in the future. This point is clearly reflected by the history of cognitive rehabilitation. What exactly, however, is the useful past?

First, Sheppard Ivory Franz' contributions highlight the importance of the fact that recovery is a slow arduous process. It requires ongoing repetition and practice. There are very few 'short fixes' in cognitive rehabilitation.

Second, cognitive rehabilitation requires sustained effort and motivation. Therefore, the personality characteristics of both therapist and patient may be crucial ingredients to the success of cognitive rehabilitation.

Third, normal brain function may lose its normal physiological activity. Therefore, cognitive deficits might be reversible if we knew specifically how to 'deblock' these inhibitory activities. This is the tradition of von Monakow and Luria.

Fourth, recovery is seldom complete (Kolb 1990, 1995). The problems of partial recovery and possible deterioration of function with the passage of time must be studied systematically by students of cognitive rehabilitation (see Prigatano 1999). As Geshwind (1985) pointed out, there is no such thing as a static lesion of the brain. The central nervous system changes either for the better or for the worse. We must determine when cognitive rehabilitation not only aids recovery during the first few years after brain injury, but equally important, when it helps to avoid deterioration several years after brain injury.

Fifth, until the organization of higher cerebral functions and how deficits affect those functions (i.e., Luria's influence) are understood, we will be unable to plan systematic cognitive rehabilitation. As a corollary, until the processes underlying recovery (von Monakow, John Hughlings-Jackson, Lashley's influences) are understood, we also will be unable to improve outcomes systematically.

Finally, our most practical efforts focus on teaching patients to compensate for cognitive deficits rather than on reversing the deficits that are present (Wilson 2002).

The practical present, evidence-based practices, and cost-outcome research

The cost of health care is an unavoidable concern. Since the mid 1990s, there has been a systematic attempt to determine the cost of different forms of medical care and to measure the costs associated with different outcomes. The world of economics has entered the field of medicine and health care. Neuropsychologists can respond to this demand (Prigatano and Pliskin 2003). Cost–outcome studies as they relate to cognitive rehabilitation can be performed. We are not only being asked to determine the efficacy of our treatment, we are also being asked to identify the cost-effectiveness of those treatments. Cost-effectiveness always implies a comparison of treatments rather than the effectiveness of a given treatment in and of itself. Efficacy includes not only relief of symptoms but the dollars spent or saved.

At the heart of evidence-based medicine and cost–outcome research, however, is the issue of value. Value has both objective and subjective markers (Prigatano *et al.* 2003). From an economic perspective, value often implies paying less for a service than it is worth. Subjective markers of value, however, relate to quality of life and the willingness to pay for a service. In terms of cognitive rehabilitation, patients' and family satisfaction with an intervention becomes extremely important in determining its cost-effectiveness.

For the first time, we are not only asking how effective cognitive rehabilitation is (Sackett *et al.* 2000), we are asking the worth of cognitive rehabilitation from the perspective of patients, families, and society. Those of us in the field must take a much broader view of our work. We must continue to place our efforts in the perspective of past work that continues to influence our current scientific and clinical efforts. We must pay homage to those who have shown us the way: Constantine von Monakow, John Hughlings-Jackson, Shepard Ivory Franz, Karl Lashley, Walter Poppelreuter, Kurt Goldstein, A. R. Luria, and Oliver Zangwill.

2 Cognitive rehabilitation and its relationship to cognitive-neuropsychological rehabilitation

Max Coltheart, Ruth Brunsdon and Lyndsey Nickels

Abstract

We draw attention in this chapter to the differences between cognitive-neuropsychological rehabilitation and cognitive rehabilitation. Three of the major differences are (a) that cognitive-neuropsychological rehabilitation relies on cognitive models of the impaired processing system for assessment and for treatment definition whereas cognitive rehabilitation does not; (b) cognitive-neuropsychological rehabilitation emphasizes restoration of function rather than compensation whereas cognitive rehabilitation does not; and (c) cognitive rehabilitation is used only for treating acquired cognitive disorders (those acquired through brain damage) whereas cognitive-neuropsychological rehabilitation is applied also to developmental disorders of cognition. The methods of cognitive-neuropsychological rehabilitation are illustrated by description of a treatment study of developmental surface dysgraphia.

Two approaches to the rehabilitation of cognitive impairments are *cognitive-neuropsychological rehabilitation* (Coltheart 1983; Coltheart and Byng 1989) and *cognitive rehabilitation* (Sohlberg and Mateer 1989, 2001). We begin this chapter by considering what each of these two approaches consists of, and how they differ, if they do.

What is cognitive-neuropsychological rehabilitation?

This approach is discussed in detail by Coltheart, Bates and Castles (1994, p. 20). They begin by noting that 'Cognitive-neuropsychological rehabilitation ... by definition refers to the use of models of normal processing as an aid to rehabilitation' and they go on to point out that there are three different kinds of contribution to rehabilitation that models of normal cognitive functioning *could* make to the treatment of disorders of such functioning:

(a) A model can serve as a basis for the development of rational assessment techniques
(b) Model-based assessment can be used to define what the specific focus of treatment should be
(c) A model might serve as a source of ideas about specific treatment *methods*.

The first of these aims is achieved by, for example, the PALPA battery for assessing language disorders (Kay, Lesser and Coltheart 1992) and the BORB battery for assessing disorders of visual perception and visual object recognition (Riddoch and Humphreys 1993). Both batteries are based on explicit modular models of a cognitive processing system (the language-processing system and the visual processing system respectively).

Such model-based assessment allows the clinician to determine which modules of the relevant information-processing system are functioning abnormally and which have been spared. That allows the second of the three aims listed above to be pursued: since the components of the system which are not functioning normally have been identified, the clinician knows what abilities should be targeted by the treatment program.

This second aim involves a commitment to a particular conception of rehabilitation – to *restoration* rather than *compensation*. 'Restorative training focuses on improving a specific cognitive function, whereas compensatory training focuses on adapting to the presence of a cognitive deficit' NIH Consensus Statement 1998, cited by Sohlberg and Mateer (2001, p. 16). Clinicians adopting the restorative approach might hope that treatment will improve the functioning of impaired components of a particular cognitive system, so that the effect of treatment will be to move this system in the direction of normality – to partly or even wholly restore normal functioning in that system. Alternatively, clinicians might decide that the damage to the cognitive system is permanent and irreversible; here the aim of treatment might be to find a way in which to reduce or eliminate the impact of this permanently reduced ability on the person's life For example, a memory impairment might be dealt with by training in the use of memory aids such as pagers or diaries rather than by seeking to improve the performance of the memory system itself.

There may be domains of cognition in which an impairment caused by brain damage is such that restoration of normal processing is impossible. It is conceivable that face processing is one such domain. Face processing depends on a specific brain region and this region may have a particular kind of structure that is specialised for the specific types of computations needed for recognising the unique stimulus that faces are. Here if the damage to the face-processing regions is permanent then an impairment in the ability to process faces (prosopagnosia) may be permanent, i.e. restoration may be impossible. We know of four published studies reporting attempts to treat prosopagnosia (De Haan *et al.* 1991; Ellis and Young 1988; Polster and Rapcsak 1996; Wilson 1987). All were unsuccessful. Thus it is conceivable that, for some cognitive impairments, approaching them with a view to restoration rather than compensation will always fail, and compensation is the only practical possibility.

However, we do know already that in at least some cognitive domains restoration is possible after acquired impairments of cognitive processing, because such restoration has been achieved by cognitive-neuropsychological rehabilitation. Cognitive domains where this has been demonstrated include reading (Coltheart and Byng 1989), writing (Behrmann 1987), sentence comprehension (Byng 1988), sentence production (Jones 1986) and naming (Nickels 1992).[1] Total commitment to a compensation approach and complete disregard for the possibility of successful restoration is thus unjustified.

We have so far discussed two of the three possible ways in which models of normal cognitive functioning can be used in rehabilitation – for developing assessment techniques and for defining treatment focus with attempts at restoration in mind – and have described successes in both cases. The third way in which models could conceivably help is as a source of ideas about actual treatment methods. Ten years ago, Coltheart *et al.* had this to say concerning this third possible contribution of cognitive neuropsychology to rehabilitation:

> There seems to be some ground for optimism about future contributions from models vis-à-vis treatment methods, but so far such contributions have been minimal. After the specific sub-ability

---

[1]In all of this work, particular care was taken to design the treatment study in such a way that specific effects of treatment could be measured separately from nonspecific treatment effects and from general effects such as spontaneous recovery, etc. All studies showed specific treatment effects.

to be treated has been specified, it has usually been up to the therapist's ingenuity to work out methods by which performance of this impaired sub-ability might be improved.

Coltheart *et al.* (1994, p. 27)

This remains the case, and we think there are two reasons why.

First, models of cognitive processing systems which explicitly describe the functional architecture of the system – what the modules of the system are and what pathways of communication between them exist – may not be explicit about the exact ways in which the modules do their job, because nothing may yet be known about this even if there is good agreement as to what the functional architecture of the system is. As Coltheart *et al.* (1994) wrote, a modular model of language processing:

> allowed Coltheart and Byng (1989) to pinpoint E.E.'s processing impairment, and his treatment was targeted at this impairment. But the treatment method used was not suggested by the model. No attempt was made to deduce, from anything known about how the visual word recognition system actually works, what methods might be efficacious in getting the system to work again. The mnemonic technique used for treatment was a product of the ingenuity of the therapist, not of insights provided by the model.

Model-based assessment allowed Coltheart and Byng (1989) to determine that a major cause of E.E.'s acquired reading impairment was either loss of information within the orthographic lexicon, or an impairment of the pathway from letter identification to orthographic lexicon, or both. If it had been possible to decide between these three possibilities, there could have been implications for choice of treatment methods; but it wasn't possible, since the model of reading was not sufficiently explicit about how access to the orthographic lexicon actually occurs to suggest assessment techniques which could decide whether a particular patient's problem is in access to a system of representations or arises because of damage to the representations themselves. Models of cognitive functioning are becoming more and more detailed and explicit, and as this happens the ideal of model-suggested treatment *methods* may be approaching.

The second reason why models have contributed little to the choice of treatment methods for rehabilitation so far is that modellers have in general said very little about the specific ways in which a mental information-processing system could behave abnormally after an acquired impairment of cognition, and little about the specific ways in which the acquisition of such a system could be abnormal in cases of developmental disorders of cognition. The sole exception to the latter point is the connectionist approach to modelling, in which models are created via a connectionist learning algorithm such as back-propagation, applied to some database of linguistic information (see e.g. Plaut *et al.* 1996). However, back-propagation is not regarded as a psychologically plausible learning mechanism; there's no reason to believe that the way children acquire language abilities is in any way like the way neural networks acquire language abilities when trained using back-propagation, and so there's no reason to believe that this approach to modelling as currently practiced will provide insights into developmental disorders of cognition.

What is cognitive rehabilitation?

> A systematic functionally-oriented service of therapeutic cognitive activities, based on an assessment and understanding of the person's brain-behavior deficits. Services are directed to achieve functional changes by (1) reinforcing, strengthening or reestablishing previously learned patterns of behavior or (2) establishing new patterns of cognitive activity or compensatory mechanisms for impaired neurological systems.

Official statement by the US National Academy of Neuropsychology (May 2002)

It isn't exactly clear from this statement what is particularly *cognitive* about cognitive rehabilitation. Is the approach called 'cognitive' because the therapeutic tasks given to the patients are cognitive tasks, or because the approach is for use with patients who have cognitive impairments?

This issue is dealt with somewhat more clearly in one of the standard texts on cognitive rehabilitation, Sohlberg and Mateer (2001). They write:

> The term *cognitive rehabilitation* was perhaps always too narrow, and focussed too heavily on remediating or compensating for decreased cognitive abilities. The term *rehabilitation of individuals with cognitive impairment* probably better captures the emphasis on injured individuals that has and always will be the target of cognitive rehabilitation.

(2001, p. 3)

From this it seems that the reason cognitive rehabilitation is called 'cognitive' is because the deficits at which it is aimed are deficits in cognition. Since that is also true for cognitive-neuropsychological rehabilitation, are there actually any differences between the two approaches?

There are in fact at least two major differences. The first concerns the role played by models of cognitive processing in rehabilitation. Sohlberg and Mateer (2001) suggest that such models do have a role in cognitive rehabilitation:

> We hold that disorders need to be understood before they can be rehabilitated. Working from a taxonomy or model of a cognitive process helps clinicians to organize assessment and treatment activities and practices [and] rehabilitation specialists need to apply current knowledge from the fields of cognitive psychology and the neurosciences.

Sohlberg and Mateer (2001, p. 10)

We agree with these tenets whilst pointing out that in the actual practice of cognitive rehabilitation they are rarely if ever followed. For example, Sohlberg and Mateer (2001, p. 21) list thirteen 'Principles of cognitive rehabilitation': none of these principles refer in any way to the use of models of cognitive functioning in rehabilitation, nor to applications of current knowledge from cognitive psychology. In the same text, Sohlberg and Mateer (2001, p. 117) list ten principles which they say 'should guide the assessment of individuals with cognitive impairment'. None of these principles is related in any way to the use of models, or of other input from cognitive psychology, for assessment. More generally, in this book and in its predecessor (Sohlberg and Mateer 1989), which are the standard texts on cognitive rehabilitation, there is almost no material on the relationship between models of normal cognitive processing and the understanding, assessment and treatment of disorders of cognition.

Another way of exploring what role models play in practice in work on cognitive rehabilitation is to examine the literature in this area. The only journal specifically devoted to cognitive rehabilitation is the *Journal of Cognitive Rehabilitation*. Not one of the papers published in this journal in the period 1998 through 2003 mentioned any specific information-processing model of any cognitive function. One can also examine the annotated review by Martin and Pauly (2000) of 54 articles on cognitive rehabilitation published in the period 1986–2000; again, none of these articles mentions any specific information-processing model of any cognitive function.

Here, then, is a very clear difference between cognitive rehabilitation and cognitive-neuropsychological rehabilitation. Although the use of models of normal cognitive functioning is not ruled out in cognitive rehabilitation, this use is not required, and in practice does not happen. In contrast, such use of models is required by definition in the cognitive-neuropsychological approach. Thus cognitive-neuropsychological rehabilitation is directly connected to cognitive psychology in a way that cognitive rehabilitation is not.

There's a second and equally clear difference between the two approaches. Cognitive neuropsychology distinguishes between two types of cognitive disorder. *Acquired* disorders of cognition are those in which a person suffers a brain injury which causes an impairment of a cognitive system or systems which before the injury were normal. *Developmental* disorders of cognition are those where a cognitive system or systems has never attained a normal level over the course of cognitive development. The cognitive-neuropsychological approach to treatment is not confined to acquired disorders but is also intended to be applicable to developmental disorders such as specific language impairment or developmental dyslexia (see e.g. Temple 1987; Jackson and Coltheart 2001). In contrast, the cognitive rehabilitation approach does not apply to developmental disorders of cognition; it concerns only acquired disorders, those due to damage to the brain in a person who previously was cognitively normal. There is no material on developmental disorders of cognition in Sohlberg and Mateer (1989) or Sohlberg and Mateer (2001); no articles on developmental disorders of cognition have appeared in the *Journal of Cognitive Rehabilitation* in the period 1998 through 2003; and there were no articles on developmental disorders of cognition in the annotated bibliography by Martin and Pauly (2000) of 54 papers on cognitive rehabilitation appearing in the period 1986–2000.

The distinction between proximal and distal causes of disorders of cognition

As soon as one is committed to model-based understanding, assessment, and treatment of acquired and developmental disorders of cognition (that is, to cognitive-neuropsychological rehabilitation), one is also committed to distinguishing between proximal and distal causes of such disorders. The proximal cause of a disorder of cognition is whatever is wrong with the relevant mental information-processing system that is responsible for the patient's difficulty in performing the relevant cognitive task. Something will have cause that abnormality of the cognitive system, and that is the distal cause of the disorder. Indeed, there may even be a chain of distal causes, with the last link in the chain being what gave rise to the proximal cause.

This distinction is of special interest in the case of developmental disorders of cognition. Take, for example, the view that phonemic awareness is crucial for young readers, and that poor phonemic awareness causes poor reading in children. Let's suppose this is true. Is this an instance of proximal or of distal cause? Well, is the poor phonemic awareness an abnormality of the relevant mental information-processing system, the reading system? The answer is no: we do not use phonemic awareness online as we carry out an act of reading. If phonemic awareness has an influence, it is on the process of *learning to read,* not on the process of *reading itself.* If this argument is accepted, then we are led to ask the clinically critical question: if poor phonemic awareness is the distal cause of poor reading in some children, what's the proximal cause here?

That's a critical question for the cognitive-neuropsychological approach, since that approach by definition seeks to target proximal causes.

Commitment to the single-case study approach

Figure 2.1 shows a model (from Jackson and Coltheart 2001) of the reading and writing system which was used for assessing and treating a case of developmental dysgraphia (discussed later in this chapter). This system has 19 arrows and 9 boxes, i.e., 28 components. If these are individually impairable by brain damage, or if a child can have difficulty in acquiring any one of them, then the number of possible different patterns of impairment to this system (whether this be an acquired or a developmental impairment) is $2^{28}-1$. The probability that in his or her lifetime a clinician will see two patients with exactly the same pattern of impairments is therefore $1/(2^{28}-1)$, which is effectively zero.

So no two patients will be the same; hence each patient must be treated as an individual case. What allows one to generalize from one patient to another is not that both patients have the same impairment: it is that both patients have impairments to the same system. The assumption that the functional architecture of any cognitive system is uniform across people is therefore required for cognitive neuropsychology; but it also required for all of cognitive psychology as that subject is currently practiced.

An illustrative case study

We'd like to illustrate how cognitive-neuropsychological rehabilitation works in practice, and to highlight the differences between this approach and the cognitive rehabilitation approach, by describing some work on the rehabilitation of developmental writing and spelling difficulties (developmental dysgraphia). MC is a 12-year-old boy with a full scale IQ of 112 and a history of severe difficulties in learning to read and to spell.[2] Our aim was to apply cognitive-neuropsychological treatment methods to these difficulties. The first step in applying such methods is always to define a model of the relevant cognitive functions which will provide a framework for assessment and treatment, and the model we used was that shown in Figure 2.1.

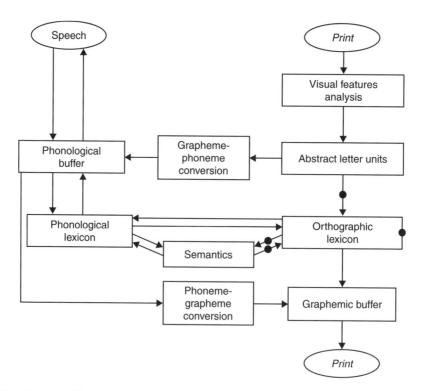

Figure 2.1 A model of the language processing system (Jackson and Coltheart 2001). Black dots indicate imperfections of the system identified in MC.

---

[2]Full details of this work can be found in Brunsdon, Coltheart and Nickels (in press).

The first use for this model was assessment, and in this context assessment means determining which components of this model are functioning normally given the child's age and which are not. This was done as follows:

1. Reading aloud of nonwords was normal for age using the nonword reading test and norms of Coltheart and Leahy (1996). This indicates that the pathway *print* → Visual Feature Analysis → Abstract Letter Units → Grapheme-Phoneme Conversion → Phonological Buffer → speech is intact in this child.

2. Writing nonwords to dictation was judged to be normal for age using the nonwords from the reading test of Coltheart and Leahy (1996); there are no age norms for the task of writing these nonwords to dictation. This indicates that the pathway *speech* → Phonological Buffer → Phoneme-Grapheme Conversion → Graphemic Buffer→ *print* is intact in this child.

3. Comprehension of spoken language was assessed by Spoken Word to Picture Matching test from the PALPA battery (Kay *et al.* 1992) on which performance was appropriate for age. This indicates that the pathway *speech* → Phonological Buffer → Phonological Lexicon → Semantics is intact in this child.

Production of spoken language was assessed by a picture naming test on which performance again was appropriate for age. This indicates that the pathway Semantics → Phonological Lexicon → Phonological Buffer was intact in this child. The child's conversational speech appeared entirely normal, confirming this interpretation.

Visual word recognition was assessed via the visual lexical decision test from the PALPA battery (subtest 27). He performed worse than 9–10 year old normal readers on this task. The pathway *print* → Visual Feature Analysis → Abstract Letter Units → Orthographic Lexicon is used to perform this task. Since his nonword reading aloud was normal, we can infer that the pathway print → Visual Feature Analysis → Abstract Letter Units is intact. Hence the poor performance on visual lexical decision implies a deficiency of the orthographic lexicon or of the pathway to it from the abstract letter units in this child.

The next assessment task required MC to read aloud printed irregularly-spelled homophones such as *queue, pear, their* or *steak*, and also to indicate his comprehension of them by using them in a phrases or sentence. On a number of occasions, MC correctly read aloud such words yet defined them wrongly as the other member of the homophone pair. For example, all four of the irregular words listed above he read aloud correctly, but when asked what they meant he said 'the actor needed a cue', 'socks – pair of them', 'there is a ball' and 'I stuck a stake in the ground'. Since these words were read aloud correctly, they must have been correctly accessed in the orthographic lexicon. Given that MC's spoken word comprehension is normal, we assume that these words are represented normally in his semantic system. If he could recognize the printed forms of these words, and if the words are represented in his semantic system, why could he not understand them from print? We infer that this was because the pathway of communication from orthographic lexicon to semantics is imperfect, since it is this pathway that is essential for the reading comprehension of such words. When the pathway fails, the only route from print to Semantics is *print* → Visual Feature Analysis → Abstract Letter Units → Orthographic Lexicon → Phonological Lexicon → Semantics. But since *cue* and *queue*, or any pair of homophones, have the same representation in the phonological lexicon, this pathway cannot discriminate between homophones in reading comprehension; hence MC's homophone errors.

Lastly, we carried out a spelling-to-dictation test involving homophones. Since the items were homophones, we used phrases to disambiguate them, such as 'Bred … They bred cattle carefully' or 'Bare … The desert landscape was bare'. Despite this disambiguation, MC sometimes wrote down the wrong member of the homophone pair and produced an irregularly-spelled words as this response (bread and *bear* respectively, in these two examples). Since these responses are spelling-irregular and so could not have been produced by phoneme-grapheme rules, the spellings are coming from the orthographic lexicon. Since MC's spoken word comprehension is normal, we assume that the correct entries are being accessed in his semantic system in this task. Hence his production of irregularly-spelled words as homophone errors here indicates impairment of the pathway from semantics to the orthographic lexicon.

The result of this detailed assessment process is that we may say that all of the modules and pathways of the system shown in Figure 2.1 are intact except those in and around the orthographic lexicon. The two pathways from orthographic lexicon to semantics and from semantics to orthographic lexicon are functioning imperfectly, and so is the orthographic lexicon itself (or the pathway to it from the abstract letter units). These imperfections are the proximal causes of MC's difficulties with reading and spelling. These imperfect components of the system are indicated by the black dots in Figure 2.1; our assessments have indicated that all of the remaining components of the system were normal for age in MC.

Having completed a detailed model-based assessment which succeeded in precisely localizing the sources of MC's reading and spelling difficulties, we then embarked on a treatment study aimed at remediating his spelling difficulties.

As is characteristic in cognitive neuropsychological rehabilitation, we designed this study so that if there were any improvements from pretest to posttest in MC's reading we would be able to tell whether these (a) would have happened even if there had been no treatment or (b) were a consequence of simply being treated or (c) were a consequence of the particular treatment method we adopted. Unless this is done, claims re treatment efficacy cannot be justified.

We selected 308 irregular words and asked MC to spell them to dictation twice on different occasions. 222 of these words were misspelled at least once in these two tests, and these words were used in the treatment study. We divided them into three sets of 74, Sets A, B and C, matched on spelling accuracy in the pretreatment tests and on word frequency.

The design was as follows:

1. First pretreatment baseline of spelling to dictation for Sets A, B and C.
2. Second pretreatment baseline of spelling to dictation for Sets A, B and C.
3. Treat Set A
4. Test spelling to dictation for Sets A, B and C.
5. Treat Set B
6. Test spelling to dictation for Sets A, B and C.
7. Treat Set C
8. Test spelling to dictation for Sets A, B and C.
9. Post-test spelling to dictation for Sets A, B and C 2 months after cessation of treatment
10. Post-test spelling to dictation for Sets A, B and C 4 months after cessation of treatment.

The treatment was as follows:

1. MC was shown a flash card showing the word
2. MC copied the word
3. Then the word was removed and MC wrote it after a 10-second delay
4. Then the word was spoken to him and he wrote it to dictation
5. Home practice: Parents were instructed in this. MC practiced writing to dictation with them at home, with feedback from them, until he could correctly write 68 of the 74 words in the set being trained.

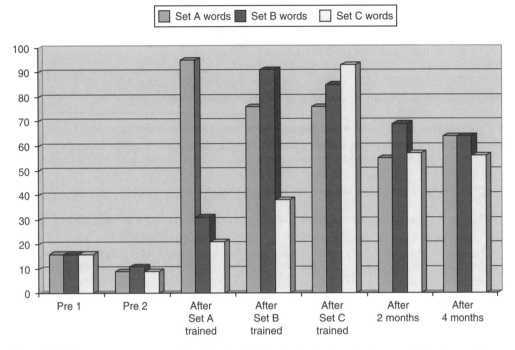

Figure 2.2 Percentage correct word spelling to dictation in the treatment of a case of developmental surface dysgraphia (Brunsdon, Coltheart and Nickels in press).

The results are shown in Figure 2.2.

Note the following:

1. The three sets of words were equally difficult for MC to spell prior to treatment, since accuracy across the three sets did not differ in the first pretreatment baseline, nor in the second pretreatment baseline.

2. MC was not improving in spelling prior to treatment, since performance was no better in baseline 2 than in baseline 1.

3. After Set A words were treated, accuracy of their spelling was vastly higher than in the pretreatment baselines and also vastly higher than spelling of the not-yet-treated Sets B and C.

4. Although at the assessment stage following the completion of Set A treatment, Sets B and C had not yet been treated, they were nevertheless being spelled slightly (but significantly) more accurately than they had been in the two pretreatment baselines. We discuss this generalization effect further below.

5. After Set B words were treated, accuracy of their spelling was vastly higher than in the pretreatment baselines and also vastly higher than spelling of the not-yet-treated Set C.

6. Although at the assessment stage following the completion of Set B treatment, Set C words had not yet been treated, they were nevertheless being spelled slightly (but significantly) more accurately than they had been in the two pretreatment baselines.

7. While the Set B words were being treated, treatment was withdrawn from the Set A words. Their spelling accuracy nevertheless remained far higher than it had been in the two pretreatment baselines, though it declined slightly compared to the level achieved at the end of Set A treatment. The treatment effect was thus durable.

8. After Set C words were treated, accuracy of their spelling was vastly higher than in the pretreatment baselines.

9. While the Set C words were being treated, treatment was withdrawn from the Set B and Set A words, but their accuracy of spelling remained at high levels.

10. Two months after cessation of all treatment, accuracy had declined somewhat but was still far higher than it had been prior to treatment.

11. There was no further loss of accuracy between two and four months after cessation of treatment.

We can conclude that this method of treating developmental dysgraphia:

- is efficacious (since treated words improved more than matched untreated words);
- is relatively durable (since even four months after cessation of treatment treated words were being spelled with about 55 per cent accuracy compared to about 12 per cent accuracy prior to treatment); and
- produces some degree of generalization to the spelling of untreated words.

In addition to demonstrating an effective treatment for a child's spelling problems, these data allow one to investigate a number of interesting scientific questions, of which we will mention just two.

First, why did spelling improve somewhat for words which had not yet been treated? A similar effect occurs even when what's being treated is surface dyslexia rather than surface dysgraphia and even when the disorder is an acquired one: Coltheart and Byng (1989) used a similar design in a treatment study of acquired surface dyslexia and found some improvement in the reading of not-yet-treated words, though not as much improvement as in treated words. Weekes and Coltheart (1996) obtained exactly the same result.

We noticed with MC that the degree to which his misspellings resembled the correct spelling varied greatly. We therefore analysed how similar his misspellings of untreated words were to the correct spellings, and found that the higher this similarity the more likely the word was to be spelled correctly after other words had been treated. In other words, the degree of generalization of treatment effects to untreated words depends upon how close the original misspellings of these words were to the correct spellings. Not only does this have implications for the design of treatment studies, but it also has implications for models of reading and spelling since different models will define orthographic similarity in different ways. Which of these definitions is the one which best captures the kind of similarity that is responsible for generalization here?

Second, what effect on word reading does this treatment of word spelling have? Whilst MC's word spelling was being treated and assessed, his reading of these and other words was also being continually assessed, so as to determine whether the treatment of his developmental surface dysgraphia would spill over and affect his developmental surface dyslexia. Preliminary analyses suggest that the reading of words treated for spelling improves relative to pretreatment baseline accuracy, but that the spelling generalization effect (spelling of untreated words improves somewhat when other words' spellings are being treated) does not occur for reading: the accuracy of reading for words not treated for spelling remains at pretreatment baseline level. This pattern of carryover effects from spelling treatment to reading accuracy also has interesting clinical and theoretical implications.

We conclude by noting what is especially characteristic of the cognitive-neuropsychological approach, and especially different from the cognitive-rehabilitation approach, in this study:

- there was extensive use of an information-processing model for the purposes of assessment and of treatment focus;
- this was a developmental case – and note that the approach was nevertheless just the same as taken with acquired cases such as those of Coltheart and Byng (1989) and Weekes and Coltheart (1996);
- the study involved a detailed investigation of a single case;
- the study was designed so that unambiguous evidence of treatment efficacy could be obtained.

3 Fundamentals of cognitive rehabilitation

Catherine A. Mateer

Abstract

The field of cognitive rehabilitation draws from many traditions, including neurology, neuropsychology, cognitive psychology, physical rehabilitation, education, and psychotherapy. This chapter provides a brief overview of general principles for the practice of cognitive rehabilitation, and identifies important elements for enhancing successful functional outcomes that make a real difference in the lives of individuals affected by brain injury. It describes the major approaches to working with individuals with acquired cognitive impairments, and provides guidelines for selecting effective intervention strategies. It briefly describes environmental interventions, implementation of compensatory devices, restorative approaches to improving attention, and the use of specialized instructional techniques. It also emphasizes the need to address the emotional needs of individuals and families that commonly arise as a function of living with persistent cognitive impairments.

The rehabilitation of individuals who have suffered neurological disease or trauma has received increasing interest in the last two decades. Several factors have contributed to this. Survival rates from even very severe neurological injury have been increasing since the mid 1970s with greater understanding of the effects of trauma, the advent of more responsive emergency care, and more sensitive and sophisticated diagnosis of acute injury and disease. Coupled with this growing population of 'survivors' of neurological injury is a much more optimistic view with respect to the potential for reorganization and recovery of function than had been previously held (Kolb 1996; Robertson and Murre 1999). Considerable experience-dependent neuroplasticity, particularly at the level of the synapse, has been demonstrated in adult mammalian brains. Finally, advances in cognitive neuroscience have increased our understanding of cognitive processes and the nature of acquired cognitive impairments. These developments have occurred in the context of medical care and management systems that emphasize functional outcomes and the use of empirically validated approaches to treatment and intervention. This chapter reviews some of the basic tenets and primary approaches used in the rehabilitation of cognitively impaired individuals.

The field of rehabilitation has a long history (see Chapter 1). Some of the earliest rehabilitation 'specialists' appear to have been neurologists who worked closely with young soldiers injured in the first two World Wars in Germany, Russia, and England. Prominent early figures in neurology such as Kurt Goldstein, Alexander Luria, Richie Russell, Henry Head, and Henri Hecaen wrote extensively about their experiences with wounded soldiers. Their observations of individuals with focal brain injuries contributed greatly to our understanding of acquired disorders of language, perception, memory, and executive functions (Luria 1966). They also left a legacy in rehabilitation in which recovery was not viewed simply in physical terms, but in a social context. It was not enough to assist individuals in being able to walk, talk, and care for their immediate physical needs. Rather, rehabilitation was seen as involving families, communities, and the ability to integrate into home, school, and work. (For a review of rehabilitation's early history, the reader is referred to *Neuropsychological Rehabilitation*, vol. 6, 1996). Rehabilitation professionals recognized early on that impairments in cognitive and self-regulatory abilities contribute significantly to functional limitations and poor integration into home, school, and work environments.

Consistent with this early perspective, cognitive rehabilitation can be conceptualized as the application of techniques and procedures, and the implementation of supports to allow individuals with cognitive impairment to function as safely, productively, and independently as possible in their environment (Ponsford *et al.* 1995; Sohlberg and Mateer 2001). Although physical therapy aimed at restoring or improving postural stability, balance, and mobility is a key element of most rehabilitation programs, this chapter will primarily focus on interventions designed to address acquired impairments in cognitive abilities, and concomitant alterations in behaviour, mood, and emotional regulation. Impairments in these domains can negatively affect a wide range of adaptive abilities, including the ability to care for one's own needs, to maintain personal and social relationships, to achieve in school, and/or to engage in gainful employment.

A substantial literature has developed in the area of cognitive rehabilitation, and while many questions remain, the issues are better understood and the intervention procedures and approaches are better articulated. There are now a number of peer-reviewed journals that focus on the rehabilitation of individuals with brain injury and on interventions for impairments in cognitive ability. Recently, there have been a large number of new texts devoted to this topic (Finlayson and Garner 1994; Mills *et al.* 1997; Ponsford *et al.* 1995; Rosenthal *et al.* 1999; Sohlberg and Mateer 2001; Stuss *et al.* 1999). Review papers and meta-analyses evaluating the efficacy of cognitive interventions have also begun to appear (Carney *et al.* 1999; Chesnut *et al.* 1999; Cicerone *et al.* 2000; Coelho *et al.* 1996; Hall and Cope 1995; Park and Ingles 2001).

As a result of this body of research and clinical practice, clinicians working in the field are better able to identify the cognitive characteristics of patients who will likely benefit from different types of interventions. It is no longer appropriate or useful to ask the question 'Does cognitive rehabilitation work?' That would be akin to asking 'Does surgery or pharmacotherapy work?' The appropriate questions now ask what particular types of interventions are effective in addressing a variety of functional goals or outcomes in individuals with different profiles of cognitive ability.

General practice principles for cognitive rehabilitation

Following are a list of general principles for the practice of cognitive rehabilitation. Some of these derive from rehabilitation practice in general, including the need to take an individualized approach, involvement of clients and caregivers in all aspects of the rehabilitation process, and the importance of clear and realistic goal-setting. Others derive from the newness of the field and the critical need to evaluate both the short-term efficacy and long-term outcome of particular approaches and procedures. Still others derive from the common impact of cognitive impairments on emotional functioning, and emphasize the need to integrate cognitive interventions with interventions that can ameliorate emotional responses that interfere with response to treatment, increase adaptive functioning, and improve long term emotional adjustment.

1. *Cognitive interventions must be tailored to the individual.* A number of variables have been shown to be important in selecting appropriate and effective rehabilitation strategies in the heterogeneous TBI population (Sohlberg and Mateer 2001; Ylvisaker and Feeney 1998).

These include a variety of pre-injury factors, the client's level of insight and awareness, their ability to self initiate and regulate behaviour, the nature and severity of cognitive impairments in particular domains, the needs of the family, and the goals for rehabilitation with respect to personal care and home and community involvement.

2. *Cognitive interventions are most effectively viewed as a collaboration between the client, the client's family or caregivers, and the therapist.* Cognitive rehabilitation is not something that is done 'to' someone, but rather done in a collaborative partnership, to the extent that the client's cognitive deficits and level of awareness allow (e.g., Sohlberg *et al.* 2001; Ylvisaker and Feeney 1998).

3. *Cognitive intervention should be focused on mutually set and functionally relevant goals.* The World Health Organization defines four levels that need to be considered in working with individuals who are challenged by disability (for information about the current WHO classification scheme please see www3.who.int/icf/icftemplate.cfm. as well as Wade's contribution to this text, Chapter 4). The first level, *pathophysiology,* refers to the underlying disruption of physical functioning (e.g., a tumour or stroke). The second level, *impairment,* refers to the specific losses or alterations relative to normal functioning that occur as a result of the pathophysiological injury or disease (e.g., loss of ability to speak or to remember new information). The third level, *activity/functional limitation,* refers to changes in routine or daily functioning that occur as a result of the *impairment* (e.g., inability to communicate with others, safely care for oneself, or to take public transportation). The fourth level, *participation,* refers to the effect of activity and functional limitations on the person's ability to engage in age-appropriate social activities and roles (e.g., working, parenting, ability to live independently). While rehabilitation is not traditionally viewed as altering the underlying pathophysiology, it seeks to reduce functional limitations and increase and normalize participation; for example, by improving or implementing compensations for specific impairments. Within the domain of cognitive rehabilitation, much greater emphasis has been placed on the need to address goals and measure outcome and efficacy at the level of disability, and not just impairment. The therapist should seek to work with the individual and family to set clear objectives and goals that have relevance to the person's everyday life. It is not sufficient or appropriate to set improved test scores as a target goal, although changes in test scores may serve as one indicator of change or responsiveness to an intervention.

4. *Evaluation of efficacy and outcome should incorporate and capture changes in functional abilities.* A wide range of outcome measurements and approaches has been identified. Functional changes can be identified through a variety of assessments tools that identify the frequency of everyday successes and failures in particular domains (e.g., taking medication), the quality of behaviour, and the amount of assistance, supervision, or support needed to accomplish a task. Outcome assessments now include performance-based measures (e.g., Wilson *et al.* 2001), and questionnaire and/or rating scales completed by the client and/or caregivers (e.g., Cicerone 2002).

5. *Most successful cognitive interventions are eclectic and involve multiple approaches.* Given unique individual profiles and the likelihood of multiple areas of disability, many intervention plans will incorporate several approaches (Ylvisaker *et al.* 2002). Specific treatment tasks are typically arranged hierarchically so that treatment activities change over time as clients make progress in skills and toward reaching functional goals. For example, a client with severe anterograde memory disorder and executive impairments may require cues for initiation and prospective memory, and an external memory aid for recording past events, accessing new information, and looking to future scheduled events. Implementation of these external supports might be accompanied by a behavioural or cognitive-behavioural program for reducing anxiety and frustration, and by family or caregiver counselling to provide education and support.

6. *Interventions should address the affective and emotional components of cognitive loss or inefficiency.* There has been increasing recognition of the role that emotional response to changes in one's ability plays in contributing to, and in some cases maintaining disability. While there has been recognition of the high frequency of depression and anxiety after acquired brain injury, there is greater appreciation that fear, frustration, and loss of self-regulation of cognitive abilities often results in withdrawal from cognitive challenges and the development of negative self-expectancies. Increasingly, efforts are being made to avoid separating the treatment of cognitive and emotional difficulties, and instead provide integrative treatment that acknowledges the interdependence of these domains (e.g., Ben-Yishay and Daniels-Zide 2000).

7. *Interventions should be self-evaluative.* Although it is important to be aware of the theories and the support for efficacy related to a specific intervention, it is also important to evaluate the utility of that intervention in the individual case in which it is used. Ultimately the strongest evidence of efficacy is from patient-specific hypothesis testing (Ylvisaker *et al.* 2002). Baseline data, regular monitoring of progress in terms of changes in performance or behaviour, and measurement of outcome and goal attainment should be an essential part of any rehabilitation treatment plan.

A review of the literature suggests that a number of critical elements are important for successful rehabilitation planning, implementation, and evaluation (Sohlberg and Mateer 2001; Ponsford *et al.* 1995; Rosenthal *et al.* 1999). These include:

- An understanding of the underlying disease process or injury and its natural course.
- An appreciation of the individual's premorbid strengths, weaknesses, and lifestyle.
- A comprehensive assessment of the individual's cognitive strengths and weaknesses.
- An assessment of the person's current and projected living environment, including the demands on them and supports available to them.
- An assessment of the person's awareness of their situation, and their ability to self-regulate behaviour and emotion.
- An assessment of the person's emotional response to cognitive challenges and/or failures, and general coping style.
- An assessment of the person's ability to learn and the identification of teaching strategies to which they best respond.
- An assessment of the family's understanding of the cognitive and/or behavioural difficulties, the nature and degree of support they provide, and their expectations for treatment.

Establishing a process for gathering and assimilating the above information increases the likelihood of identifying and implementing effective interventions. The ability to consider each of these elements usually requires a multidisciplinary team with a capacity for sharing information and coordinating services.

Selecting an intervention strategy

The selection of a particular intervention approach for a client demands careful consideration of a number of different factors. One of the more important individual client characteristics is the level of self-awareness a client demonstrates with respect to recognizing current cognitive and physical difficulties, and the implications of those difficulties for aspects of everyday functioning. For clients with little insight, and a low capacity for self-regulation, effective interventions will likely target factors external to the individual. This includes a wide array of behavioural strategies, facilitation/ training of task specific routines, and the implementation of environmental modifications that provide substantial cues and supports for prompting and guiding behaviour. Much of the intervention at this stage can be considered compensatory, but it tends to involve more passive compensations to which the individual is trained to respond, rather than to self-initiate or regulate. The strategies implemented with such clients are often very situation- and task-specific, and generalization to other contexts is often not anticipated (Mateer 1999).

For individuals with higher or emerging levels of insight into changes in their ability, and who have more capacity for initiation and self-regulation, other techniques are likely to be effective. Such individuals may benefit from training to increase processing efficiency, from implementing and practising a wide variety of active compensatory strategies, from awareness training, and from approaches that help them cope with emotional responses to cognitive difficulties that serve to further reduce their

coping and efficiency (Mateer 1999; Sohlberg and Mateer 2001). In many cases, therapists will adopt new approaches as clients gradually increase in their awareness and self-regulatory capacity.

Additional factors important to consider when selecting an intervention include the nature and severity of the cognitive impairments. For example, clients with a severe anterograde memory impairment will usually be unable to recover any significant memory ability, and will almost certainly be dependent on memory aids or compensations (e.g., Donaghy and Williams 1998). In contrast, clients with forgetfulness secondary to attentional difficulties, or poor spontaneous use of memory strategies may benefit from attention training (e.g., Sohlberg et al. 2001), and training in mnemonic or other meta-cognitive strategies (e.g., Fasotti et al. 200z0), as well as training in the use of external memory aids.

Commonly used intervention strategies

Once client-specific information has been obtained, a treatment plan can be developed. Although many specific examples of techniques for working with cognitively impaired adults and children have been articulated, the following are three broad approaches to rehabilitation: (1) *environmental modification*; (2) *implementation of compensatory strategies*; and (3) *restorative approaches*. These approaches are distinguished by the agent that is targeted for change, though in fact, they are often used simultaneously. Environmental manipulations seek to change the physical environment, including the actions of other people, to accommodate impairments. The use of compensatory strategies focuses on training or teaching clients and/or caregivers to adopt behaviours that will circumvent difficulties caused by cognitive impairments. Restorative approaches also focus on the client, but specifically target the underlying neuropsychological impairment with the goal of improving the deficit function. Additional approaches involve the use of special instructional techniques that have been shown to be useful for individuals with learning and memory impairments. All of these are integrated with approaches designed to manage common but potentially maladaptive emotional reactions to cognitive limitation (see Table 3.1).

Following a description of these general approaches is a discussion of treatment techniques that have relevance regardless of the specific intervention approach that is adopted. These are the adoption of specialized learning and teaching techniques, education, awareness training, and the integration of treatment for emotional response to impairment. In most situations, a combination of therapies and approaches is selected. For example, the literature suggests that restorative approaches for the rehabilitation of attention impairments are most effective if paired with awareness training (Cicerone et al. 2000). Primary in all effective rehabilitation plans is the importance of collaborating with clients and families, and of setting functional outcomes that are measurable and meaningful to the client.

Table 3.1 Commonly used cognitive intervention strategies

Environmental interventions
Implementation of compensatory devices and strategies
Restorative techniques
Adoption of specialized instructional techniques
    Direct instruction
    Errorless instructions
    Fostering procedural learning
Managing emotional reactions to cognitive limitations
Client, family and caregiver education
Cognitive-behavioural interventions

Environmental interventions

Environmental modifications involve changing aspects of the injured individual's environment so as to reduce behavioural and functional impairments. In the acute stage after injury, most environmental interventions are designed to keep the person safe (e.g., locked doors to stairwells, temperature controls on taps), and to minimize overstimulation (Ducharme 1999). Bright lights, noisy environments, and rapid movement can exacerbate confusion and distress. Rehabilitation specialists, in concert with family members, control the environment in order to limit fatigue, and to reduce frustration during treatment tasks.

In the more chronic stage, environmental modifications are tailored to areas of specific functional impact. One type of environmental modification involves organization of physical space. Individuals with significant memory or executive function deficits may benefit from such manipulations as labelling cupboard contents, establishing a clutter-free zone, and setting up a family message centre on the refrigerator (Sohlberg and Mateer 2001). An extension of organizing the physical space is to post prompts or cues to increase adaptive behaviour. A number of researchers have described the utility of using posted checklists to help individuals complete activities (e.g., Martelli 1999). Checklists can be used to remind someone of the steps in a daily routine (e.g., grooming, dressing, laundering), or to provide cues for completing an activity (e.g., conversation prompts). Similarly, the environment may contain posted reminders to assist with task initiation and orientation to time (e.g., calendars to monitor passage of days and target activities). Thompson and Kerns (1999) describe a number of different types of environmental modifications specifically for classrooms, that can be helpful for students with brain injuries. Examples for students with attention impairments include clearing clutter from workspaces, providing earplugs or a headset during independent work, seating students away from noises such as windows or clocks, and posting information or task expectations on cue cards. Family carers also play an important role in fostering an environment conducive to effective functioning by providing cues, reminders, encouragement, and support. Although the aforementioned interventions can be thought of as environmental or physical supports, there is usually an associated educational or training component. The injured person and care providers may need to be oriented to the aids, and may require training and practice to use them appropriately.

Implementation of compensatory devices and strategies

The literature contains a number of experimental and case reports suggesting that the use of external compensatory aids is effective in managing cognitive difficulties (e.g., Kim *et al.* 1999; Wilson *et al.* 2001). Within the realm of cognitive rehabilitation, compensatory aids may take many forms. Probably the most effort has gone into the study of compensatory memory devices. Compensatory memory aids, in the form of calendars, alarms, watches with the date, memory books or organizers, and personal computers are widely used by many people who are not injured. The complexity of daily life often requires assists for memory and retention of information and detail that could not otherwise be managed. For individuals with any decrement in new learning and memory, such aids can be invaluable and are often essential.

The results of experimental reports support the effectiveness of this rehabilitation approach (Wilson *et al.* 2001; Wright *et al.* 2001). Wright and colleagues compared two different styles of pocket computer memory aids. The authors concluded that people with brain injury could effectively use a computer-based external aid, and that they found them useful. Wilson and colleagues (2001) provided paging systems to people displaying a wide variety of cognitive difficulties. The pagers reminded them to carry out self-selected functional tasks. The results indicated a significant increase in the initiation of functional tasks (e.g., taking medication) that for some subjects continued beyond the removal of the paging systems.

Several training protocols based on cognitive and instructional theory have been specifically developed for teaching individuals with cognitive impairments to utilize external aids (e.g., Donaghy and Williams 1998; Sohlberg *et al.* 1998). In general, reports of using external aids suggest that it is important to conduct a needs assessment of the learner and environment in order to match the external aid to the individual. Effective implementation of the aid is dependent upon systematic instruction, incorporating care providers, and monitoring the effects of using the aid. Instructional issues are described in a later section in this chapter.

New technological advances designed mainly for use by the general public have opened up new opportunities for people with disabilities. For example, some pharmacies provide electronic reminders that patients wear to remind them to take medications. Alarms on watches can also provide reminders. Some watches (e.g., the Timex Data Link) interface with personal computers via simple programs and a barcode reader on the watch to provide detailed information about scheduled appointments, medication reminders, etc. Alphanumeric pagers can interface with either telephone or computer programs allowing individuals to be reminded about things to do. Some Internet web sites offer customized paging and notification systems that interface with pagers, cell phones, and personal organizers. Rehabilitation specialists should review available or potential systems with the injured individual and family. Such factors as initial and ongoing cost, ease and flexibility of programming, and type of notification (auditory, visual, or vibratory) can be considered. Even more important is an analysis of what sort of supports the injured person needs, who is available for ongoing support if the person needs it, and how the person will be trained to use the system effectively. A recent case study describes the development, implementation, and functional efficacy of an Internet-based paging system to improve markedly reduced initiation of behaviour (adynamia) in a severely amnestic subject with associated impairments in executive function (O'Connell *et al.* 2003). This client was prompted to engage in everyday activities, such as playing the piano, walking the dog, and taking medication, all activities of which he was capable, but failed to initiate independently.

Restorative approaches

Another approach to working with cognitive problems is to engage the person in systematic activities that are designed to improve some underlying cognitive capacity. The cognitive ability that has probably received the most attention in this regard is attention. Attention is a multifaceted capacity that underlies many other aspects of cognitive functioning (Posner and Peterson 1990; Van Zomeren *et al.* 1984). For example, limited attention can result in poor learning or memory of new information, difficulty following a conversation or movie, and ineffective problem-solving. Underlying this approach is a belief that systematic practice and exercise of certain cognitive skills will result in a strengthening of those skills.

Further detailed review of the outcomes of this line of research is provided in later chapters of this volume. In general, the evidence suggests that to maximize the effects of attention training, clinicians should: (1) combine it with strategy training and feedback; (2) use hierarchically sequenced tasks that address complex attention and working memory as opposed to simple vigilance or reaction time tasks; (3) select exercises that target the specific attention impairments of individual clients, rather than administering a standard program; and (4) be explicit in establishing and measuring outcomes by asking what the client/clinician/payer expects to change as a result of attention training (Park *et al.* 1999; Cicerone 2002; Cicerone *et al.* 2000).

Specialized instructional techniques

The rehabilitation of individuals with cognitive impairment often involves teaching new information and skills, a challenge in clients who typically demonstrate fundamental difficulties with memory and new learning. There is, however, a growing body of instructional literature describing techniques that have been shown to be effective in working with individuals with brain injury.

Direct instruction techniques

Direct instruction is a systematic approach to the design and delivery of curricula to build and maintain basic academic skills (Sohlberg and Mateer 2001). Examples of some of the principles of direct instruction include:

- Breaking a skill into component parts and teaching all component parts
- Careful selection of teaching examples so clients can build on prior learning
- Instructional pacing using high response and success rates
- Sufficient practice with guided assistance followed by independent practice
- Use of distributed vs. mass practice
- Cumulative review.

A number of researchers have used direct instruction techniques with success for people with brain injuries. Glang *et al.* (1992) reported success in teaching three students with brain injury using direct instructional techniques. The skills that were targeted included academic skills (e.g., math), language, and behavioural self-monitoring. Sohlberg and Mateer (1989) used elements of direct instruction to teach an individual with severe memory impairment to utilize a memory notebook.

Errorless instruction

One feature of direct instruction is the notion of errorless learning. This has been explored in the brain injury population in some detail. Errorless learning techniques have been shown to be effective when working with individuals with severe memory impairments (Wilson *et al.* 1994). When using this technique, correct answers or strong cues for correct answers are provided to the memory-impaired individual until they establish the new information. By avoiding incorrect guesses (errors), confusion in memory is reduced while the new information is consolidated and stored. Errorless learning techniques have been shown to be superior in learning name and face associations, orientation information, short sequences of behaviour (such as entering information into a memory device or organizer), and routes around a hospital in severely memory-impaired individuals. Such approaches do not in any way change or correct deficiencies in the memory system, but they allow individuals with impaired memory systems to learn new information more effectively. The techniques also tend to reduce stress in learning new skills and information as frustrating errors are decreased. For many brain-injured individuals, such approaches are helpful and an important part of rehabilitation treatment planning.

Procedural learning

Another distinction in memory relates to the conscious or unconscious nature of memory. Recall of biographical information, word lists or stories, discussions with friends or family, television shows, and books one reads are all examples of explicit, conscious recollections, or what is termed *declarative memory*. Traditional neurological and neuropsychological tests typically sample this kind of memory for which we are consciously aware. However, there are other ways to demonstrate that one has been affected by experience and some kinds of learning are considered unconscious or implicit (Squire 1992).

Sometimes referred to as *procedural memory*, this kind of memory typically involves learning that occurs over time with repetition. Importantly for rehabilitation, this type of learning is often relatively spared. The potential effectiveness of this kind of learning can be used to train new skills and procedures in individuals with otherwise very impaired new semantic learning ability.

Specialized instructional techniques such as those briefly described above have provided new tools and approaches to addressing rehabilitation goals. Their effectiveness reinforces the need for rehabilitation specialists to draw from a broad literature base, including learning theory, behaviorism, and cognitive neuroscience.

Meeting the emotional needs of individuals with brain injury

Increasingly, rehabilitation specialists have identified the importance of addressing the client's emotional response to changes in their functioning and the reactions and concerns of families and caregivers. Education about the nature of neurobehavioral changes is a crucial part of rehabilitation, allowing the individual and others involved in their care to interpret symptoms more accurately and manage the environment more effectively to foster adaptive functioning. Many individuals who experience cognitive difficulties also develop a range of fears, frustrations, and anxieties around cognitively demanding activities. Individuals with a limited sense of self-control with respect to their cognitive functions may avoid or withdraw from activities that they perceive as demanding or stressful.

One concern is that rehabilitation has for too long compartmentalized components of rehabilitation, with various specialties working in single domains. Most textbooks on the topic of cognitive rehabilitation have separate chapters for working with cognitive disorders and emotional responses, when in fact they are often linked. More specificity with respect to the role of the 'adjustment piece' of rehabilitation is needed. Cognitive-behavioural and educational approaches to assist individuals in achieving a more balanced response to cognitive difficulties, and to feel more confidence in their ability to self-regulate both emotion and cognition appear to have significant utility. Fostering a sense of empowerment and emphasizing self-management and feelings of self-efficacy are often a critical component of treatment (Sohlberg and Mateer 2001).

Summary

Over the last decade, there has been increasing interest in identifying how best to work with individuals who are challenged by cognitive impairments. Over this time, there has been substantial additional research, clarification of major principles underlying such interventions, and greater specification with respect to training procedures and teaching techniques that are effective. Cognitive rehabilitation specialists recognize the need to be skilled in a number of different types of interventions. It is becoming clearer what techniques will work for particular individuals based on their cognitive profiles, level of insight, and capacity for self-regulation. Cognitive rehabilitation is eclectic, functionally oriented, and involves a partnership with clients, families/caregivers, and professionals. While much remains to be learned, this has certainly been a decade of progress and innovation.

4 Applying the WHO ICF framework to the rehabilitation of patients with cognitive deficits

Derick T. Wade

Abstract

Models of illness are important. They facilitate a systematic and logical analysis of clinical problems and hopefully thereby allow for a more coherent plan of treatment to be devised and implemented. The World Health Organization's International Classification of Functioning (WHO ICF) is a descriptive system that can be transformed into a powerful way of analysing illness. In relation to cognitive deficits, it highlights the fact that cognitive impairments are conceptual constructs that are derived from behavioural observations, and that the associated disability or disabilities are not in themselves specifically attributable to a single 'cognitive' deficit. It also highlights that rehabilitation for patients with cognitive losses may well involve many different interventions at many different levels, not simply attempting to reverse the loss itself.

Introduction

Ideas often constrain action more effectively than any physical barriers. For example, when people did not believe that flying in 'heavier than air' machines might be possible, then attempts that questioned this were ridiculed and serious research was delayed. In the same way, the rehabilitation we offer our patients with brain damage and cognitive deficits might be constrained by our rehabilitation paradigm or model and also our understanding of brain damage. Indeed most conferences and texts refer to 'cognitive rehabilitation', immediately constraining action to those interventions that might somehow reduce the deficit. In this chapter a wider view will be developed.

Most healthcare professionals and most health care activities are based on an unspoken and poorly described biological or 'medical' model of illness that assumes that all illness can be traced back to some single prime cause or disease (the diagnosis). They further believe that disease leads to symptoms and signs which may in turn limit the patient's ability, causing 'disability'. Interestingly the model and its assumptions are rarely if ever described or taught, and it is difficult to find any serious discussion of the topic in most medical and para-medical texts. This is unfortunate, because the pervasive nature of the dominant model of illness may in fact seriously limit the effectiveness and efficiency of most health interventions.

One alternative related model that is gaining popularity is the bio-psychosocial model (Engel 1977, White 2005), and its particular emphasis on the importance of social factors in the genesis of disability. It is certainly an advance on the standard biomedical model of medicine. There are of course many other models of more or less general applicability (Waddell 2002, Wade 2001a).

However, another model of illness can be derived from the descriptive framework that underlies the World Health Organization's International Classification of Functioning (WHO ICF) (WHO 2000), which was developed from the WHO International Classification of Impairments, Disabilities and Handicaps (WHO ICIDH). The WHO ICF, as it stands, is simply a way of categorising the various aspects of ill health, but it is based upon an implicit model of how ill health arises. This chapter will first describe briefly the WHO ICF and how it forms a model of illness. It will then use this model to explore how the many problems faced by patients with cognitive deficits (usually but not inevitably secondary to brain damage) may be analysed rationally so that patients can be helped to have a fuller range of activities and a fuller level of participation in society.

The WHO ICF framework

The World Health Organization's International Classification of Functioning (WHO 2000) was developed as a means of describing the totality that is the experience of illness. In fact it is only complete if coupled with the WHO International Classification of Diseases (ICD), but this is a minor point. There are hundreds of articles published about the WHO ICIDH and ICF, but few consider its use in the process of rehabilitation or the power of the underlying model. This section will describe my understanding and interpretation of the framework and how it can be used as a model to analyse illness.

In essence the framework states that any patient with an illness can be described using four levels, and that to gain a fuller understanding three contextual factors also need to be taken into account (see Table 4.1). It should be noted that in practice this model applies perfectly well to people who are not ill, and indeed might profitably be used when considering criminal behaviour and how it is managed by society (Wade and Halligan 2003). Table 4.1 also shows how the framework relates to systems, and how this might help analyse illness.

The first level is that of (abnormal) structure and/or function of an organ or organ system and the words usually used are *disease* or *diagnosis*. Another word is *pathology*, and problems at this level are generally classified using the ICD. Of course a more detailed description can be given, such as specifying the biochemical (genetic) abnormality, or electron microscopic changes within cells. For example one may state that someone has had a *stroke* (more correctly a *cerebral infarction*), but one could add that this was located in the *internal capsule* on the left, and that it was associated with *hypertension*, and *hypertensive vascular disease* of the perforating arteries. A second example might be *Huntington's chorea*, where it is known that changes occur in the *caudate nucleus* and that an *expansion of ITI5 gene DNA* within chromosome 4p16.3 is the ultimate cause.

The second descriptive level is that of abnormal structure or function of the whole body or parts of the body, and the words used are *symptoms* and *signs*. Another word is *impairment* (usually of some bodily skill or bodily function). Examples in neurology include hemianopia, aphasia, spasticity, wasting of muscles, pain, depression, fatigue and weakness. Other examples might include hepatomegaly (a large liver), absence of a limb, reduced range of movement at a joint, and swelling of the ankles.

Cognitive impairments, and indeed all neurological impairments, are of especial interest because they are no more than conceptual constructs used to explain and make sense of observed clinical phenomena. Usually clinical staff either simply observe a pattern of behaviour (such as bumping into objects on the left) or they may structure a formal test where certain behaviours may be observed (such as crossing out all the small stars in a cancellation test), and they then deduce that the construct

Table 4.1 Rehabilitation model – the WHO ICF Framework

Term	Level of description		
	System	*Synonym*	*Comment*
Pathology	Organ within body	*Disease/diagnosis*	Refers to abnormalities or changes in the structure and/or function of an **organ or organ system**
Impairment	Person, body as a whole	*Symptoms/signs*	Refers to abnormalities or changes in the structure and/or function of the **whole body** set in **personal context**
Activity (was *disability*)	Person in the physical environment	*Function/observed behaviour*	Refers to abnormalities, changes or restrictions in the interaction between a person and his/her environment or **physical context** (i.e. changes in the **quality or quantity of behaviour**)
Participation (was *handicap*)	Person in social environment	*Social positions/roles*	Refers to changes, limitations, or 'abnormalities' in the **position** of the person in their **social context**

Contextual factors			
Domain	Characteristics	Examples	Comment
Personal	Internal, abstract constructs	*Previous illness*	Primarily refers to **attitudes, beliefs and expectations** often arising from previous experience of illness in self or others, but also to personal characteristics.
Physical	External, physical objects	*House, local shops, carers*	Primarily refers to local physical **structures** but also includes people as **carers** (not as social partners)
Social	External, abstract constructs	*Laws, friends, family*	Primarily refers to **legal** and local **cultural** setting, including attitudes and expectations of important others

Note: This model is usually prefaced with the words: 'In the context of illness, …'

of 'visual neglect' is present. In practice it is more likely that they will first make clinical observations and will then use a test to confirm (or refute) their hypothesis, but the 'test' is itself simply a set of particular behaviours that are observed. The named impairment is in fact no more than a short label used to summarise and explain a larger group of observations. It may of course also be useful predictively and in other ways. But neurological impairments do not have any physical reality; their presence has to be deduced from the subjective accounts of the patient (symptoms) and the associated behavioural evidence (signs).

The third level is that of the interaction between a person and their environment. In other words it is the person's behaviour, and problems at this level were called disabilities and are now referred to as limitations on activities performed. Several points need stressing. The behaviour may be altered in two ways: the person may simply be unable to perform the activity or may do so slowly (a quantitative change) or there may be a qualitative change, and the goal may be achieved in a different (often called abnormal) way. For example someone might be able to walk but slowly, or to walk but with a limp, or to walk but only if supported by a stick, or not to walk but able to get around in a wheelchair. It is also worth stressing that the label 'abnormal' is ill advised: the method may well be the most effective and efficient in the circumstances; it is not abnormal for the person concerned; and in many circumstances the range of statistical normality (i.e. 95 per cent of the population) may include the quality observed.

In contrast to impairments, behavioural performance is more objective (however, see Van Gijn and the plantar reflex 1976). Observers can see and agree on what activities are or are not being undertaken and also how. Observers may of course disagree on (a) what the underlying causes are for any changes, (b) whether the person is potentially able to behave in a different way and (c) the quality of the behaviour observed.

The last descriptive level is that of a person's social position; their roles and who they are (in the opinion of themselves and others). The word used in the WHO ICIDH classification was 'handicap' but is now, more appropriately, limitations on participation (in society).

A person's social position is deduced from their behaviour (including their statements) and an interesting contrast can be drawn between impairment and participation. Briefly we (external observers) can all see and generally agree on behaviour observed. On the one hand, we can analyse the behaviour and try to make certain deductions about the person's underlying skills or lack of skills. This might include a nebulous description of their 'personality', which simply means that we try to predict future behaviour from past behaviour. On the other hand we also interpret the behaviour in terms of its (social) meaning, thereby attributing certain roles to the person.

These four levels describe the illness both within the person (pathology and impairment) and in terms of its external consequences (behaviour observed by others, and interpretations placed upon that behaviour by others). In order to understand the description one also needs contextual information, and the WHO ICF recognises three major contexts of importance: personal, physical, and social. To a limited extent these might be considered to affect the interactions between pathology and impairment, impairment and activities, and activities and participation.

The personal context refers to the relevant mental characteristics of the patient as an individual. It is their expectations, beliefs, attitudes etc. These may have come from past experiences and from more general cultural factors as well as being intrinsic to the individual. They are internal, and again are conceptual constructs created for the purposes of communicating interpretations and explanations from observed behaviour and known events.

The physical context refers to the significant environmental objects around the person, both peri-personal and more distant. It also includes the availability of other people as helpers (but not as social contacts). Factors in the physical context are external, and can be observed by anyone (although an external observer may not appreciate how important or otherwise any specific object is to the patient).

The social context refers to the culture, primarily the local culture affecting the patient. Of course this also includes national and even international laws etc. These are also external. Some can be known to external observers – such as the laws, and the general attitudes of society – but others can only be known to the patient and their immediate social contacts.

Developing the WHO ICF framework

The WHO ICF framework has some deficiencies. It does not cover quality of life, probably best conceived of as well-being on a separate axis (Post *et al.* 1999). It does not explicitly distinguish between the perception of the patient/subject and the perception of others. It does not take into account the importance of time in an illness, but within a descriptive system this does not matter. However, if it is used as an explanatory model it does matter. An expanded model which includes quality of life and two points of view (external and internal) is shown in Table 4.2.

The WHO ICF framework was developed as a means of categorising different components of illness. As such it is a static system of classification: however it can also be considered as a systems analytic approach for understanding illness. Briefly one may postulate that there are relationships between the different levels, and these relationships are causal. For example it seems likely that complete paralysis

Table 4.2 Expanded model of illness (WHO ICF plus) A way of describing someone's situation

'Location' of description	Subjective/internal	Objective/external
	Experience, attributions and beliefs of the patient	Observations made by, and implications drawn by others
Level of description: term used		
Organ within person:	Disease	Diagnosis
Pathology	Label attached by person, usually on basis of belief and experience	Label attached by others, usually on basis of investigation
Person:	Symptoms	Signs
Impairment	Somatic sensation, experienced moods, thoughts etc	Observable abnormalities (absence or change), often elicited explicitly; and deficits assumed from observations
Person in environment:	Perceived ability	Activities undertaken
Behaviour/'activities'	What person feels they can do and cannot do, and opinion on quality of performance	What others note person does do, quantification of that performance (not what others think *should* do)
Person in society:	Life satisfaction	Participation, roles in society
Roles/'participation'	Person's judgement or valuation of their own role performance (what and how well)	Judgement or valuation of important others (local culture) on role performance (what and how well)
Context of illness		
Personal context	'Personality'	'Past history'
	Person's attitudes, expectations, beliefs, goals outlook, reasoning style etc	Observed/recorded behaviour prior to and early on in this illness. Known experiences of illness in others
Physical context	Personal importance	Resources
	Person's attitude towards specific people, locations, objects etc.	Description of physical (buildings, equipment etc.) and personal (carers etc.) resources available
Social context	Local culture	Society
	The people and organisations important to person, and their culture; especially family and people in same accommodation	The society lived in and the laws, duties and responsibilities expected from and the rights of members of that society
Totality of illness		
Quality of life:	Contentment/well-being	Social involvement
Summation of effects	Person's assessment of and reaction to achievement or failure of important goals. Or sense of being a worthwhile person	Extent of positive interaction with society, contributing to social networks. Or apparent happiness

and loss of sensation affecting both legs (after a spinal cord injury) is in fact the cause of a person's inability to walk. Indeed we all make such assumptions as part of our daily life.

An overall model based on the WHO ICF framework is shown in Figure 4.1, showing some possible relationships with and causes of limited activities (disability). This model will be used to explain, communicate, and understand illness. We will consider first the relationship between cognitive losses and disability, and then the totality of interventions that might be involved when faced with disability

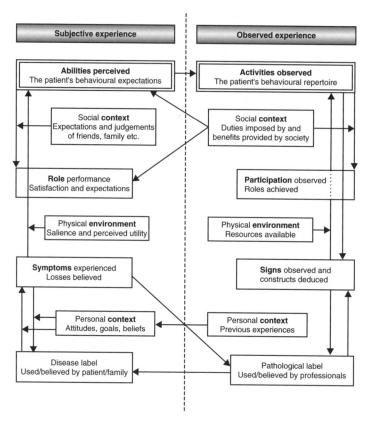

Figure 4.1 Observed (limitations on) activities and some influences thereon.

associated with cognitive deficits. In general, evidence will not be reviewed in detail, because this chapter only aims to set a broad framework and does not aim to discuss whether interventions are effective.

An impairment of cognition, not a 'cognitive disability'

It has become quite common to refer to cognitive disabilities, supposedly contrasted with physical disabilities. However, this shows a failure to understand the distinction between impairment and disability in the WHO ICF framework. A patient may need assistance in getting around the environment (i.e. have a 'mobility disability') for many reasons such as: complete spinal cord transaction at T6, stroke with severe motor weakness on the right, loss of sensation in both legs due to peripheral neuropathy, amputation of both legs at the hips, loss of all vision, severe amnesia, marked visuo-perceptual losses and neglect, agoraphobia or other fears, etc. Thus the so-called 'physical disability' of being unable to walk unaided can arise in many ways, many of which are not 'physical' (i.e. motor) impairments.

   As another example, consider a patient who has had a head injury and fractured right ankle with a mild right hemiparesis. He may be continually getting up, walking short distances slowly and sometimes falling. This disability is walking that is slow and unsafe. This may arise from the right-sided weakness and some associated sensory loss, or pain from the fractured ankle, or forgetting that he should not walk, or a lack of insight into his own problems, or impulsiveness etc. Note that many of the quite usual 'explanations' assume impairments that involve mental constructs or capacities, such as 'lack of insight' or 'impulsiveness', and even 'sensory loss' cannot be proven in the same way as structural pathology.

In practice a person's activities depend upon a whole range of intact underlying skills or functions (there is no good word implying the opposite of impairment), and most activities can still be undertaken in the absence of a single skill. It is usually the combination of impairments that limits activities, and this in itself demonstrates how people can learn to overcome impairment. For example a person with a more-or-less fixed (immobile) knee can walk provided they have no other loss.

Naturally some impairments tend to disrupt some activities more than others. However, there are few, if any, one to one correspondences or mapping between impairment and disability. Motor loss in the legs tends to reduce mobility (unsurprisingly) and visual impairments tends to reduce reading. Therefore it is reasonable to state that some activities are more (or less) likely to be affected by certain cognitive impairments than other activities. For example impaired language disrupts communication; amnesia disrupts complex community activities such as shopping; visuospatial impairment may disrupt many activities including dressing; confusion disrupts continence etc.

However, it is vital to remember that combinations of impairment are usually more disabling. For example poor memory can be overcome by writing lists but if writing (or reading) is disrupted (or if the person was anyway illiterate) then the disability associated with the amnesia is much more dramatic. And, in terms of rehabilitation, this means that the best way to reduce the limitation on activities might be to enhance another impaired function (such as motor function in the right arm to allow writing) rather than focusing on the impairment itself.

Figure 4.2 attempts to show this. One activity is limited through a combination of three cognitive impairments and two other impairments, whereas a second activity which may rely on cognitive function 'C' is nonetheless normal and a third activity is disrupted by a single non-cognitive impairment.

In summary the WHO ICF model of illness suggests that:

- Cognitive impairments are abstract constructs that usefully summarise observed behavioural data and may usefully predict performance of other activities.
- A cognitive impairment may affect some activities more than others, but does not in itself cause 'cognitive disability'.
- Most disability arises from the specific combinations of cognitive and non-cognitive impairments experienced by the patient.
- Improving an activity limited in part by a cognitive impairment might depend primarily upon ameliorating an associated non-cognitive impairment.
- The links between specific (cognitive) impairments and specific activities is probably weak.
- Aspects of the context may have an important moderating function.

Rehabilitation for patients with cognitive impairments

The section above has already suggested that even at the level of impairment, treatment for a patient with cognitive deficits might best be targeted at another, non-cognitive impairment. This section will review the potential to intervene at all four levels and also in the three contexts. This is shown in a general way in Table 4.3, but this section will focus specifically on potential interventions for patients with cognitive deficits.

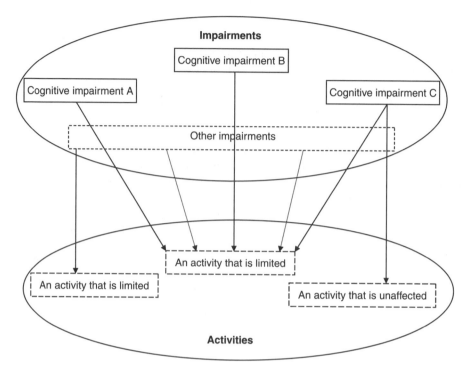

Figure 4.2 Separation of impairments and activities.

Reducing pathology

While it is accepted that currently one cannot revive or replace dead neurons, nonetheless there is sometimes scope for reducing pathology within the central nervous system and thereby improving cognitive losses.

First there may be scope for slowing down or stopping a pathological process. For example it seems likely that treatment with beta-interferon ameliorates the cognitive losses experienced by most patients with MS. Similarly, protecting the brain from additional anoxic brain damage after traumatic brain injury may have dramatic cognitive benefits. There may be drugs that slow down or limit the damage in more diseases in future.

Next, patients with one diagnosis may be at risk of secondary pathological processes that may cause cognitive losses. Hydrocephalus developing after subarachnoid haemorrhage or traumatic brain injury is one specific cause; the late development of a subdural haemorrhage is another; recurrent vascular episodes after stroke are a third. All may be avoidable or treatable and some dramatic recoveries can be seen.

Last, patients may simply develop an incidental second disease. A patient who has had a stroke may also later develop carcinoma with cerebral secondaries. It is important to detect this, both so that specific treatment can be given if available and also so that decisions are based on an appropriate prognosis.

Consequently, an accurate diagnosis of the underlying disease and undertaking specific actions to prevent avoidable damage are both vital. Any rehabilitation service seeing patients with neurological

Table 4.3 Some examples of rehabilitation interventions within the WHO ICF

Level/term	Intervention	Comment
Level of illness		
Organ	Prevent Reverse or remove Replace lost physiological function (e.g. insulin) Give information and advice	Important to know pathology for prognosis and likely impairments. 'Cure' often not possible. NB pathology is not always present in an illness
Person	Prevent occurrence or worsening of impairment Reverse or improve impaired skill Replace lost skill or part	May use therapy, drugs, orthoses, prostheses etc. Note that impairment may improve secondary to functional practice
Person in environment	Prevent patient learning abnormal behaviours Teach how to undertake activities in presence of immutable impairments Practice activities, advising on risks, techniques etc.	Involves altering behaviour in one way or another. Will often also involve changing the environment. May involve changing patient goals or goals of others. Takes time, and depends upon learning
Person in society	Prevent loss of social contacts and roles Help identify new roles, and how to develop them Ensure has opportunities to develop or maintain roles	Will almost always involve other people Takes a long time
Context of illness		
Personal context	Prevent development of maladaptive beliefs and expectations Alter beliefs and expectations if necessary, usually through giving information and psychological therapy	Beliefs and expectations are major determinants of behaviour; but consequences of behaviour may also affect beliefs and expectations
Physical context	Avoid loss of familiar environment if possible Adjust environment physically, including through providing care	Could include orthoses etc.
Social context	Adjust or help patient find new social context; or help adapt to new social context	Usually strongly linked to accommodation and work
Totality of illness		
Quality of life	Full rehabilitation	Depends upon interventions at many levels

Note: Almost all interventions depend upon active involvement and participation of patient and/or family.

diseases must have a specialist doctor familiar with the diagnosis and treatment of neurological diseases as an integral part of the team.

Reducing impairment

This is the first treatment considered by many professional staff and patients, drawing on the analogy (likely to be invalid) that cognitive processes are like muscle, and that exercise or use will increase strength or function. This is at least part of if not all of cognitive rehabilitation as commonly understood; training to overcome neglect is one example. The evidence relating to this will be reviewed in depth elsewhere in this book.

However, there may be other ways of reducing cognitive impairment. Many if not most patients undergoing rehabilitation after brain injury are on drugs that sedate or in other ways affect the function of the central nervous system. Indeed there is some evidence that some drugs may actually reduce (Goldstein 1998) or increase (Walker-Batson *et al.* 2001, but see Sonde *et al.* 2001) cerebral plasticity after brain damage in humans. Reducing and stopping medication may have a dramatic effect.

In addition cognitive function can be adversely affected by mood disturbance, and control of low or unstable mood (without too much sedation) may well improve cognitive function considerably. Further, as mentioned earlier, reducing other impairments may allow the patient to overcome cognitive losses using alternative strategies.

Consequently, an accurate appraisal of all of the impairments that may be contributing to limitation of activities is also vital if a rational effective treatment plan is to be instituted, and any rehabilitation team treating any patients with neurological disease must have a range of specialists familiar with all aspects of neurological impairment as integral members of the team, including not only clinical neuro-psychologists but also physiotherapists, orthoptists, nurses, occupational therapists, speech and language therapists etc.

Practicing activities

The brain, even when damaged, is an adaptive organ that is responsible for all goal-directed behaviour and often it will achieve activities in ways that are effective given the residual functions. Therefore one way to overcome limitation in activities that are or may be secondary to cognitive losses is simply to practice undertaking the activity, usually in the most relevant environment compatible with safety. In patients with reduced mobility secondary to MS it seems that task-related therapy (i.e. practicing walking) is as good as impairment-focused therapy at reducing motor impairment in the leg (Lord *et al.* 1998). Indeed there is a growing literature to support the effectiveness of a task-related approach to rehabilitation (Dean and Shepherd 1997; Dean *et al.* 2000).

This approach, focused on the limited activities, has the advantages of maximising patient motivation and not depending upon an accurate analysis of the deficits within an accurate theoretical framework. In other words, therapy focused on an impairment assumes that the therapist has correctly identified the impairment that is the key to the limitation on activities. This in turn depends upon having an accurate model of what skills are needed to perform the activity. We do not generally have information of this accuracy or detail; for example there are several cognitive models of language or memory processes.

This approach does not mean that proper analysis of the situation is not necessary. This is only one potential treatment method, and often an intervention elsewhere may be more effective. Further, without a clear understanding of the underlying impairments the team may not know what risks may be present when undertaking treatment. For example, if cooking is difficult due to neglect then the therapist will specifically look out for one set of dangers, but if ataxia or amnesia is the primary impairment then different risks will need to be considered.

Increasing social participation

This is similar to practicing activities, except that the focus has moved from the activity itself to the meaning of the activity. It is the difference between practicing cooking a dinner, and practicing being a host to a dinner party. Again this approach may enhance patient engagement and motivation, both of which facilitate learning. There is relatively little research into this sphere, the nearest being research into the rehabilitation of leisure activities after stroke (Parker *et al.* 2001). However even that research focused on the activities more than on actual participation in social leisure activities. One specific problem with this approach is that social activities are generally considered to be outside the remit of health rehabilitation services. This artificial barrier may in fact limit the effectiveness of rehabilitation.

Altering personal context

The potential benefits of acting on a patient's personal context have been discussed before (Wade 2000). Although we are not in the position to alter a person's experiences, or what they have been taught up to this point, it is possible to try and alter their attitudes, expectation and beliefs.

There is some evidence that interventions aimed at increasing self-efficacy can be effective, and there is a strong evidence base behind cognitive behavioural therapy. However it should be recognised that standard cognitive behavioural therapy may be of limited applicability in patients with cognitive deficits. Given the central role of beliefs in many illnesses, especially such illnesses as back pain, it is surprising how neglected this area of intervention is.

Interventions aiming to alter attitudes, expectations and beliefs are just as relevant for patients with cognitive deficits as for patients with other problems. A 'hidden' cognitive deficit can have major effects upon a patient's self-confidence, especially when other people are unaware of the deficit. Intervening to teach coping strategies and increase self-efficacy may well reduce the patient's self-imposed limitations on activity.

Altering physical context

Changing the environment is an obvious treatment for patients with motor impairments – for example providing a wheelchair, or environmental controls, or adapted cutlery. However it may also be effective in some instances for people with cognitive deficits.

One common practice in many rehabilitation units is to place signs about, telling the amnesic patient where their room is. This is an alteration in the physical context. Another quite common practice is to place a ruler or line on the left side of a page to help a patient with neglect read. In the same vein, patients with a right hemianopia sometimes find that turning the book upside down allows successful reading.

There are many other ways that changing the physical environment may help, including teaching carers how to act so that a patient's performance of activities is improved.

Altering social context

This is a less obvious area for intervention, but it too may be effective. The social context may be altered in three ways to help a patient with cognitive deficits; two will apply to all patients with illness and one is specific.

Changing the general laws and culture of a society may, over time, improve the activities and participation of people with impairments and disabilities. Research has shown this for back pain (Wade 2001b), and it is common experience in Western countries that enacting laws has slowly increased the ease of participation of disabled people in society. Examples include increasing accessibility to public buildings for people in wheelchairs, use of hearing loops, provision of more official documents in forms for people who are blind, support for people with disability to work, and provision of day centres and transport to facilitate more social interaction.

Next it may sometimes be possible and appropriate to act on the person's local culture, for example changing the way that friends and family act towards the patient and involving local groups in increasing social participation. Examples might include educating family members that disability is not reflective of immorality, encouraging a church group to take the patient to church, and educating family members that it is reasonable not to do everything for the patient.

Finally, and specific to patients with cognitive deficits, it may be appropriate and possible to structure the social environment in a way that increases activity performance. This includes the setting up of routines so that a patient who has difficulty in planning or remembering when to undertake activities is more likely to achieve them alone. This is the equivalent of altering the physical environment, and involves adapting the social environment to their needs.

Conclusion

A person who is ill might be compared to a house in need of repair. Sometimes the problem is minor, and a small action such as mending a broken pipe can stop further damage and no other action is needed. Often, however, there are many problems and simple small repairs are not enough. Then several specialists are needed, and the renovation of the house will only succeed if there is an overall plan. Even if a leaking pipe was the original cause of all the subsequent problems, the repairs will not succeed if the only intervention is aimed at the pipework by a plumber.

In this analogy, a rehabilitationist is not simply a carpenter, repairing a broken-down house. Rather he (or more usually she) is part of a team working with the remaining sound structures to create a new house, different from but neither better nor worse than before. Of course carpenters are needed, but so are plumbers, electricians etc. The team rehabilitating a house works on the whole house, not simply one part, and often the team will need to devise new solutions to particular problems. Sometimes an architect may be needed to help plan the new house and how it is achieved, but in rehabilitation this role is often also undertaken by the team itself. Furthermore in rehabilitation the patient is an active member of the team; he or she owns the house!

This chapter has hopefully shown that the rehabilitation of patients with cognitive deficits should be undertaken by a team that analyses the situation and considers a whole range of interventions, only a few of which will specifically target the cognitive deficits themselves.

5 Methodological issues in evaluating the effectiveness of cognitive rehabilitation

Keith D. Cicerone

Abstract

The rehabilitation of cognitive deficits following acquired brain injury has shown tremendous growth over the last three decades. This period of development has been accompanied by increased demands that cognitive rehabilitation demonstrate its maturity, and expectations that the field evaluate itself and provide scientifically sound evidence of its clinical effectiveness. In the absence of scientific evidence, claims for the effectiveness of any medical or rehabilitation practice rely upon clinical 'expert opinion,' typically reflecting the judgments and beliefs acquired by individual clinicians through their professional experience and clinical practice. As a field matures, it should become more common to utilize evidence from systematic research to inform clinical practice. The practice of evidence-based rehabilitation is based on the 'integration of individual clinical experience with the best available external clinical evidence from systematic research' (Sackett *et al.* 2000, p. 2).

Methodologies and classes of evidence

Evidence-based evaluation of the available research typically requires the classification of individual studies according to their methodological design and rigor. Three levels of evidence are frequently considered, reflecting different degrees of experimental control.

Single-subject designs and uncontrolled group studies

Studies reporting results from one or more single cases using appropriate single-subject methodology and studies reporting a clinical series without concurrent controls are considered Class III evidence. The early published reports of cognitive rehabilitation for persons with acquired neurocognitive impairments often described the treatment of individual cases using single-subject methodology (Glasgow *et al.* 1977; Gianutsos and Gianutsos 1979). Single-subject investigations often follow the traditional logic of clinical interventions in which the patient is started on a treatment and monitored to determine whether the patient's deficits improve or not. This continues to be the most common method of evaluating cognitive rehabilitation interventions, based on recent evaluations of the current literature. Well conducted, single-subject investigations may be particularly useful for describing an innovative treatment approach and its direct clinical application. However, the interpretation of findings is tempered due to the large number of possible confounding factors that can influence the results. For example, it may be difficult or impossible to isolate the effects of the treatment from the natural course of recovery from the illness or injury. Even if this is addressed by studying a patient who is far enough after injury so that the effects of spontaneous recovery are considered small, the effects of repeated practice or test administrations and normal fluctuations in performance (especially regression to more average or normal scores) may obscure the treatment effects. Finally, non-specific effects such as patient or investigator expectancies are more likely to influence the results of single subject or uncontrolled studies. While all of these factors may operate in studies that utilize more sophisticated designs, they are likely to be most evident in the absence of control subjects, who are presumably also subject to the same factors. Sackett *et al.* (2000) describe a method for applying the logic of randomized clinical trials to single-subject investigations, referred to as an N of 1 randomized trial. This approach, which resembles the more traditional behavioral ABAB design, requires that the patient and therapist/investigator agree to evaluate the treatment under investigation, compared with no treatment or an alternative treatment. The patient then receives paired treatment periods in which one period consists of the treatment under investigation and the other period consists of the alternative treatment condition, which may subsequently be repeated. The order of the two treatment periods within each pair is determined at random (e.g., by coin toss). The N of one randomized trial may have utility when evaluating interventions that require their active use within the confined treatment period, such as the use of external compensations. This approach may be less useful when the intervention is expected to result in the maintenance and generalization of treatment effects to untreated periods. To my knowledge, this design has not been utilized in the evaluation of cognitive rehabilitation.

Controlled, observational studies

Studies providing Class II evidence consist of prospective, non-randomized cohort studies or retrospective, non-randomized case-control studies. These observational studies consist of two (or more) well defined groups of patients that, ideally, are similar in all ways other than the type of treatment that was received. This design may be used when there are naturally occurring groups of patients that receive different treatments due to external factors. Examples of external factors that produce naturally occurring groups could be variations in the differential use of the treatment due to regional differences, or the introduction of a new treatment protocol, particularly when the disease prevalence remains constant and patient characteristics are well defined and stable (Whyte 2002). In the latter case, patients currently receiving the novel treatment are compared with a similar group that received treatment prior to implementation of the novel treatment protocol (a retrospective design using 'historical' controls). Unfortunately, it is difficult to ensure that the groups of subjects are in fact identical, other than the treatment received, in these designs. Observational studies also consist of prospective studies in which the patients are assigned to treatment conditions neither by randomization nor by factors presumed to be unrelated to the treatment itself. Instead, the groups of patients (or cohorts) are formed by the decisions of clinicians and/or the preferences of patients to receive one of the treatment conditions. In these cases, it is hard to assume that the cohorts are in fact identical other than the treatment, since treatment decisions and group assignments may be influenced by clinical factors such as time after injury, severity of impairments, patients' motivation, or a host of other considerations. In addition, the factors that determine clinician's decisions regarding the assignment of patients to treatment are frequently difficulty to measure or unknown. Under these circumstances, the influence of non-comparable groups on treatment effects is difficult to overcome, even with the use of sophisticated statistical techniques that attempt to correct for such biases (Powell *et al.* 2002; Vogel *et al.* 2002).

One evidence-based review (Cicerone *et al.* 2000) also classified clinical series with well-designed controls, which permitted between-subject comparisons of treatment conditions, (e.g., multiple baseline across subjects) as Class II evidence. Well designed multiple baseline across subjects studies do allow a direct comparison across treatment conditions, and therefore conform to the general intent of other Class II designs. Within a typical clinical setting, the 'best available' treatment may be the combined application of standardized treatment protocols and individualized treatments dictated by clinical experience. Controlled multiple-baseline designs may provide an approximation of the clinical application of interventions and may be intuitively attractive to clinicians for that reason. There is currently no evidence that would answer the question of whether multiple-baseline studies and other non-randomized observational designs are equivalent methodologies and produce comparable results.

Prospective, randomized controlled studies

Randomized controlled trials, in which the appropriate patients are randomly allocated to treatment and non-treatment conditions, are generally considered to provide the strongest, Class I evidence for the effectiveness of an intervention. This is based largely on the assumption that the process of randomizing patients to treatment conditions makes it more likely that the groups receiving alternative treatments are comparable in all aspects other than the nature of the intervention. The use of randomized, controlled trials should therefore reduce effects due to bias in selecting subjects for different treatment conditions. Randomized controlled trials of rehabilitation effectiveness can be difficult to conduct, not only due to the time and expense involved but because of the belief that it is unethical to withhold treatment that is strongly believed by clinicians to be of benefit. Several recent reviews of the medical literature have suggested that estimations of treatment effect sizes from well-designed observational studies are comparable with those obtained from randomized controlled trials, providing some support for the use of observational studies in rehabilitation (Concato *et al.* 2000; Benson and Hartz 2000). The randomization of patients to avoid selection biases is assumed to underlie the superiority of randomized controlled trials. However, there is some indication that the adequate concealment of treatment allocation (Kunz and Oxman 1998; Schulz *et al.* 1995), double-blinding (i.e., the degree to which both patients and clinician were unaware of the treatment condition; something that would be hard to accomplish in a trial of rehabilitation) (Schulz *et al.* 1995) and restrictiveness of eligibility criteria (Horwitz *et al.* 1990) all make significant contributions to the size of treatment effects.

Randomization of patients helps to ensure the internal validity of intervention studies (i.e., the likelihood that the results reflect the effects of the treatment itself), but randomized controlled trials may also suffer from subject selection biases that limit the external validity of the study (i.e., the ability to generalize results to clinical samples). Since patients who consent to participate in clinical trials are by definition a self-selected group, they may not be representative of patients who either fail to meet enrollment criteria or refuse to participate. Sackett (cited in Silverman 1998) has described an example of this 'volunteer participant problem' in a large scale randomized trial of breast cancer screening. The study demonstrated a marked reduction in breast cancer mortality among women who underwent screening, compared with controls. Mortality from other causes was equivalent between the groups, confirming the comparability of groups and internal consistency of the study. At the recruitment stage, one-third of eligible patients refused to participate but continued to receive their typical medical follow-up. Compared with the patients who refused participation, the volunteer participants in either arm of the breast cancer screening trial were about half as likely to die from other causes. This is not an isolated example, and Sackett goes so far as to suggest that patients who volunteer for clinical research trials are, in general, 'a strange and healthy lot, and we cannot generalize from them to other patients'

(Silverman 1998, p. 34). In a study comparing structured neuropsychological treatment with an alternative treatment (computer games, relaxation training, small group discussion and didactics) for persons with traumatic brain injury (TBI), Ruff *et al.* (1989) screened a group of patients living in the community for the evidence of neuropsychological impairment and neurosurgical or radiological evidence of a brain contusion. The resulting subset of potential participants were then further screened to ensure that they had functional expressive and receptive language abilities, at least one functional hand, at least 25 per cent intact visual fields, no premorbid history of neuropsychiatric disturbance, no history of other neurologic disorder that might affect cognitive functioning, and were motivated to participate in treatment. Previous treatment for TBI is not reported, but it is reasonable to consider that these patients from the community, without neurologic or psychiatric comorbidities, who were motivated to volunteer for treatment might not reflect the general population of patients with TBI who are referred for cognitive rehabilitation. Both groups showed significant improvements from the respective treatments, with marginal differences between the groups on neuropsychological measures. While Ruff *et al.* (1989) interpreted the results as supporting the relative benefits of the neuropsychological intervention on specific cognitive measures, it is clear that both the experimental and control patients who volunteered for the study benefited from treatment. In their analysis of effect sizes from both randomized trials and observational studies, Concato *et al.* (2000) noted that patients in the experimental treatment groups had similar outcomes regardless of the study design; however, the control patients in observational studies had worse outcomes than the controls in randomized trials. In other words, when smaller differences between groups are evident in randomized, controlled trials, this may be due to the tendency for both treated and untreated groups to improve. In a randomized trial of cognitive rehabilitation for traumatic brain injury, Salazar *et al.* (2000) compared cognitive rehabilitation with a low-intensity home program and found no significant differences between groups on neuropsychological functioning, psychological adjustment, return to work, or fitness for duty at one year after treatment. Participants were still in the acute stage of recovery at the time of treatment and all were in the military healthcare system. The selective nature of the population represents a potentially important limitation. For example, Glenn *et al.* (2001) noted that the patients in this study were highly atypical of most patients admitted for inpatient rehabilitation with respect to severity and recovery; only 2 of 643 (0.3 per cent) patients enrolled in a national TBI database during the time-frame of the Salazar *et al.* (2000) study were far enough recovered to have met the entrance criteria. The authors of the study also noted that both groups had 'extraordinarily high return-to-work rates' (Salazar *et al.* 2000, p. 3079).

Efficacy, effectiveness, and practical clinical trials

While randomized, controlled trials of cognitive rehabilitation should have a prominent role in evaluating the effectiveness of cognitive rehabilitation, there appears to be a clear role for observational studies, and probably even for single subject designs. In addition to consideration of the hierarchy of research designs in evaluating the evidence for cognitive rehabilitation, an additional distinction should be considered. Intervention studies may be considered either as studies of treatment *efficacy* or as studies of clinical *effectiveness*. Efficacy studies are often designed to evaluate the effects of a highly constrained treatment, provided to a strictly defined sample, under ideal conditions of use. In contrast, many studies of clinical effectiveness evaluate the effects of a typical treatment, provided to an existing clinical group of patients, under usual conditions of use. The distinction between efficacy and effectiveness studies may parallel the distinction between randomized trials and observational studies, but may be dissociated. Efficacy studies are particularly suited for determining whether a treatment can work, while effectiveness studies may illustrate whether a treatment does work in a clinical setting. Observational studies of clinical effectiveness may provide the basis for subsequent, more rigorous analyses using randomized controlled trials. Efficacy studies may also allow investigation of the potential utility and feasibility of interventions in clinical practice. For example, Levine *et al.* (2000) conducted a randomized trial in which 30 patients with TBI received a single 4 to 6 hour session of either goal management training for the remediation of executive functioning, or motor skills training. The goal management training was demonstrated to be efficacious in improving performance on 'everyday paper and pencil tasks' compared with the motor skills training. The external validity of these findings is limited by several factors. First, the length of intervention probably does not reflect the typical clinical treatment needs for patients with executive dysfunction. Second, there is some question as to how well these patients represent the patient with dysexecutive syndrome seen in clinical settings. Levine *et al.* (2000) note that TBI is associated with ventral frontal and anterior temporal lesions and none of the 30 patients had frontal lesions on CT scan. However, there is no indication that these patients actually exhibited significant executive dysfunction, although all were impaired on a strategy application test that resembled the demands targeted by the goal management training. Finally, there was no assessment of the effect of training on actual dysexecutive impairments in these patients' lives, and the likelihood of generalization after a single training session may well be slight. In order to demonstrate the clinical application of goal management training to practical, real-life situations, these investigators did describe the treatment and follow-up of a single patient, five months after of an episode of meningo-encephalitis causing attention and executive deficits.

Some studies with demonstrated efficacy in controlled settings may have practical restrictions in their clinical application. For example, constraint-induced movement therapy has been demonstrated to be feasible and efficacious in reducing arm impairment during acute rehabilitation for ischemic stroke (Dromerick *et al.* 2000). However, a subsequent investigation found that 68 per cent of patients in the community indicated that they would not be interested in receiving the treatment, due to the restrictive schedule of daily use, and therapists also cited concerns about patient adherence, safety and the ability to comply with the protocol within their treatment setting (Page *et al.* 2002).

Recently, Tunis, Stryer and Clancy (2003) have described the role of *practical clinical trials* (PCTs) that may bridge the gap between efficacy and effectiveness studies, and provide direct value and relevance to clinical decision-making. According to Tunis *et al.* (2003), the characteristic features of PCTs are that they (1) compare and evaluate clinically relevant alternative interventions, that (2) include a diverse population of participants (3) referred from representative, heterogeneous practice settings, and (4) assess the effects of treatment using a broad range of outcome measures. While explanatory clinical trials are designed primarily to understand why and how an intervention might work, practical clinical trials are attempts to formulate hypotheses and study designs based on the information needed to make decisions in clinical practice. Thus, PCTs may provide a means to combine scientific rigor with clinical relevance.

Evidence-based analyses of cognitive rehabilitation

Any attempt to systematically evaluate the evidence regarding the effectiveness of cognitive rehabilitation needs to consider a host of factors ranging from the methodological rigor and quality of research to the clinical feasibility and utility of interventions to its cost-effectiveness. There have been a number of evidence-based reviews of cognitive rehabilitation published in the past several years, all varying somewhat in their approach. The Cochrane Collaboration has conducted reviews of cognitive rehabilitation for attention deficits (Lincoln *et al.* 2001), memory deficits (Majid *et al.* 2001) and spatial neglect (Bowen *et al.* 2003) following stroke. These reviews typically rely solely upon high quality, randomized controlled trials to reach their conclusions. The review of rehabilitation of attention deficits identified two trials with 56 participants. The reviewers concluded that there was some indication that training improves alertness and sustained attention, but no evidence to support or refute the effects of cognitive rehabilitation on functional independence. The review of memory deficits considered only one trial with 12 participants that failed to show any benefit of strategy training on memory deficits or subjective memory complaints after stroke. There were 15 studies with 400 participants considered in the review of treatments for spatial neglect. There was evidence to support the beneficial effects of cognitive rehabilitation on some impairment measures, but insufficient evidence to confirm or exclude an effect of cognitive rehabilitation on disability or status following hospital discharge.

In 1999, an independent, nonfederal group of investigators presented their findings before an NIH consensus panel regarding the scientific basis of common therapeutic interventions for the cognitive and behavioral sequelae of TBI (NIH Consensus Panel 1999). This review included an evaluation of 32 studies of cognitive rehabilitation for TBI, including 11 randomized, controlled studies (Carney et al. 1999). Their review noted that data on the effectiveness of cognitive rehabilitation programs was limited by the heterogeneity of subjects, interventions, and outcomes studied. It was noted specifically that efficacy had been demonstrated for the use of compensatory devices, such as memory books, to improve particular cognitive functions and to compensate for specific deficits. It was also noted that comprehensive, interdisciplinary programs that included individually-tailored interventions for cognitive deficits were commonly used for persons with TBI. Although this personalized approach led to difficulty in the scientific evaluation of effectiveness, several uncontrolled studies and a non-randomized clinical trial supported the effectiveness of these approaches.

The Brain Injury-Interdisciplinary Special Interest Group (BI-ISIG) of the American Congress of Rehabilitation Medicine reviewed 171 studies of cognitive rehabilitation following TBI or stroke (Cicerone et al. 2000). This review considered 29 Class I randomized controlled trials, 35 Class II studies, and 107 Class III studies. Following the initial review, articles were assigned to one of seven categories reflecting the primary area of intervention: attention, visual perception and constructional abilities, language and communication, memory, problem-solving and executive functioning, multimodal interventions, and comprehensive-holistic cognitive rehabilitation. Of the 29 studies, 20 provided some evidence to support the effectiveness of cognitive rehabilitation for subjects with acquired TBI or stroke. Eight studies were considered to provide evidence to support the use of visuospatial remediation of visual scanning deficits resulting from right hemisphere stroke, and four studies were considered to provide evidence supporting the use of language remediation following left hemisphere stroke. Twelve Class I studies evaluated the effectiveness of cognitive remediation primarily for persons with TBI. Eight of these studies provided clear support for the effectiveness of cognitive remediation for impairments of attention, functional communication, memory and problem-solving following TBI.

Differences in conclusions across evidence-based reviews may be due to variations in methodological rigor as well as biases in the interpretation of study results (McCormack and Greenhalgh 2000). With the increasing emphasis on evidence-based medicine, methods have been developed to evaluate the quality of different practice guidelines (i.e., there are now guidelines to evaluate the guidelines) (Cluzeau et al. 1999; Graham et al. 2000) (Table 5.1).

The quality of intervention studies is determined by a number of factors that operate across the hierarchy of research designs, and will affect both the integrity and applicability of the findings. These factors include the adequate specification of the intervention being investigated, complete description of the sample being studied and analysis of relevant patient characteristics, the use of outcome measures that are appropriate and congruent with the intended effects of the intervention, and the equivalence of alternative treatment conditions. The following discussion of these factors is based largely on the findings from the Cicerone et al. (2000) review.

Table 5.1 Suggested domains for the evaluation of practice guidelines (based on Cluzeau *et al.* 1999)

Scope and purpose: the overall aim of the guideline, specific clinical questions, and the target population

Stakeholder involvement: the extent to which the guideline represents the views of its intended users

Rigor of development: the process used to gather and synthesize the evidence, and methods to formulate the recommendations

Clarity and presentation: appropriateness of the language and format of the guideline

Applicability: the likely organizational, behavioral and cost implications of applying the guideline

Editorial independence: the independence of the recommendations and acknowledgement of possible conflict of interest from the guideline development group

Specification of interventions for cognitive deficits: what are the effective ingredients in cognitive rehabilitation?

Despite the increased efforts to evaluate the effectiveness of cognitive rehabilitation, we still lack an adequate understanding of the exact nature of many interventions (see Section 6). Unlike pharmacologic or surgical interventions, rehabilitation is likely to involve multiple, simultaneous treatment components. An adequate understanding of the nature, theory, and rationale for cognitive rehabilitation is necessary to conduct the relevant studies of efficacy and effectiveness (Whyte and Hart 2003).

In order to evaluate the effectiveness of cognitive rehabilitation, studies need to specify not only the nature of the specific interventions provided, but also the underlying assumptions of the intervention. In reviewing the literature, it is striking to note how frequently the rationale for the intervention is not explicitly indicated. Cicerone *et al.* (2000) noted that specific interventions intended to rehabilitate cognitive functioning may represent a variety of approaches. These approaches include (1) reestablishing previously learned skills or patterns of behavior, perhaps reflecting restoration of function; (2) establishing new patterns of cognitive activity through the development of internal cognitive compensations for impaired neurological systems; (3) establishing new patterns of activity through external compensatory mechanisms such as the use of assistive technology or environmental structuring and support; and/or (4) efforts directed toward enabling persons to adapt to their cognitive disability, even though it may not be possible to directly modify or compensate for cognitive impairments, in order to improve their overall level of functioning. While these approaches do not have to be mutually exclusive, the specification of a rationale is necessary to identifying the relevant level of outcome and success of the intervention. Disagreements regarding the interpretation of the literature may result from ignoring distinctions between these different approaches. This is central to the question of the construct validity of cognitive rehabilitation, i.e., whether the effects of cognitive rehabilitation are consistent with the intentions of cognitive rehabilitation.

Treatment integrity

Even when the rationale for interventions is specified and evaluated, it is necessary to evaluate the integrity of the intended treatment. For example, Dirette *et al.* (1999) compared the effects of remedial (restorative) versus compensatory interventions for visual information processing deficits after TBI. The compensatory intervention consisted of instruction in the use of three compensatory strategies (verbalization, chunking, and pacing). The restorative intervention was of equivalent intensity, but remedial computer activities were substituted for instruction in the use of compensatory strategies. Both groups improved, with no evidence of a differential treatment effect.

Actual use of strategies was examined through self-report and observation. Despite the different intended effects of the interventions, 80 per cent of the patients used compensatory strategies whether or not they were instructed to do so.

Simultaneous treatment components

Many treatments for cognitive deficits are likely to consist of a combination of task demands and therapist interventions, although this distinction has been largely ignored. Niemann *et al.* (1990) conducted a randomized controlled trial to evaluate the efficacy of a computer-assisted attention retraining program after moderate to severe TBI. The attention training was divided into three components: visual, auditory, and divided attention (i.e., simultaneous audiovisual stimulus presentation). These components were further divided into task demands intended to reflect focused and alternating attention. Considerable attention was devoted to systematically varying task demands along the dimensions of number of targets and distractors, similarity of targets and distractors, interstimulus intervals, shifts in target dimensions, and the location of the stimulus display. All of the tasks were computerized and six 2-hour sessions were allocated for each component. Within each session, the authors note that at least 30 to 40 minutes was devoted to practicing the task, with the remaining 80 to 90 minutes was allocated for 'feedback and strategy training,' although the nature of the strategy training was not described further.

Unfortunately, there have been few attempts to assess the activities of the therapist in cognitive rehabilitation or to evaluate the relative contribution of task demands and therapist interventions to treatment effectiveness. Ponsford and Kinsella (1988) evaluated a program for the remediation of speed of processing during acute recovery from TBI. The study failed to demonstrate a treatment effect when the effects of spontaneous recovery were controlled, but the authors noted that three of the 10 subjects appeared to benefit from the addition of feedback and reinforcement to the computer-mediated training. Wilson and Robertson (1992) incorporated highly personalized therapeutic interventions in treating a single patient for attentional slips during reading, including therapist feedback and monitoring the subject's emotional reactions to deficits. They note that the rationale for the treatment was based on 'reducing capacity-occupying thoughts about poor performance, which themselves sabotage performance, i.e., the exercise was one largely of confidence building.'

Unless the nature of interventions are adequately specified, it is difficult to compare the results of different studies. Park and Ingles (2001) did conduct a meta-analysis of attention rehabilitation after acquired brain injury, although they noted that many of the relevant studies did not provide enough detail to determine the specific nature of the treatment methods. The primary objective of this analysis was to evaluate the efficacy of interventions that attempted to directly retrain attention, and compare these effects with interventions intended to retrain specific, functional skills. Studies of direct attention retraining typically used a series of repetitive exercises or drills with improvement determined on psychometric cognitive tests. The studies of specific-skill training attempted to compensate for or retrain skills of practical significance, such as driving or activities of daily living, although this analysis also included studies where the attention outcome measures were highly similar to the training tasks. The analyses also compared studies with pre-post assessment of effects only, with those using pre-post assessment with a control condition. The effect size for studies with a control condition were smaller than those with pre-post assessment only, suggesting that the latter effect sizes were inflated by practice effects. The studies of direct retraining generally produced small effects, whereas the studies that attempted to rehabilitate specific skills that required attention showed considerably larger, significant improvements. The authors also suggest that therapist activities such as breaking down complex tasks and structuring the patients' responses to task demands were a critical aspect of successful interventions, a process they refer to as 'neuropsychological scaffolding' (cf. Cicerone and Tupper 1991).

Effective for whom?

The relevance and clinical utility of research on cognitive rehabilitation is also limited by the adequacy of description of the persons who received the intervention, and for whom it is intended. The range of relevant patient factors is extensive, but includes: patient demographics; premorbid social, neurologic, and psychiatric history; nature of the illness or injury; severity of illness or injury; chronicity; severity of impairment; description of how the presence of the impairment under study was determined; presence of concurrent cognitive impairments; and factors influencing treatment compliance. A number of studies have identified participants based on a specific neurologic diagnosis, e.g., traumatic brain injury, assuming the disorder in question to be present. Given the variability in nature and severity of deficits within a given population, the failure to assess and identify participants based on the presence and severity of the impairment being investigated will reduce the probability of detecting an effect, even if the treatment is effective. In reviewing the area of visual-perceptual remediation, Cicerone et al. (2000) noted that the studies that identified, and directed the intervention at, a specific impairment (e.g., visual scanning for neglect) were more likely to result in significant improvements than studies directed at improving general visuospatial functioning after stroke. There was also evidence that treatment was most effective for patients with severe impairments during the acute period of recovery. Evidence for the effectiveness of visuospatial remediation was much less certain when deficits are mild, chronic, or when the treatment was evaluated with diagnostically diverse groups.

Stage of recovery

In reviewing the evidence regarding effectiveness of remediation for attention deficits after TBI and stroke, Cicerone et al. (2000) also reported evidence from two randomized controlled studies and two observational studies to support the effectiveness of attention training, beyond the effects of nonspecific cognitive stimulation, during the post-acute phase of recovery and rehabilitation. In contrast, there was insufficient evidence to distinguish the effects of specific attention training from spontaneous recovery or more general interventions during the acute period after injury, due to the effects of spontaneous recovery or the more general effects of acute brain injury rehabilitation.

Severity of deficits

The evidence regarding the effectiveness of compensatory strategies for memory deficits is mixed, but appears to depend on the severity of patients' memory deficits. Cicerone et al. (2000) reviewed four randomized, controlled trials of memory rehabilitation for persons with TBI. The four Class I studies addressed the effectiveness of training compensatory strategies in memory rehabilitation. Berg et al. (1991) compared memory strategy training with a 'pseudo-treatment' and no treatment conditions. All of the patients were living independently and about half were working in their previous vocation, although at a reduced level, suggesting that they exhibited a relatively mild degree of memory impairment. Results of objective memory testing showed improved memory function in the strategy training group only. Kerner and Acker (1985) demonstrated enhancement of memory skills using computer based memory retraining software for patients with 'mild-to-moderate' memory impairment at least three months post injury. Schmitter-Edgecombe *et al.* (1995) evaluated notebook training relative to supportive therapy for rehabilitation of memory disturbance in eight patients with traumatic brain injury who were more than two years post injury. The degree of memory impairment in all subjects appeared to be relatively mild. Patients who received the notebook training reported fewer observed, everyday memory failures than the supportive therapy subjects. Ryan and Ruff (1988) compared memory retraining employing rehearsal and visual imagery strategies with an alternative treatment, including computer games and psychosocial support. Both groups improved on neuropsychological measures of memory functioning, independent of the type of treatment. In a post hoc analysis, the groups were divided based on severity of initial neuropsychological functioning, and the data were re-analyzed. Differential benefit of the memory retraining was observed only in those subjects who had mild memory impairment prior to treatment. Cicerone *et al.* (2000) also cited several Class III studies indicating that this form of memory remediation is effective for subjects with mild impairments and not for subjects with severe memory impairment. Both Carney *et al.* (1999) and Cicerone *et al.* (2000) concluded that there is evidence for the effectiveness of compensatory memory training for subjects with mild memory impairments after TBI.

In contrast, several observational studies have suggested that patients with severe memory deficits may benefit from the use of external, compensatory aids (which should be distinguished from interventions that attempt to promote the use of internalized, compensatory memory strategies). Sohlberg and Mateer (1989) reported the effective use of a memory notebook to facilitate performance of daily activities by a patient with severe memory impairment. They also noted that the successful use of the notebook required extensive, highly structured training. Zencius *et al.* (1990 compared the effectiveness of three memory retraining strategies (verbal rehearsal, written rehearsal, and acronym formation) with the use of memory notebook to improve recall of specific, functional material over a 24-hour period. The memory notebook (which was available to subjects at the time of recall) was superior to all of the retraining techniques. The benefits of using the memory notebook were most apparent for the subjects with more severe memory difficulties, for whom the retraining techniques were largely ineffective. Wilson *et al.* (1997) demonstrated the effectiveness of a portable paging system to circumvent specific, everyday memory failures, such as remembering to take medication on time or remembering to shut off appliances. In a subsequent randomized controlled trial Wilson *et al.* (2001) confirmed the benefits of using a pager for carrying out everyday activities by persons with memory, planning or organizational problems. The authors note that many of the patients in the study had been referred by their therapists 'in desperation ... when all else had failed' (p. 481), although they also indicate that the patients had to have some insight into their memory problems and be motivated to use the paging system.

Co-morbid cognitive impairments

As noted by Wilson *et al.* (2001), patients receiving cognitive rehabilitation for specified deficits (e.g., memory) frequently have cognitive impairments in other areas (attention, executive functioning). Lawson and Rice (1989) described one patient with a traumatic brain injured whose ability to benefit from training on memory strategies was hampered by the presence of executive deficits which limited his ability to initiate strategy use. The independent use of the previously learned memory strategies was increased following a period of training for the executive dysfunction that explicitly addressed the initiation and self-monitoring of strategy use. Cicerone and Giacino (1992) reported improvement in executive functioning for five of six patients with the use of a self-verbalization strategy. The remaining patient exhibited severe memory deficits that interfered with his ability to apply the strategy independently. The impact of co-morbid cognitive impairments on the effectiveness of rehabilitation has received little explicit attention or direct investigation. The careful consideration of individual differences in the nature and severity of impairments, chronicity, and other unique patient characteristics is central to effective clinical assessment and treatment. In contrast, large-scale clinical trials and evidence-based guidelines generally tend to obscure individual patient characteristics, by their nature. This may be one of the primary reasons why clinicians fail to find these research findings to be useful (Caplan 2001).

Can we match patients to interventions?

In an appropriate use of an observational research design, Malec and Degiorgio (2002) described the patient characteristics and outcomes of successful and unsuccessful completers of three intervention pathways within a post acute brain injury rehabilitation program. The patients were referred for differing levels and intensity of treatment (specialized vocational services alone, specialized vocational services plus a group addressing community integration issues, or comprehensive integrated day treatment) on the basis of the judgement of a team of rehabilitation providers, the patient, and significant others. Patients who were less impaired and earlier post injury were able to benefit from limited intervention, while those with more extensive disability many years after injury were more likely to benefit from comprehensive treatment. Factors influencing successful participation at all levels of service included the time since injury, premorbid educational level, specific cognitive limitations, and patients' self-awareness. The authors note that many factors have to be considered in developing specific rehabilitation plans for specific patients, and further research of this type may help to specify the appropriate rehabilitation pathways for individual patients with increased accuracy.

Specification of outcomes: what are the effects of cognitive rehabilitation?

In reviewing the evidence for the effectiveness of cognitive rehabilitation, it is important to consider whether the level of outcome being assessed is specified a priori, whether the outcome measures are consistent with the intent and rationale of the intervention, and whether the specified outcomes are consistent with the intervention pathway being investigated. The outcomes of an intervention may be assessed at varying levels of functional analysis. Development of the *International Classification of Impairments, Disabilities and Handicaps – 2* has identified four levels of functioning relevant to rehabilitation outcome measurement (Gray and Hendershot 2000). Impairments are assessed at the level of bodily structure and function. Activities represent the performance of tasks by the person as a whole, such as moving around, communicating, learning and applying knowledge, and performing simple to complex tasks of everyday living. Participation reflects the person's involvement in life situations, including home life, social relationships, work and education, and involvement in community activities. The individual's social participation may be qualified by their subjective satisfaction. Finally, outcomes may be influenced by contextual factors such as environmental obstacles, social attitudes, and personal attributes such as coping and motivation. In principle, assessment of treatment effects after cognitive rehabilitation may reflect one or more of these dimensions (Table 5.2), representing focal or global outcomes (Whyte 1997). In practice, it may be difficult to relate outcomes to these discrete, conceptual dimensions (e.g., inability to learn to perform a task needed for a new job).

Neuropsychological functioning as an outcome of cognitive rehabilitation

A majority of studies of cognitive rehabilitation have utilized measures of neuropsychological functioning to assess the effectiveness of treatment. In many instances, a large number of neuropsychological tests

Table 5.2 Potential levels of outcome measurement for cognitive rehabilitation

Dimension of functioning	Relevant outcome measures
Impairment	Neurophysiological function (e.g., fMRI) Experimental neurocognitive function Clinical neuropsychological measures
Activity	Subjective complaints that limit activities Simple to complex tasks of daily living Use of compensations in everyday life Observations of behavioral functioning Need for assistance or supervision
Participation	Engagement in household activities Interpersonal relationships Socialization Leisure activities Academic participation Community-based employment
Quality of life	Satisfaction with functioning Subjective well-being
Contextual factors	Environmental barriers Social supports Secondary health conditions (mental or physical) Coping style Perceived role limitations

have been administered before and after treatment, with little or no specification of the expected effects of the treatment on the various measures. The use of a large number of varied neuropsychological outcome variables in hope of detecting a significant treatment effect is best avoided, since the findings are likely to be spurious or uninterpretable.

When there is a conceptual basis for using multiple outcome measures, statistical techniques may be used to evaluate whether the number of significant changes on multiple neuropsychological outcome measures exceeds that which would be expected by chance (Ingraham and Aiken 1996). However, it is probably preferable to address this problem at the stage of research design, through the adequate specification of planned comparisons and the prediction of expected effects of treatment on different outcome measures. For example, within the domain of attention training, Sturm *et al.* (1997) evaluated the benefits of different interventions directed at four specific components of attention. The evaluation of treatment effects allowed for the comparison of the expected benefits of specific components of training on the relevant outcome measure, as well as an assessment of non-specific effects of training across components. Kaschel *et al.* (2002) used a large number of psychometric measures in a randomized controlled trial comparing structured training in imagery mnemonics with 'pragmatic' memory retraining. Different predictions were made for both the imagery and pragmatic group in relation to both the type of material where effects should occur and the temporal pattern of expected improvements. Despite the use of multiple outcome measures, the investigators were able to analyze the results in accordance with specific predictions to determine the specificity and generalization of treatment effects.

Congruent outcome measurement

It is difficult to determine the effectiveness of an intervention unless the outcome measures reflect the intended effects of the intervention, which Whyte (1997) has termed 'congruent outcome measurement.'

In the study of notebook training for memory impairment conducted by Schmitter-Edgecombe *et al.* (1995), the effects of training were assessed through a number of outcome measures, including a laboratory-based measure of verbal recall, a laboratory-based measure of everyday memory, self and other report of retrospective memory failures, and recording of observed everyday memory failures. Patients who received the notebook training reported fewer observed everyday memory failures (with the use of the notebook), although there were no significant treatment effects for the laboratory-based tests of memory (which did not allow use of the notebook). The findings are noteworthy since the reduction in everyday memory failures is presumably the goal of memory rehabilitation. However, a clinically beneficial treatment effect would not have been detected if the investigators had relied solely on laboratory-based memory measures. Failure to find a significant effect of cognitive rehabilitation due to the use of incongruent outcome measures may therefore lead to the unfortunate conclusion that the treatment is ineffective.

The longitudinal assessment of outcomes can help to demonstrate the functional benefits (or limitations) of cognitive rehabilitation. For example, Milders *et al.* (995), conducted a follow-up of the patients treated by Berg *et al.* (1991) in which training in memory strategies was initially demonstrated to be superior to pseudo-treatment and no treatment conditions. Maintenance of the benefits of this treatment was assessed four years after training. There were no differences between the three groups on overall memory performance or subjective memory complaints, which reflected both continued improvement in the pseudo- and no-treatment groups and a return toward baseline in the strategy training group. The investigators also noted that the maintenance of improvements in memory functioning in some subjects was directly related to their continued use of compensatory strategies.

Cicerone *et al.* (2000) have emphasized that, regardless of the specific approach or area of intervention, cognitive rehabilitation should be directed at promoting changes that improve persons' functioning in areas of relevance to their everyday lives. There is now a fair amount of evidence to indicate that the effect sizes from cognitive rehabilitation are largest when the training closely resembles the outcome measure, suggesting task-specific or skill-specific effects (cf. Park and Ingles 2001). Even when it can be demonstrated that a cognitive intervention results in significant, clinically meaningful improvements on neuropsychological functioning, concerns may be expressed as to how well neuropsychological measures relate to, or predict, changes in functioning in everyday life. Although most studies of cognitive rehabilitation have relied upon neuropsychological measures to evaluate the effectiveness of treatment, there is some evidence that comprehensive treatment can produce improvements in patients' productivity, even in the absence of major changes in specific cognitive abilities (Cicerone *et al.* 2000; Malec and Basford 1996). It remains difficult to compare these results across studies due to variations in injury variables, subject characteristics, length of follow-up, and lack of a standard outcome measure.

Participation as an outcome of cognitive rehabilitation

Relatively few studies of cognitive rehabilitation have directly assessed the benefits of cognitive rehabilitation in terms of community integration and social participation, other than return to work. Malec (2001) reported improvements in social participation following comprehensive TBI rehabilitation, assessed with the Mayo Portland Adaptability Inventory (MPAI), despite the fact that primary cognitive functions showed relatively little improvement over the course of treatment. Following a comprehensive TBI rehabilitation, Seale *et al.* (2002) reported clinically significant improvement on the Community Integration Questionnaire (home integration, social integration, and productivity) for about half of their patients. Neither of these studies included a comparison group, limiting the interpretation of results. Cicerone *et al.* (2002) conducted an observational study comparing intensive-holistic cognitive rehabilitation with a 'standard' program of neurorehabilitation for persons with TBI. While both groups improved, the participants receiving intensive-holistic cognitive rehabilitation were over twice as likely to demonstrate clinically significant improvement in community integration as those receiving standard neurorehabilitation, despite being further post injury and having slightly worse community functioning prior to treatment.

Although the assessment of quality of life after cognitive rehabilitation would appear to be an important concern, this is a neglected area of research. It is interesting to note that there appears to be a marginal relationship, at best, between measures of community integration and life satisfaction for persons with TBI who have completed rehabilitation and are living in the community (Burleigh *et al.* 1998; Cicerone *et al.* 2002; Smith *et al.* 1998). There is a strong need to develop the appropriate instruments to measure health-related quality of life in a manner that is relevant to persons with neurologic disabilities (Bullinger and TBI Consensus Group 2002).

Effective compared to what?

In a mature clinical science, the effectiveness of a given intervention is typically determined through a comparison of an unproven treatment with the best available practice in that area. Despite recent developments in evaluating the effectiveness of cognitive rehabilitation, this is often not possible as there are few established best practices. Controlled trials do at least allow a comparison between a remedial cognitive intervention and alternative treatment approach. Of the 64 controlled Class I and Class II studies reviewed by Cicerone *et al.* (2000), only two studies failed to demonstrate improved functioning among subjects receiving cognitive rehabilitation. Several studies demonstrated an advantage of cognitive rehabilitation over conventional forms of rehabilitation. In essentially all of the controlled studies with negative or equivocal results, the intervention in question was compared with an alternative form of treatment (in some instances, an alternative form of cognitive remediation), all but one study demonstrated significant improvement even though there was not evidence of a *differential* treatment effect. In no study was there evidence that cognitive rehabilitation was *less effective* than an alternative treatment. These latter findings provide indirect support for the use of cognitive rehabilitation, while raising questions regarding the role of non-specific factors in determining treatment effects. The results of such comparisons also appear to vary depending on the nature of the alternative treatment condition (Table 5.3).

In order to examine the differential effectiveness of cognitive rehabilitation, the 29 Class I studies reviewed by Cicerone *et al.* (2000) were classified according to the nature of the alternative treatment condition. This resulted in 30 study comparisons, since one study included two alternative treatment conditions. Conventional rehabilitation comparisons consisted of routine physical, occupational, or speech therapies. Pseudo-treatment was defined as the provision of non-therapeutic attention,

Table 5.3 Differential treatment effects of cognitive rehabilitation compared with alternative treatment or control conditions based on 29 Class I studies (Cicerone *et al.* 2000).

Percent showing benefit of cognitive rehabilitation				
Alternative treatment	Studies	Patients	Studies (%)	Test comparisons (%)
Cognitive/psychosocial	7	235	47	44
Pseudo-treatment	8	333	63	57
Conventional rehabilitation	10	399	90	61
No treatment	5	169	100	76

recreational activities, computer games, or repetitive 'drill and practice' on tasks that were not anticipated to produce significant benefit. Treatments comparing different forms of cognitive rehabilitation
and those comparing cognitive rehabilitation with a psychosocial intervention were considered
together. A number of studies included a large number of outcome measures, making it difficult to
interpret the results and make a discrete determination as to whether cognitive rehabilitation was more
effective than the alternative treatment condition. Therefore, the total number of test comparisons for
each study was also considered. Based on this analysis, it is clear that providing cognitive rehabilitation is superior to not providing treatment. Cognitive rehabilitation also appears to be more effective
than conventional rehabilitation therapies for the type of deficits investigated. It is of some interest to
note that the benefits of cognitive rehabilitation compared with 'pseudo-treatment,' while still relatively substantial, were not striking and less apparent than the benefits of cognitive rehabilitation
compared with conventional rehabilitation. Most of the 'pseudo-treatment' interventions were apparently delivered in the context of providing treatment for the patients' cognitive deficits. In all of these
studies, patients in both the treatment and 'pseudo-treatment' conditions improved; thus, these findings may reflect the Hawthorne effect, i.e., the tendency for patients to improve solely due to the
increased attention from caretakers (Silverman 1998). A specific benefit of cognitive rehabilitation
compared to an alternative form of cognitive intervention (usually for a different deficit area) or psychosocial intervention was apparent in less than half of the studies examined. This appears to be
equally true when cognitive rehabilitation is compared separately with an alternative cognitive intervention or psychosocial intervention. This again suggests that 'non-specific' therapeutic factors play a significant role in cognitive rehabilitation, which should not be surprising. Rattok *et al.* (1992)
conducted a controlled observational study comparing cognitive and interpersonal components of
holistic neuropsychological rehabilitation. They found that improvements in neuropsychological
functioning were associated with cognitive remediation, improvements in psychosocial functioning
(e.g., affective regulation and self appraisal) were associated with small group interpersonal training,
and the greatest benefits were associated with combined cognitive and psychosocial treatments.

Translating evidence into clinical practice

Clinical decision-making involves the selection of the most appropriate treatment for a particular
patient from a number of possible alternative, at a particular point of recovery and time in the
patient's life, with consideration of possible coexisting conditions, social supports, environmental barriers, and the patient's own preferences and goals. Some considerations in applying the evidence for
the effectiveness of cognitive rehabilitation to clinical practice are listed in Table 5.4., based on the
suggestions given by Sackett *et al.* (2000).

Table 5.4 Application of evidence to clinical practice

- Is the patient sufficiently similar, in most important ways, to the patients described in the clinical trial or practice guideline?
- Is the nature of the cognitive impairment similar to the impairment targeted by the clinical trial or practice guideline?
- Are there coexisting cognitive impairments that are likely to influence the effectiveness of the intervention?
- What are the expected benefits and potential costs of applying the intervention?
- Is the treatment feasible to apply the intervention in this clinical setting?
- Is the intervention consistent with the patient's own preferences, values, and expectations?

Even when there is convincing evidence from well designed, controlled studies, the application of that evidence to clinical practice may not be straightforward (Caplan 2001; Woolf 1993). Barriers to the implementation of clinical practice guidelines include the lack of knowledge and familiarity with guidelines, lack of agreement and differences in the interpretation of the evidence, lack of clinician self-efficacy in the implementation of guidelines, the inertia of previous practice, and external limits on implementation (e.g., lack of time or resources) (Cabana *et al.* 1999). Clinicians' attitudes are among the most common reasons for the failure to apply evidence-based guidelines in clinical practice. Clinicians are often hesitant to adopt practices that contradict their own experience and 'expert opinion,' particularly if they feel that their autonomy or the integrity of the patient-therapist relationship is threatened.

As noted in the introduction, an evidence-based approach to cognitive rehabilitation integrates the clinician's experience and judgement with the best available information from systematic research. Well-designed, randomized clinical trials will continue to provide the strongest evidence for the efficacy of cognitive rehabilitation. Controlled, observational studies can demonstrate the clinical effectiveness of interventions, and help to determine the patient characteristics and treatment algorithms that contribute to successful outcomes. Small observational studies and well-designed single-subject research can advance the development of innovative treatment approaches that promise to be effective. The efforts to conduct research that demonstrates the effectiveness of cognitive rehabilitation must be matched by efforts to interpret and apply that evidence in clinical practice.

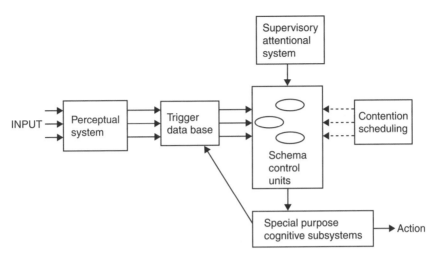

Figure 6.2 Simplified version of the Norman and Shallice model based on Shallice *et al.* (1989) by permission of Oxford University Press.

it up and write with it. However, we could choose to use the pencil in a different way if we had the goal of unblocking a small hole.

This model can account for both normal performance and the behaviour of patients with frontal lobe damage, who show deficits in planning, goal directed behaviour and the inability to maintain attention in the face of distraction. Although the model demonstrates the links between memory and attention, it does not explain how the SAS is itself controlled. Jahanshahi and Frith (1998) propose a willed action system based on known frontostriatal circuits to account for cognitive, motor and motivational deficits observed in patients with frontal damage, schizophrenia and Parkinson's disease. Issues of attentional control are developed, in this volume, by Paul Burgess in Chapter 19. It is important to remember that what attention is, or does, cannot easily be separated from how it is directed, divided or controlled. The SAS has been likened to the central executive of working memory by Baddeley (1986), and loading short-term working memory can interfere with maintaining the focus of attention on task relevant stimuli (DeFocket *et al.* 2001).

As there are many varieties of attention, it is more appropriate to consider varieties of attention in terms of the different behaviours it is said to be involved with. Reviewing twenty-five years of research into attention, Allport (1993) emphasised that the important question is 'What is attention for?' The basic answer is that attention, in some form or other, is necessary for maintaining coherence of behaviour in the face of multiple, competing sources of information, possible actions and conflicting goals. We should accept that the term 'attention' refers to a set of cognitive processes and involves many brain areas.

Varieties of attentional tasks

Research on attention can be broadly divided into different areas defined by task demands: Selective, or focused attention; divided attention; sustained attention and vigilance, and executive control of goal-directed behaviour. In the area of selective attention most work since the 1970s has been on visual selection, particularly spatially selective speeded detection tasks such as Posner *et al.*'s (1980) visual orienting experiments. Another variety of task is one requiring visual search and selective report of one object from many, depending on specific object attributes such as colour, shape and location, or a conjunction of at least two of these. Work on visual focal attention by Treisman and Gelade (1980) is of this kind. More recently there has been revived interest in auditory selective attention (Scharf 1998), and the attentional processes involved in selective reaching, grasping (Tipper *et al.* 1999), and cross modal attention (Driver and Spence 1999). Divided attention tasks require the combination of, or monitoring and response to, more than one source of information. In general the limits on combining tasks or dividing attention between them depends on task similarity, level of skill (i.e. how much of the task is automatic) and the input/output relations between the tasks (McLeod 1978). Given that some tasks appear to be able to be combined without cost, this could imply modality-specific attentional processes or resources but there may still be supra-modal attentional systems (Farah 1989), and a review of evidence suggests that there is always some dual task interference (e.g. Passingham 1996; Pashler 1998). Other applications of the term attention apply to tasks of vigilance and sustained attention. Here the cognitive system needs to be maintained in a state of readiness to respond, and is related to the control of attention and levels of arousal (see Parasuraman 1998).

How to research attention?

Despite the complexity of theoretical issues surrounding attention a great deal is known about some aspects of attentional behaviour. Evidence comes from several related disciplines. First, cognitive psychology contributes detailed, quantitative empirical knowledge from experimental studies of healthy participants and seeks to generate functional models that will account for task performance. Some of these models may be implemented as computer simulations to test their viability. Second, cognitive neuropsychology seeks to explain the behaviour of patients with brain damage in terms of models from cognitive psychology: see Styles (1997) for an overview. One approach to understanding cognitive functioning is founded in the belief that the human brain is an information processing device, and that it is modular (Fodor 1983). In a modular system specific processes are computed by specific modules and these modules operate independently such that if one is damaged the processing specific to that module may be lost, but the remaining system continues to operate. Careful neuropsychological testing can reveal which particular process is damaged: see for example Chapter 2 in this volume by Coltheart. This approach not only clarifies the nature of the patient's deficit, but also contributes to clarifying the functional model of normal behaviour. Third, advances in cognitive neuroscience and the development of *in vivo* imaging techniques provide a means of linking localised brain activity to cognitive functions: see Gazzaniga (2000) for a useful collection of papers.

These three approaches offer different levels of explanation of the same behaviour. Cognitive psychology and cognitive neuropsychology provide explanations at what Marr (1982) termed the computational and algorithmic levels. These levels define the 'software' or program for what has to be done and the rules and procedures for how it is done. Neuroscience attempts to provide explanations at the level of the 'hardware' on which the programs run. This is the implementational level. The program might be implemented by a computer, but in the case of human task performance, it is implemented in the brain. Marr believed that theories and understanding at one level could help understand and constrain theories and understanding at another level (see Table 6.1).

The joint contribution of cognitive psychology, cognitive neuropsychology and cognitive neuroscience to understanding both normal performance and the deficits observed in patients with brain damage can be appreciated in the examples that follow.

Visual orienting

One task, developed by Posner and his colleagues (Posner *et al.* 1980), has come to dominate research on the orienting of attention. The task was originally applied to visual orienting, but has subsequently

Table 6.1 Summary of the three approaches to studying cognitive processes, which include attention

	Cognitive psychology	Cognitive neuropsychology	Cognitive neuroscience
Goals	To produce functional models of performance in cognitive tasks.	To explain the cognitive behaviour of brain damaged patients.	To map the functional anatomy of cognitive and processes.
Methods	Controlled experiments, computer modeling.	Case studies and careful testing within framework of normal cognitive behaviour.	*In vivo* scanning of healthy and brain damaged patients, and animal models.
Theory	Humans can be thought of as information processors.	The mind is modular, and is an information processor.	Identifying anatomical components involved in tasks inform theory.
Subjects	Healthy human participants.	Patients	Patients and healthy volunteers.
Level	Computational and algorthimic levels	Computational and algorithmic levels	Mainly the implementational level

been extended and applied to the auditory and tactile modalities e.g. Driver and Spence (1999). We know that the spatial location of eye fixation is not necessarily coincident with the location to which attentional processing is directed. While reading this page, and without an overt eye movement, the colour of the wall or the presence of another person can be covertly attended. The original experiments examined the benefit of providing a cue for the visual location where a to-be-detected target would appear. Two types of cue were used: central or peripheral. A central cue is an arrow presented on fixation indicating that the target will arrive to the left or right of visual space. It is central in two senses, first it is centred in the visual field, but second, it requires the transformation of a symbolic representation into a representation that can specify the direction in which visual attention is oriented. A peripheral cue is presented in peripheral vision on the side of visual space where that target will appear and is usually a brief change in luminance. On control trials neither cue is given. Results revealed that without the participant making an eye-movement, targets at the cued location were responded to more quickly than targets arriving at a different location. This showed that visual attention can be covertly oriented in the absence of overt eye movements and led Posner *et al.* (1980) to propose that 'Attention can be likened to a spotlight that enhances the efficiency of the detection of events within its beam.' Further experiments manipulated the likelihood that the cue was a valid indicator of target location. Performance on trials with a central cue indicated that the participant could ignore cues likely to be invalid and direct attention to the other side of visual space. However, peripheral cues known to be improbable indicators of upcoming target location produced reaction costs, as if they could not be voluntarily overruled. The pattern of data suggested to Posner *et al.* (1980) that there is a distinction between the endogenous, internal intentional control of visual attention by the participants interpretation of the central cue, and the exogenous, or stimulus-driven capture of attention by the peripheral cue.

Unilateral visual neglect

Posner *et al.* (1984) examined the effect of parietal lobe injury on covert orienting in patients with the neuropsychological deficit of unilateral visual neglect (see Chapter 7). In daily life such patients tend to bump into objects in the left side of visual space, copy only the right side of a drawing, turn only to the right and so on. However, despite appearing 'blind' to the neglected side they have no visual field defects. Patients usually have posterior parietal lesions in the right hemisphere. When tested on Posner's orienting task these patients were found to have difficulty orienting attention to the neglected side of space, contralateral to the lesion. In particular, when attention has previously been cued to the right visual field but the target is in the neglected left visual field. On the basis of this evidence together with that from cognitive neuroscientific studies of event related potentials, (ERP's), positron emission tomography (PET) data and experiments on alert monkeys, Posner and Petersen (1990) proposed three separable but interacting attentional systems. The *posterior*, covert orienting system directs attention to stimulus locations using the operations 'engage' which involves the pulvinar nucleus of the thalamus, 'disengage', which involves parietal regions, and 'shift' which involves the superior colliculus. Information at the attended location is enhanced in comparison to unattended locations. A second *anterior* system is involved in overt orienting and controls the detection of events and additionally involves frontal areas. Posner and Petersen (1990) also included the proposal that a right hemisphere arousal system was involved in modulating selection and maintaining enhancement.

Posner and Badgaiyan (1998) provide a recent overview of the evidence, which now includes data from functional magnetic resonance imaging (fMRI). They summarise the role of posterior attentional system: 'In terms of cognitive theories, this network mediates disengagement, engagement and amplification of the attentional target' (1998, p. 64.). The second attentional system is involved in overt, intentionally controlled orienting. Areas involved in this network are the midprefrontal cortex, including the anterior cingulate gyrus and the supplementary motor area, which is involved in making eye movements. This anterior network

> is involved in attentional recruitment and it controls the brain areas that perform complex tasks. It exerts general control over the areas involved in target detection and response ... and ... is also responsible for anticipation of the target location.
>
> Posner and Badgaiyan (1998, p. 65)

Posner and Dehaene (2000) discuss PET data which support the asymmetric involvement of the hemispheres in attention functions. Blood flow increases are evident in the right parietal lobe for attention shifts in both fields, but blood flow in the left parietal region only increases for right field shifts. They suggest that this asymmetry might account for unilateral neglect following right parietal damage.

A number of other proposals from the cognitive neuroscience perspective have been put forward that relate visual orienting behaviour to brain mechanisms. LaBerge (2000) assumes that the selective property of attention is expressed by the amplification of neural activity in cortical columns. This expression can be controlled by the stimulus, 'bottom-up', or by intention 'top-down'. Laberge identifies many triangular circuits of connections between the parietal areas of brain in which attention is expressed, frontal areas involved in control and thalamic areas involved in amplification. There is a direct pathway between the parietal lobe and the frontal area and an indirect pathway between parietal and frontal areas via the pulvinar nucleus of the thalamus. The direct frontal-parietal pathway is involved in selecting parietal neural structures, in which attention will be expressed and the indirect pathway, via the thalamus, has the function of modulating the intensity of expression in the selected parietal areas. LaBerge (2000) assumes that an abrupt onset initiates, bottom-up, brief activity in the parietal areas, which an be considered an expression of orienting. If this activity is to be prolonged, then top-down activity is required.

Simultanagnosia and visual extinction

Patients with unilateral visual neglect may also display further visual attention deficits. Simultanagnosia is characterised by the inability to 'see' more than one object concurrently. Visual extinction is a deficit in detecting the more contralesional of two stimuli. Although the contralesional stimulus can be detected when presented on its own, with simultaneous presentation only the ipsilateral stimulus is detected. However, a number of observations demonstrate that although the patient is apparently unaware of the extinguished stimulus they have nevertheless encoded attributes of that stimulus which can affect the processing of other related stimuli (e.g. Berti *et al.* 1992) or allow a judgement to be made as to whether the stimuli are the same or different (Volpe *et al.* 2000).

Some theoretical explanations that can account for not only normal visual attention, unilateral neglect, but also simultanagnosia and extinction, involve the argument that attentional behaviour is a result of an integrated brain state. Duncan (1999) proposes a distributed view of attentional functions in which ' ... generally, attention is seen as a widely distributed state, in which several brain systems converge to work on different properties and action implications of the same, selected object' (p. 126). The hypothesis is that the multiple sources of information activating different brain systems responsive to visual input are subject to competitive processing. If one source of information is enhanced, than another is inhibited and the most active pattern of activity gains dominance, or control. Following consideration of lesion studies, Duncan proposes that the attentional bias observed in unilateral neglect and the phenomenon of extinction can be explained in terms of damaged areas losing the competition to dominate processing. Duncan argues that lateral bias is a widespread consequence of lateralised brain injury and that right parietal lesions are not the sole predictor of bias in neglect, simultanagnosia and extinction.

Another approach to explaining neglect that relates to more general, non-lateralised attentional deficits has been proposed by Robertson and Manly (1999). According to this view there is evidence that the right hemisphere is more important for sustaining attention than shifting it, and that contributions to neglect, extinction and simultanagnosia may result from a more general effect of arousal, impaired spatial attention and reduced attentional capacity.

Cross-modal attention and spatial orienting

While most work on attentional orienting had concentrated on visual stimuli, attention can also be oriented in other modalities. Driver (1996) and Spence and Driver (1996) have investigated cross-modal links in both overt and covert attentional orienting. Using adaptations of Posner's orienting tasks, they have demonstrated strong spatial links between auditory and visual attention. When conversing, the face we see speaking provides both visual and auditory information that we expect to be integrated. The ventriloquism illusion is an illustration of how orienting in one modality facilitates processing in the other (Driver 1996). Attending to the visual location at which the moving lips synchronise with the words being spoken, gives the illusion that the sound is emanating from the moving lips, even if the sound is localised elsewhere. Thus orienting attention in the visual modality allows the listener to compensate for poor auditory localisation in a noisy environment. In a review of cross-modal attention, Driver and Spence (1999) argues that this facilitation can only arise if cross-modal spatial links are pre-attentive.

Selecting what, where and how

For effective interaction with the environment it is necessary for the brain to encode and make available for the control of perception and action, all source information about the properties of objects. We perceive and act on objects not only on the basis of where they are, but also according to their sensory and semantic properties. For example, if we grasp a raspberry to pick it we know it is small and soft so grasp it differently to an apple which we know is large and hard. In vision there are two parallel streams of information analysis projecting from V1 (Ungeleider and Mishkin 1982). The first, a ventral stream, projecting to the inferior temporal lobe, is responsible for analyzing *what* an object is, for example 'It is a pencil'. The other, a dorsal stream, projecting to the parietal lobe, is responsible for analyzing where an object is located, for example, 'there is something on the'. Rather than a 'what' and a 'where' stream, the streams might be better considered as a 'what' and a 'how' stream, where the 'how' stream specifies how to act on what is detected. For example, how to grasp the pencil. Milner and Goodale (1995) identify selective links to separate areas of pre-motor and pre-frontal cortex. There are functionally and anatomically distinct, cross-connected circuits for eye movements, grasping and coding for short-term memory. The three routes between V1 and posterior parietal cortex contain different information involved in the transformation from visually-based to motor-based coordinates. In addition different brain areas code for colour, orientation and other properties of objects. The problem that arises from this division of coding labour is how attributes belonging to the same object are accurately combined to control response. Unless the brain can accurately bring together the knowledge from all streams behaviour will not be accurately controlled. This is known as the 'binding problem'. We have already met one interpretation that could account for this in Duncan's (1999) integrated field theory of attention. Another approach is Feature Integration Theory (FIT), proposed originally by Treisman and Gelade (1980).

Feature integration theory (FIT)

Since its inception FIT has undergone revisions to take account of new experimental and neurological discoveries. It is concerned with explaining how information about different perceptual attributes is brought together to allow an object to be recognised. Typical experiments involve the observer in searching a visual display for a predesignated target embedded within a number of distractor stimuli. The target in a visual search task is at an unknown location, and is therefore different from the orienting experiments discussed above. When the target is uniquely defined by a feature, say 'red' and is set amongst distractors all of another colour, say 'green', search times are independent of display size. The target is said to 'pop out' without the necessity of searching every display location in turn. Features are automatically detected, in parallel, without the need for attention. On the other hand, if the target is defined by a conjunction of features, say it is a 'red X' and the distractors are a mixture of red O's and green X's, then search time is dependent on the number of items in the display. The target does not 'pop out', but must be found, according to Treisman and Gelade (1980), by serial search of display locations with focal attention. Focal attention is said to be the 'glue' that binds features at the same location together. Features are coded independently on their respective feature maps, and if the target is defined only by a feature it can be detected on its own map. The difficulty with searching for a conjunction is that the information from more than one feature map must be combined. This is achieved by mapping features located on separate maps onto a master map of locations over which focal attention moves, binding together features at the same location. Once bound the features are entered into an object file and the object can be identified by matching with memory representations.

Patients with Balint's syndrome have bilateral parietal lesions, but have normal acuity, stereopsis, colour vision and contrast sensitivity. They have no fundamental visual deficits, but show neglect, fail to orient head and limbs and make gross errors in reaching. Treisman (1999) tested patient RM on a variety of tasks requiring feature integration and found that even in when there were only two differently coloured letters he made binding errors, reporting one letter in the colour of the other. Treisman concluded that RM had lost the master map of locations and was therefore unable to form a stable representation of integrated objects. RM knew *what* things were, but not *where* they were. This difficulty meant that RM was unable to combine relevant object space features for everyday functional performance.

Attention and neglect in different spatial and representational frames

Space is not only defined in terms of where objects are on the retina. Objects are distributed in reaching space, parts of a single object are spatially arranged relative to each other and different objects may be grouped together or separated. The evidence presented so far has concentrated on visual attention in retinotopic space, but there is evidence for selective attention operating on the basis of objects, and within other spatial and representational frames such as memory. There are a number of demonstrations of 'pop out' for conjunctions, and Duncan and Humphreys (1992) suggest pop out can be mediated by grouping effects in the display, and therefore selective visual attention may be object based. Humphreys *et al.* (1994) studied another Balint's patient, G.K. who demonstrated extinction even when two objects were presented one above the other, and even when one object was on fixation. Extinction was dependent on properties of the objects such as closure. For example, pictures extinguished words, a complete square extinguished an incomplete square. However, decisions on object location were at chance. Although information about spatial location has been lost in this individual, selection or neglect can be based on object properties. Humphreys *et al.* (1994) argue that even when spatial selection and localisation are poor, object properties can mediate selection and that 'there is normally coordination of the outcomes of competition within the separate neural areas coding each property, making shape, location and other properties of a single object available concurrently for the control of action' (p. 359). A study by Driver and Halligan (1991) provides more evidence of object-based attention. They found that patients with unilateral visual neglect still ignored the neglected side of an object, even when it appeared in the non-neglected side of environmental space. Thus neglect can be of one side of an object's principle axis, not simply of the side of space occupied by that object, and if the problem for the patient is attentional, then attention also can operate on object-centred space.

Rizzolati and colleagues (1994) have demonstrated that, in monkey, lesions in different pre-motor areas can produce different, dissociable, forms of neglect. Neglect may be of 'reaching' space, when the animal makes no attempt to reach for an object, of oculomotor space when no eye movement is made toward objects, or orofacial space, where the animal will not lick juice from around the mouth. Space and the operation of attentional orienting must therefore be considered in terms of the type of action that is appropriate in different spatial frames. In humans, Guariglia and Antonucci (1992), demonstrated a dissociation between neglect of personal and extrapersonal space. Attention can operate not only on representations derived from perceptual input, but also on internal representations generated from memory. Bisiach and Luzzatti (1978) asked another neglect patient to report, from memory, what could be seen if they stood in the cathedral steps in Milan, a view with which they were familiar. The patient reported all the buildings on one side and ignored those on the other side. Then the patient was asked to imagine crossing the square to face the cathedral and report what they could see now. All the buildings previously ignored were reported. Clearly the memory was intact, but one side of representational space was being neglected. All this evidence suggests a complex variety of 'spatial' and representational systems within which attention can operate and that conscious awareness breaks down the same way.

Conclusions

Posner and Petersen (1990) suggest that a major challenge for the future was to determine how multiple attentional systems operate in a coordinated manner to maintain unity of behaviour. This challenge still remains. Attentional behaviour emerges from the activity of a number of complex anatomical networks, pathways and circuits. Within these networks each area has its own specialised computations. As a consequence of the widely distributed nature of attentional functions, attentional deficits are diverse and can result in the loss of normal attentional behaviour in a number of spatial and representational frames. The inability to attend can also give rise to a dissociation of processing from conscious awareness and the breakdown of coherent activity. An additional challenge, then, is to link attention and consciousness. At the neurobiological level, one account is that consciousness emerges from the synchronised activity across different brain areas (Crick and Koch 1990). If particular brain areas are damaged, they will not be synchronised and will not contribute to conscious experience.

Glossary

Automatic processing. Processing that happens unintentionally and requires little or no attentional resources. It cannot be prevented and is not interfered with by other processes.

Blindsight. The ability to respond appropriately to a visual stimulus despite having no conscious awareness of that stimulus due to a damaged primary visual cortex. Patients with blindsight have no confidence in their judgements, yet are accurate.

Central executive. A supervisory system involved in allocating attention and integrating information from other cognitive systems. Similar to the Supervisory Attentional System (SAS).

Contention scheduling. A process of weighing up the relative importance of tasks if concurrent performance is not possible.

Controlled processing. Processing that requires attention and is intentional. It is open to interference from other attention demanding tasks.

Divided attention. A situation that requires the simultaneous performance of more than one attention demanding task.

Extinction. A disorder of attention in which a stimulus presented on the opposite side to the brain damage can be seen alone, but becomes undetectable when a stimulus is presented on the other side.

Neglect. A disorder of attention in which objects or parts of objects are ignored or not responded to when presented on the opposite side to the brain damage. Usually affects vision, but may also affect images in memory or auditory and tactile stimuli.

Schema. An organized packet of information, stored in long term memory that contains knowledge about the world, objects, people and events, what they are and how to behave towards them.

Selective attention. A system that allows one source of information to be processed from amongst many. It involves having to ignore other irrelevant sources. This mechanism may select information for perceptual processing, for semantic processing or response processing. It requires focal, or focused attention.

Semantic processing. Processing that delivers the meaning and associated knowledge of a stimulus.

Simultanagnosia. A disorder of attention in which only one stimulus can be detected at a time.

Supervisory Attentional System (SAS). A system that uses attentional biasing to allow schema for intended actions to be made in the face of competition from other active schema. Without the action of the SAS, environmental stimuli trigger familiar actions automatically.

7 Testing speed and control

The assessment of attentional impairments

Adriaan H. van Zomeren and Joke M. Spikman

Abstract

This chapter argues that it is fruitful to look at attentional impairments, their assessment and their remediation within a simple theoretical framework: the distinction between speed of processing and attentional control (the executive aspects of attention). Although this distinction is not absolute, it has two major advantages: it is empirically based in factor analyses of performance on attention tests by normal control subjects and patients, and it brings some order in the enormous collection of attention tests available to clinicians and investigators. Last but not least, the approach chosen here signals a need in the clinical assessment of attention: as increased mental fatiguability and loss of concentration are frequent complaints in brain-damaged patients, assessment should focus on tests of sustained attention that demand a greater cognitive effort from the patient and that consist of timeblocks enabling the assessment of abnormal time-on-task effects. Finally, for cognitive rehabilitation the distinction between speed and control suggests that psychologists might try to reduce time pressure and improve structure in tasks that patients have to face. In addition, strategy training might focus on time pressure management and dealing with poorly structured task situations.

Relevant impairments

For two reasons, assessment of attentional impairments is necessary in a rehabilitation setting. First, these impairments hinder and prolong the processes of both physical and cognitive rehabilitation. Second, the deficits themselves should be targets of rehabilitation, as they have negative effects on the patient's social reintegration and resumption of roles. In our view, there are four main kinds of potential impairments. First, *hemi-neglect* is a disturbance in a basic biological aspect, our symmetrical orientation on the outside world. Next, *mental slowness* is a very frequent sequel to brain damage or diseases that has important consequences for dealing with this outside world – in particular when it is offering a lot of relevant information. Third, *impairments of attentional control* can be observed, i.e. deficits in focused and divided attention. Finally, *impaired sustained attention* is often seen in subjects with brain damage. The concept is related to mental fatigue and should be operationalized as time-on-task effects.

Theoretical background

Hemi-neglect

Neglect consists of a range of phenomena related to the high level representation of, and attention to, space (Robertson and Heutink 2002). For visual hemi-inattention, Heilman *et al.* (1985) presented a neuro-anatomical model with an extensive network: these authors view neglect as an attentional-arousal disorder, caused by dysfunction of a cortico-limbic-reticular loop. Thus, lesions on various levels can cause neglect. Robertson and Heutink (2002) likewise assume that 'neglect is merely the result of a disruption of a large network of anatomically distinct yet functionally connected cortical and subcortical structures which are all (partially) involved in attention and spatial cognition'. Still, chronic neglect in particular is associated with lesions in the tempero-parieto-occipital junction in the right hemisphere.

The fact that neglect is seen in particular after right hemisphere lesions is explained as resulting from a functional asymmetry between hemispheres. Heilman states that the right hemisphere is equipped for panoramic attention, which implies that it is also watching to some degree over the right half of extrapersonal space. In contrast, the left hemisphere is attending to and acting in the right half of our outside world only. Hence, differential effects of lesions in either left or right hemisphere emerge. In case of a lesion in the left hemisphere that might produce right-sided neglect, the panoramic function of the right hemisphere ensures that the right half of extra-personal space is still taken care off. On the other hand, if the cortico-limbic-reticular loop in the right hemisphere is disrupted and attention for the left half of the outside world fails, there is no compensation: the intact left hemisphere keeps attending to the right side of space only.

Mental slowness

A slowing of behaviour can be readily observed in many patients who have sustained brain damage or are suffering from degenerative brain diseases. In its severest form, the phenomenon can be characterized with the clinical terms bradyphrenia and bradykinesia. However, even in patients who are not visibly slow a certain delay in responding can usually be demonstrated with, for example, reaction time measures. Nowadays, the slowness is usually described as a slowing of information processing – probably because this sounds quasi-exact. In our experience, the expression 'slow information processing' is sometimes used uncritically. If responses are delayed, this is not direct proof of slow processing. A lack of motivation in the subject or a motor deficit (e.g. dysarthria in verbal responses) may result in delayed responses, while the rate of information processing is in fact normal.

There exists no adequate explanation for the fact that a lesion in almost any location may result in mental slowness. In the case of diffuse injury or degenerative diseases, a connectionistic view offers some kind of explanation. In a connectionistic model, the information processing systems consists of a multitude of nodes, while information is recorded in this network by strengthening of connections between nodes. If a certain proportion of nodes are lost, this has consequences that strongly remind us of clinical symptoms: the system becomes slow, it cannot activate knowledge (remember) as well as it used to do, it will not be activated as easily as before by input from outside (recognition) and its responses will become weaker and less efficient.

The slowness can be the result of three different mechanisms:

1. The detour effect. A signal travelling through the network simply no longer can use the shortest route, as this has been blocked by lacking or a-functional nodes.
2. A decreased signal-to-noise ratio. If nodes go lost, the system becomes more noisy. In a biological system, a signal is not an all-or-none or on-off phenomenon, but a growing impulse resulting

from activity in a collection of elements or nodes. In a noisy system, it will take longer before this impulse rises above the noise and can act as as a signal.

3. Desynchronization. If several subprocesses are working in concert, differential delay in the subprocesses will upset the coordination of activities with an additional slowing as a result.

The cognitive impairments caused by severe head injury might well be explained with this connection-istic view: it seems to do justice both to the cognitive impairments and to the pathophysiology of head injury. For one thing, connections in the injured brain are reduced by diffuse axonal injury. Strich (1956) originally described the mechanic version, i.e. disruption of nerve fibers in the white matter by shearing forces at the moment of impact. Recently, it has been demonstrated that in addition a sec-ondary or delayed axonotomy can occur by release of the excitatory amino acid glutamate in the injured brain (Adams *et al.* 2000).

As argued above, mental slowness will inevitably result in decreasing task performance if relevant information is presented at a rate that is too high for the brain-damaged subject. Slowness alone will already prevent the subject from attending timely to all task-relevant signals and to his or her responses. Spikman *et al.* (2000) demonstrated in head-injured subjects that their deficient perform-ance on traditional attention test such as the Stroop Colour Word Test and Trailmaking B could be explained almost entirely as resulting from slowness only.

Ponsford and Kinsella (1991) investigated impairments of attention in a rehabilitation setting, where staff used an Attentional Rating Scale to record attentional problems with 5-point scales. Two observations occurred with high frequency: mental slowness and inability to attend to more than one thing at a time.

An interesting study relevant to the question of mental slowness and divided attention was reported by Haggard *et al.* (2000). They studied *cognitive-motor interference* in patients in rehabilitation, i.e. a slowing of the gait cycle in patients with brain damage who had to do cognitive tasks while walking (category fluency, mental arithmetic). Patients showed an increased dual-task interference when com-pared with healthy controls. That is, both cognitive performance and walking showed negative effects of task combination. Haggard *et al.* concluded that dual task performance exceeded the available information processing capacity in their patients. They argue that interference arises because motor control ceases to be automatic after brain injury. Previously automatic actions such as walking may revert to the status of controlled processes. One practical consequence might be that therapists should not give instructions to patients during the course of a movement in training. Haggard *et al.* also remarked: 'We suggest that measures of dual task interference should be included in standard clinical assessment and used to inform content of therapy programs'.

Theoretically, it is important to note that information processing capacity can be translated as a reduced rate of processing, i.e. mental slowness. The idea of cognitive-motor interference is that cognitive and consciously controlled motor processes are competing for a limited central capacity. The limitation can be conceived as a slowness in basic operations: the system can only process a limited amount of information per second. Thus, both the patients in the Ponsford and Kinsella study and the Haggard *et al.* study experienced problems in doing two things simultaneously.

Impaired control over focused and divided attention

The *focusing* of attention on unusual or novel stimuli is a spontaneous biological event (bottom-up control). In contrast, the maintenance of an attentional focus demands additional top-down control. For example, we are usually not distracted by the many movements that occur in our visual field when we walk down a crowded street – and it has been demonstrated that a prefrontal mechanism is involved in this suppression of saccades towards movements (Buchtel 1987). On a higher level, our selectivity is maintained by intentions and motivation to perform well on a task. For this level of control too, the

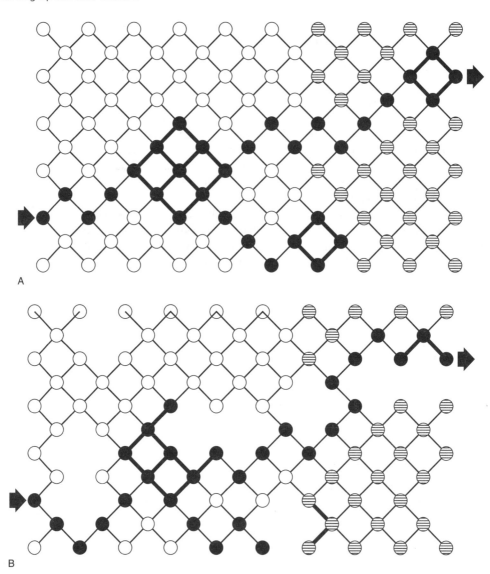

Figure 7.1 A simple connectionistic model of an information processing system with an input part and an output part (shaded nodes). The black patterns of connections indicate a concept or memory (9 nodes), a motor pattern (4 nodes, above right) and a controlling system (4 nodes, below) that can suppress the execution of a motor response. If the system is damaged diffusely, the random loss of nodes will result in slowness, failing memory and recognition, weakened control and decreased power and quality of responses.

prefrontal cortex is essential. We are talking here about the executive aspects of attention or Supervisory Attentional Control. Impairment in this control system may take the form of decreased flexibility, deficient strategy and deficient priority setting.

The ability of *dividing* attention over two sources of input or performance on two subtasks depends on two factors: processing speed and executive control. As argued in the previous section, mental slowness alone will already result in divided attention deficits. However, divided attention can also be impaired on a higher cognitive level, i.e. when control processes are not optimal. In 1988 Shallice postulated a

Supervisory Attentional System in his information processing model, and this model has greatly stimulated the interest in the executive aspects of attention. With the term Supervisory Attentional Control (SAC) we refer to these executive aspects, i.e. strategy, flexibility and priority setting. It is probable that these regulating aspects are connected with the prefrontal cortex, just as the wider concept of executive functions of which they are part. It should be noted that SAC and the Central Executive from Baddeley's model of working memory (1986) are practically identical; for one thing, a strategy and priority rules are kept active in working memory. At a certain level, flexibility is likewise an executive aspect of attention. We have distinguished three kinds of flexibility (Van Zomeren and Spikman 2003): stimulus-driven, memory-driven and strategy-driven.

Stimulus-driven flexibility occurs at a low level of control, when alternating stimuli dictate what the subject should do. For example, in our lab we use a dual reaction-time task in which subjects react manually to lights and by foot (on a pedal) to tones. Once the instruction is given, the stimuli lead the subject through the task while the cross-modal shifts require an elementary flexibility. Flexibility at this level is intact after severe head injury.

Next, flexibility in behaviour can be based on knowledge kept in long-term memory. A good example would be Trailmaking B, where the alphabet and the numerical sequence from long-term verbal memory are applied in a visual search task. The continuous switching from one series of symbols to the other requires some flexibility, and this is impaired in the most severely head-injured subjects (Veltman *et al.* 1996, Spikman *et al.* 1996).

Finally, at the highest level flexibility depends on a strategy and priority rules. This kind of flexibility is essential in unstructured task situations where the subject is not instructed by an experimenter but has to set his own priorities (Brouwer 2002). Driving one's car through the rush hour while at the same time talking with an important passenger would be an example where flexibility is required, both when the traffic presents increasing risks and the passenger (say, your employer) launches a new and heavy topic. At the anecdotal level, this kind of flexibility seems impaired after severe head injury. Unfortunately, experimental evidence is almost completely lacking in this domain.

Impaired sustained attention

Sustained attention is sustained control. In any prolonged task the subject has to spend some effort in order to stay focused on the job and to monitor their own performance. For example, the subject will be watching the rate of working and the speed/accuracy trade-off or quality level of performance. In other words, the subject will be comparing continually the actual performance with a standard set by either himself or a supervisor. If we are carrying out a routine task, this control can be marginal – but in a less familiar or more risky task, such as driving a city coach through the rush hour, attentional control will demand a much greater effort.

When studying sustained attention, the psychologist is interested in time-on-task (TOT) effects. These are gradual changes in performance, usually negative ones such as an increase of number of errors or a decrease of work pace. In order to record TOT's the test must be divided in time blocks, enabling a comparison of performance in early and later stages of the task. Further, in the domain of sustained attention a distinction should be made between low event-rate and high event-rate situations. A low event-rate situation is found in the classical vigilance task, where a subject is supposed to stay alert in a monotonous situation that offers a few target signals in a long row of non-target signals. Staying awake is the main difficulty here. In contrast, a high event-rate situation will offer a lot of task-relevant information and the subject has to do his best to keep up with the task. Thus, mental fatigue is the main difficulty in this situation. A continuous reaction time task is an example of this approach.

Assessment of attentional impairments

In our view, tests are only one means of assessing impairments of attention. The following methods of assessment should also be considered:

- Interview of patient (is the patient aware of any deficits, and if so, is there concern?)
- Interview of a close relative or caretaker
- Observation by staff
- Rating scales and questionnaires. These can also be applied in the interviews or by staff members. Several well known questionnaires contain attentional items, such as the Cognitive Failures Questionnaire (Broadbent *et al.* 1982), the Neurobehavioral Rating Scale (Levin *et al.* 1987), the Rating Scale of Attentional Behaviour (Ponsford and Kinsella 1991) and the DEX Questionnaire (Wilson *et al.* 1996).
- Tests. For most attention tests, the actual score is a time score, be it in seconds or milliseconds. Hence, slowness in performance will often be used as unjustified 'proof' that a certain aspect of attention is impaired. It should also be realized that attention tests *always* tap more functions or cognitive aspects than merely attention. Also, an attention test will usually tap more than one aspect of attention, for example both selectivity and speed of processing. The ideal attention test consists of two conditions: one that provides a baseline, and one that manipulates an additional attentional variable. Colour naming without and with interference by word meaning, as in the Stroop paradigm, is an example of this approach.

Hemi-neglect

Hemi-inattention can be assessed reliably with a variety of tests (Lezak 1995). Drawing and copying figures and line bisecting are the oldest techniques in this domain. Next, there are visual search tasks such as the Bells Test, with its seven columns in a quasi random field of stimuli (Vanier *et al.* 1990). Also useful is the indented paragraph reading text, where each line begins at an unpredictable distance from the margin, thereby provoking the patient to overlook words on the far left. The Testbattery for Attentional Performance (TAP) (Zimmerman and Fimm 2002) contains a computerized neglect test displaying three-digit numbers scattered over a computer screen. While the subject is looking at a central fixation point, one of these numbers begins to flicker and the reaction time of the subject to this event is recorded. The test may reveal an even subclinical neglect tendency, in the form of prolonged reaction times to stimuli in one quadrant or one half of the screen. Finally, the Behavioural Inattention Test was devised by Wilson *et al.* (1987). One of its attractive features is the presence of subtests with a clear ecological validity, such as telephone dialing and map navigation.

Mental slowness and impaired control: a proposal framework

We discuss the assessment of the above named aspects of attention under one heading, for reasons explained below. Although it is usual to distinguish aspects of attention such as focussed, divided and sustained attention, factor-analytic studies have failed to find these aspects in the performance of either healthy subjects or neurologic patients (Spikman *et al.* 2001). Instead, two empirical factors appeared under various names in statistical studies: a factor that could be termed *speed or processing capacity* and a second factor that could be termed *control or working memory*. In our experience, this distinction between speed and control can be quite helpful, at least in the study of attentional impairments after head injury. Thus, we propose to elaborate these concepts and to apply them to the phenomenology, the assessment and the cognitive rehabilitation of deficits of attention. In particular, we argue that performance of patients on both daily life tasks and attention tests can be described in terms of two subject characteristics: speed and control, and two task characteristics: timepressure and structure.

Time pressure and structure are important task characteristics, both in daily life tasks and tests. Structure refers to any feature of a task situation that may guide the behaviour of the subject. In terms of attention, time pressure requires speed and structure determines control. The need for control is maximal in unstructured tasks that cannot be tackled with routine responses. Control always implies activity of working memory, in which intentions and rules for performance of the task have to be kept activated. With this framework, it is possible to describe attentional performance in a model with three levels: the operational, the tactical and the strategic level derived from Michon (1979) (see Table 7.1).

At the *operational level* of attentional performance, time pressure is high and speed is the main factor. The task or test is highly structured and the amount of control required is minimal. In fact, the behaviour of the subject is largely stimulus-driven.

At the *tactical level*, being fast is no longer sufficient for satisfactory performance. Tasks are more complex and the risk of making errors exists on this level. In the case of tests, instructions are more complex and the subject chooses his own pace of working and speed/accuracy trade-off. Structure is intermediate, some control is required. As instructions and rules for performance are to be kept in working memory, the behaviour can be seen as memory-driven.

Finally, at the *strategic level* time pressure is minimal and the task is highly unstructured. Instructions do not dictate completely what should be done and subjects have to apply their own strategy, find their own priorities and estimate the cost of errors themselves. As such, tests on this level are approximations of daily life. Behaviour here is strategy-driven.

Assessment at the *operational level* is aimed at speed of information processing. Very useful are reaction time measures as found in many computerized batteries – provided that adequate norms (gender and age effects!) are available. In addition, speed of reading and colour naming in the Stroop Colour Word Test is important, and performance on the Digit Symbols from the WAIS-R. In fact, any speed test with finely-graded and age-adjusted norms will give useful information at this level.

Assessment at the *tactical level* can make use of many well-known neuropsychological tests that claim to tap focused or divided attention. In focused attention, there are weak or strong distractors in the stimulus field. In divided attention, the subject either has to attend to several related subtasks within one activity or to a dual task, i.e. the combination of two separate activities.

Assessment of focused attention may be realized with visual search tasks containing weak distractors, non-targets that in themselves do not have much attentional value. Letter cancellation tasks belong to this category, but also the visual search tasks from the Test of Everday Attention (map search, telephone search). It should be noted that the amount of control required depends partly on the structure of the stimulus field: letter cancellation requires a search that is guided by the lines of stimuli, while in unstructured quasi randomly filled stimulus fields the subject has to make sure himself that the whole field is covered by the search process. Another classic test of focused attention is the Continuous Performance Test, that presents a long series of targets and non-targets sequentially in time (externally paced). The standard example of an attention test with strong distractors is the

Table 7.1

Level	Time pressure	Structure
OPERATIONAL	High	Highly structured
TACTICAL	Intermediate	Partially structured
STRATEGIC	Low	Unstructured

Stroop Colour Word Test, where word meaning is strongly interfering through the overtrained reading response. Of all tests mentioned here, the Stroop is clearly demanding most control – as can be experienced introspectively by anyone facing the test, even someone who is quite familiar with the paradigm.

Divided attention at the tactical level can be assessed with the Paced Auditory Serial Addition Task (PASAT) (Gronwall and Sampson 1974) in which attentional capacity has to be divided over three subtasks: listening, responding and keeping track. Performance on this task is partly dependent on age and intellectual level. In the dual task approach, the Test of Everyday Attention (TEA) (Robertson et al. 1994) offers the subtest Telephone search while counting. The Test for Attentional Performance (TAP) (Zimmerman and Fimm 2002) likewise contains a useful divided attention task, a combination of a visual and an auditory task.

Although we tend to think of flexibility as a higher-order, executive aspect of attention, it can be tested in an elementary form at the tactical level too. For example, Trailmaking form B demands a memory-driven flexibility, as the subject is switching continuously between alphabet and numbers, while keeping both series activated in working memory. Bohnen (1991) devised an interesting variant of the Stroop paradigm, in which one-fifth of the coloured words are marked by boxes, randomly. Subjects have to read these words, i.e. while they are suppressing the reading response at 80 per cent of the stimuli, they have to switch back to reading every now and then. Bohnen demonstrated that this kind of flexibility is impaired after mild head injury. Unfortunately, norms and psychometric data are not available for this ingenious paradigm.

For assessment of attention at the *strategic level* the state of the art is unsatisfactory. Testing the executive aspects of attention meets with a general problem in the assessment of executive functions: the psychometric dilemma of initiative versus structure. In order to assess initiative and self-generated strategies, the test should be an approximation of real life and have little structure – but the more it resembles daily life, the more it will lack the psychometric qualities of a standardized test.

As far as we know, no clinically useful test of flexibility at the strategic level exists. That is, no dual task with adequate normative data seems to be available. Veltman et al. (1996) studied performance of head-injured patients in a simple car simulator, in which the tasks of tracking (keeping the car in lane against sidewind) and dot-counting were combined. This test had three conditions with varying instructions, in which the subjects themselves had to find their optimal way of dividing their attention over the two subtasks (Brouwer et al. 1988). Although the study demonstrated some loss of flexibility after severe head injury, the experimental set-up cannot easily be adapted to a clinical setting.

In practice, higher order impairments of attention can be assessed more or less by means of tests of executive functioning. In most of these tests, a certain aspect of attention plays an essential role. The Wisconsin Card Sorting Test and comparable tasks (Odd man out, BADS) measure some kind of flexibility, in the sense of switching to a new response mode. The Tower of London requires planning and thinking ahead, while suppressing direct and ineffective moves to the goal. The Six Elements Test in the BADS has a nice feature, in terms of ecological validity: subjects have to pay attention here to the passing of a limited amount of time. Finally, the Zoo Test from the BADS is testing, among other things, the subject's overview in a complex task situation.

Meanwhile, investigators are trying to find better ways for the assessment of executive functions in general. Spikman et al. (2001) devised the executive Route Finding Task, in which chronic head injury patients had to find their way back through the university hospital to the neuropsychology unit. Thus they were required to search for useful information, to show initiative and to develop a strategy, while the experimenter was recording their behaviour in objective categories. It was found that patients performed below the level of control subjects, and that patients with clear frontal lesions on CT did worse than patients without such signs.

Sustained attention

As observed before, tests of sustained attention should consist of time blocks that enable us to discover unusual TOT effects in patients. As a classic vigilance test, the subtest Vigilance of the TAP can be named here (Zimmerman and Fimm 2002). This is a dull visual monitoring task lasting 20 minutes, with adequate norms. Older instruments are the Continuous performance test and various continuous reaction time tests, although these tests often lack a division in time blocks – which means that the score merely reflects overall performance without saying much about the sustaining of attention.

The Test of Everyday Attention (Robertson *et al.* 1994) contains three subtests that have a loading on sustained attention: Lottery, elevator counting and telephone search while counting. Their timescale is short but the tasks have a satisfactory validity. Robertson and Manly also devised a Sustained Attention for Response Task (1997) in which subjects have to react to a random series of digits that are presented one by one on a computer screen, in a quite regular rhythm. However, subjects should not react to the digit 3. It turns out that this is very difficult, as the monotonous character of the task is luring the subject into a state of inattentive, automatic responding to anything that appears on the screen. This 'sustained selective suppressing' is impaired in head-injured patients.

In our view, what is really needed in clinical assessment is a kind of demanding cognitive task with a division in time blocks. We have found that head-injured subjects have no difficulty with prolonged visual search tasks or continuous reaction time tasks (Van Zomeren and Spikman 2003). Apparently these tasks, in which patients in fact determine their own pace of working, are too easy for them. The important thing is that these same patients are complaining about mental fatigue and loss of concentration in long-lasting daily life tasks, such as a group conversation or reading. We therefore believe that a valid assessment of sustained attention should make use of tasks that require a prolonged control and prolonged effort of our patients – just as daily life does. One could think of prolonged random letter generation or even of a prolonged PASAT of 5 × 2 minutes. In short: if sustained attention is sustained control, and if this control is the essential factor in mental fatigue in our patients, our tests should demand a greater effort of them in order to be valid.

Cognitive rehabilitation of attention

The conceptual combination of speed versus control can also be applied in the field of cognitive rehabilitation of attention (see Chapters 8 and 9). First of all, one might take a very practical approach in which one accepts that the patient with his impairments cannot be changed. Instead, one might change the situation he is facing: '*reduce time pressure, improve structure*'. With this double advice, the effects of deficits in speed of processing and attentional control could be minimized. Another practical approach might be to give the patient task-specific training. By now, it is a proven fact that brain-damaged subjects are able to learn specific tasks or skills. Hence, it is possible to train them to attend to task-relevant information in a particular situation. If the patient has trouble in dividing his attention over various pots and pans during cooking, teach him or her a system with sequences of checks; if the patient has trouble in crossing a particular intersection by car, train them on the spot and teach the patient when to attend to what. Of course, these task-specific trainings do not generalize, i.e. attention in other situations will not improve – but the practical gain of the method is obvious.

Even if we move to a more theoretical approach, the distinction between speed and control seems helpful. At the level of *strategy training*, Spikman (2001) stated that there are two targets for cognitive rehabilitation: teaching patients to deal with time pressure and teaching them to deal with unstructured situations. For the first aim, one might use the program called Time Pressure Management (Fasotti *et al.* 2000). For the second aim, the Multifaceted Program for the Dysexecutive Syndrome (Spikman 2001) offers a promising approach. This latter program is based partly on Goal Management Training as devised by Levine *et al.* (2000) and on the Problem Solving Training as proposed by Von Cramon *et al.* (1994).

8 Treating attention impairments

Review with a particular focus on naturalistic action rehabilitation

Norman W. Park and Erica Barbuto

Abstract

Treating attention impairments has received more systematic study than most other cognitive impairments because attention is frequently impaired after neurological damage, and is important in a wide variety of tasks. Results of a meta-analysis show that treatments aimed at restoring attention directly after an acquired brain injury improved performance to a limited degree, whereas treatments aimed to teach individuals functionally important skills had large effect sizes. We then review the role that attention and other cognitive processes play in the encoding and production of naturalistic actions (e.g., preparing coffee). This analysis showed that the processes mediating conceptual aspects of action and conscious aspects of attention are separable from the system responsible for timing and executing actions. Restoration-based treatments may be more effective for the treatment of motor impairments whereas treatments that focus on the treatment of functionally important skills are more effective for the treatment of consciously accessible cognitive processes. For this reason, we propose the use of a deficit-based approach to treatment. According to this approach, treatment of cognitive impairments should be based on a clear understanding of the nature of the underlying deficits, and a clear statement of the goals of treatment.

Background and conceptual overview

Over one hundred years ago, Ebbinghaus wrote that the study of memory had a long past but only a short history. The same might also be said of cognitive rehabilitation of individuals with impairments following brain disease, because systematic efforts to remediate these deficits began only well into the twentieth century. The relative youth of the field of rehabilitating individuals with cognitive deficits following brain damage has meant that the conceptual frameworks guiding these investigations are continually scrutinized, and revised in light of their shortcomings. Recently Wade (see Chapter 4) and his colleagues have proposed a model of rehabilitation of patients with cognitive deficits (Wade 2005). This model is based on the World Health Organization proposed classification of health functioning (World Health Organization, 2000). This framework, called the WHO ICF model, is useful because it highlights the possibility that rehabilitation of individuals with cognitive losses may be achieved at a variety of different levels. According to this model, rehabilitation of individuals with cognitive impairments may attempt: to improve neural functioning within the brain; to reduce cognitive impairment (e.g., visual neglect, attention deficits); to improve performance of functionally important activities; or to improve social participation.

This chapter will review treatment studies aimed at reducing the cognitive impairment of attention. Although treatments of individuals with a broad range of cognitive deficits have now been attempted (Cicerone *et al.* 2000), more effort has gone into investigating the treatment of attention than most other cognitive impairments, in part because impaired attention is a common consequence of acquired brain injury, and is functionally important. Scores on tests of attention predict return to work and performance of other functionally important life activities (Brooks 1987; Robertson *et al.* 1997; Van Zomeren and Van Den Burg 1985).

In terms of the WHO ICF model, most of the studies that we will be considering in the meta-analysis section of our review have attempted to improve attention functioning directly. For many of these studies, the reduction in cognitive impairment after treatment is hypothesized to be a consequence of restoring the neural processes that mediate attention processing. A few of the reviewed studies, however, have intervened by using compensatory approaches to train individuals with cognitive impairments to perform functionally important tasks requiring attention. In subsequent sections of this chapter, we will review studies that have attempted to improve performance of naturalistic actions, one type of functionally important activity.

Restoration versus compensation

Some of the earliest systematic work to investigate rehabilitation of individuals with cognitive impairments following brain damage considered whether treatment should attempt to restore the damaged cognitive function or whether it should focus on teaching patients compensatory strategies that enable them to perform functionally important activities (Goldstein 1942; Luria 1963; Zangwill 1947). This question, which will be considered in the present chapter, continues to be of importance because restoration and compensatory techniques require different approaches to treatment and imply that different cognitive and neural processes are being affected.

To clarify this last point, consider a patient with a hemiparetic left arm who seeks rehabilitation because the affected limb is used infrequently and its quality of movement is poor. As the WHO ICF model of rehabilitation makes clear, one could design treatments at several different levels (Wade 2005). Suppose the goal of treatment is to improve performance in activities that usually are performed bimanually. One still needs to decide whether treatment should focus on teaching compensatory strategies that enable this individual to perform bimanual actions effectively with one limb, or whether the focus should be on restoring function of the affected limb by improving the neural functioning of those regions involved in performing purposeful actions.

Research suggests that treatment can reduce the motor impairments of some patients through restoration of the underlying neural processes. One study treated 13 stroke patients, having limited movement of at least one limb, with the goal of increasing movement of the more affected limb (Liepert *et al.* 2000). These patients were treated well past the time (M = 4.9 years after stroke) when spontaneous recovery is thought to play an important role. The treatment, constraint-induced movement therapy, consisted of binding the less affected limb each day for a total of 12 days so that it could not be employed, thereby forcing patients to use the more affected limb. In addition, there were six hours of intensive therapy for eight of the days, during which a therapist used behavioural shaping procedures to improve limb functioning. Results showed a large increase in affected limb use while performing 20 activities of daily living immediately after treatment and six months later, compared to use prior to treatment. The effect size (1.5) was large (Cohen and Cohen 1983). Additionally, transcranial magnetic stimulation demonstrated that activation of the motor cortex in the affected hemisphere increased significantly after treatment.

The authors concluded that improved functioning attributable to restoration of the damaged neural processes occurred because: (a) there was behavioural improvement on motor tasks attributable to the treatment, and (b) the treatment program resulted in greater neural activity in an area damaged by the stroke and known to be involved in the performance of the tasks targeted by the treatment. In this chapter we will use these two criteria to evaluate studies that have attempted to restore attention through the restoration of the neural processes mediating attention.

Meta-analysis

One of us (NWP) completed a meta-analysis with Janet Ingles that evaluated the efficacy of rehabilitation programs administered to individuals with attention impairments as a consequence of brain damage (Park and Ingles 2001). The meta-analysis attempted to identify all studies published at the time that had treated individuals with general attention impairments as a consequence of brain damage, and to determine whether performance by these individuals improved significantly as a consequence of these programs. Most programs identified in our literature search had attempted either to restore the cognitive function of attention or to improve performance on functionally significant activities requiring attention. One objective of our meta-analysis was to determine whether these two types of programs differed in effectiveness. In addition, we attempted to identify methodological factors that contributed to the variability of improvement across studies.

Attention restoration treatment programs typically require participants to complete a series of repetitive drills in which auditory or visual stimuli must be responded to on the basis of a rule. For example, in the important and influential treatment program of Sohlberg and Mateer (1987), tasks take a few minutes to complete, feedback is presented after each task, and easier tasks are completed before more difficult ones are attempted. Treatment is usually considered to be successful when improvement is observed on psychometric tests of cognitive function. Although the use of psychometric measures is justified because the treatment programs are attempting to restore cognitive functioning, this evidence alone does not imply that the patient's level of functioning in daily living has improved (Carney *et al.* 1999). An important feature of many attention restoration programs is that they include exercises that treat different types of attention. Many psychologists and cognitive neuroscientists believe that attention can be fractionated (Posner and Petersen 1990), and it has been proposed that specific components of attention may require specific treatments (Sturm and Willmes 1991; Sturm *et al.* 1997).

Another, much less frequently studied approach to the rehabilitation of attention attempts to assist people with attention impairments by having them learn or relearn how to perform functionally significant activities. The rationale for this compensatory approach is that individuals with acquired brain damage can be trained to perform functionally significant activities, although they may use different neuropsychological processes involving different neural processes than those employed by unimpaired individuals (Backman 1989). All studies adopting a compensatory approach included in the meta-analysis focused on tasks requiring attention. For example, one study attempted to improve the driving skills of people with acquired brain injury (Kewman *et al.* 1985). Driving was conceptualized as a skill that critically requires attention. Using shaping procedures, the experimental group was trained to perform a variety of carefully designed driving-related exercises in a small electric-powered vehicle. In one exercise participants were required to divide attention and monitor a series of auditory and visual stimuli while driving. The control group of brain-injured participants drove the vehicle for the same amount of time as the experimental group, but was given no specific training.

Effectiveness of training was evaluated by having participants in both groups perform on-the-road automobile driving tests before and after training.

Method

Potential studies were identified by searching MEDLINE (from 1966–June 1997) and PsycLIT (from 1974–June 1997), by reviewing the Science Citation Index for articles that referred to several well known rehabilitation studies, and by inspecting the reference section of each retrieved article. Studies were included if:

- they evaluated the effectiveness of interventions for attentional disorders;
- participants were adults with an acquired brain injury;
- the effects of the attention treatment could be determined when the attention treatment program was part of a more comprehensive treatment program;
- at least one quantitative measure was reported in sufficient detail so that an effect size estimate could be calculated; and
- at least one outcome measure differed from the training measures.

After reviewing the retrieved articles, we were left with 30 studies involving a total of 359 participants. Of these studies, 26 were restoration-based, and 4 were compensatory. The restoration-based studies used psychometric tests of cognitive ability as their primary outcome measures, which were grouped into three broad categories – attention, learning and memory – and a residual category consisting of other cognitive tests. The tests of attention were further broken down into several different components based, in part, on the factor analytic research of Mirsky and colleagues (Mirsky 1989; Mirsky *et al.* 1991).

Quantifying study outcomes

Our general approach was to calculate separate effect size estimates for each different outcome measure, and then to aggregate these outcome measures as necessary. We did this in order to increase our ability to detect specific improvements that might have been obtained. An effect size estimate is a quantitative estimate of the effect of a treatment. It is computed in such a way that effects across studies can be aggregated.

More specifically, the effect size estimate g used in this meta-analysis is calculated by taking the difference between two means, and normalizing it (so effect sizes across studies can be compared) by dividing the difference by the appropriate standard deviation (Hedges 1982). Estimates were transformed when necessary so that positive and negative effect sizes reflect better and worse performance after training respectively. In the case of pre-post only measures, the effect size was determined by taking the difference between performance pre- and post-treatment divided by the standard deviation. If there were treatment and control groups, the pre-training effect size was subtracted from the post-training effect size (Wortman 1994). We converted g statistics into d statistics to avoid bias (Hedges and Olkin 1985). Aggregate results were reported in terms of weighted mean estimates (d_+), calculated by weighting each d statistic by the reciprocal of its variance in order to weight more reliable statistics more heavily (Hedges and Olkin 1985). A homogeneity statistic Q, which has an approximate chi square distribution with k–1 degrees of freedom, was calculated in order to determine whether the different estimates of d were consistent. A significant Q statistic, which signifies a lack of consistency across estimates, suggests that some study feature might be contributing to the differences in effect size. The relation between characteristics of the study that might be affecting performance and effect size estimates was investigated using fixed-effect categorized models (Hedges 1994; Hedges and Olkin 1985). These models partition the total variability in effect size estimates into the variability between classes or characteristics of the study (Q_B) and the variability within each class (Q_W). Significance of Q_B indicates that the study characteristic significantly determines the effect size. Q_W significance signals heterogeneity in the effect size estimates within that class.

Results

Effects of training on different cognitive functions and skills

Across the 30 studies, there were a total of 481 effect size estimates. To determine whether rehabilitation improved performance on different measures of general cognitive function, the g scores for all outcome measures belonging to the same category (e.g., attention) and type of effect size (pre-post only, pre-post with control) were averaged within a given study, and then converted to d+ statistics. Figure 8.1 shows the mean weighted effect size d+ for each cognitive function and skill assessed by pre-post measures only and by pre-post with control measures. The vertical bars represent a 95% confidence interval (CI) for each mean effect size estimate. As Figure 8.1 shows, the pre-post only effect size estimates for all cognitive functions, attention (k = 20), learning and memory (k = 12), and other (k = 11), were large and differed significantly from zero because the lower limit of the 95 per cent CI for d+ was greater than zero. In contrast, none of the cognitive functions of attention (k = 12), learning and memory (k = 7), and other (k = 5), increased significantly after treatment for the pre-post with control measures. The different pattern of findings for the pre-post only versus pre-post with control measures is most likely a consequence of practice effects inflating the pre-post only effect size estimates.

As shown in Figure 8.1, the pattern of results for the pre-post with control measures of specific skills of activities of daily living (ADL), driving, and attention behaviour were larger than the measures of cognitive function. For two of these measures, driving and attention behaviour, performance improved significantly after training.

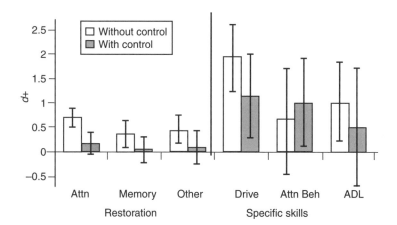

Figure 8.1 Mean Performance improvement and 95% confidence intervals after training in different cognitive functions and skills assessed by pre-post only and pre-post with control measures.

Effects of training on different types of attention

Another analysis calculated mean weighted effect size estimates ($d+$) and 95 per cent confidence intervals for different components of attention for pre-post only and pre-post with control measures. We analyzed the homogeneity of these estimates. Results showed that the Q_W statistic was nonsignificant for all measures, suggesting that no individual study estimate of any of the specific measures of attention differed significantly from the mean estimate of that measure. The pattern of results for the mean estimates ($d+$) of the different types of attention was similar to that shown for attention and the other cognitive tests shown in Figure 8.1. That is, for all types of attention, as depicted in the following list, pre-post only effect size estimates (shown first) were larger than the corresponding pre-post with control estimates (shown second): focus/execute 0.56 vs. 0.22, sustain 0.36 vs. 0.10, encode 0.47 vs. 0.32, working memory 0.78 vs. 0.12, picture completion 0.76 vs. 0.12, mental control 0.18 vs. −0.02, simple reaction time 0.89 vs. 0.17, choice reaction time 0.60 vs. 0.13, and other 0.79 vs. 0.19. Seven of the nine estimates of improvement in the pre-post only condition were significantly greater than zero, whereas none of the pre-post with control estimates differed significantly from zero.

Other analyses

To investigate the reasons for the substantial differences between pre-post only and pre-post with control measures for the restoration studies, we identified eight studies in which both types of estimates could be obtained (for further details see Park and Ingles 2001). The pattern of findings was similar to the meta-analysis results already reported for the restoration studies: pre-post only estimates were almost always significantly greater than zero and larger than pre-post with control measures, which themselves did not differ significantly from zero. These results suggest that the large effect sizes found in the pre-post only condition, but not in the pre-post with control condition for the restoration studies, are mainly a consequence of the effects of practice on the outcome measures.

Results from a comparison of effect size estimates of single-case studies and group studies showed that the effect size estimates did not differ significantly. Thus, treatment effectiveness, assessed from single case studies, provides findings that are consistent with those obtained from group studies.

Discussion of meta-analysis

In summary, the meta-analysis results show small effect sizes in those studies that attempted to restore attention when compared against conventional standards (Cohen 1977). Regardless of whether the outcome measure assessed a general cognitive function or a specific aspect of attention, the pre-post with control effect sizes were positive, small in magnitude, and not significantly different from zero. In contrast, findings from the compensatory studies that taught specific skills requiring attention, such as driving a motorized vehicle, showed medium to large effect sizes.

The meta-analysis also determined that pre-post only effect sizes were large, and significantly greater than zero in most cases. Further analyses showed that the large effects were most probably a consequence of specific practice on the outcome measures themselves. This finding shows that it is important to control for practice effects in one's experimental designs. Perhaps even more importantly, the presence of large practice effects on a large number of outcome measures demonstrates that individuals who have sustained an acquired brain injury can quickly improve their performance on a broad range of tasks after only a single trial. In turn, this provides a strong basis for being optimistic that individuals with brain damage can improve their performance on functionally important activities through practice.

The findings from the meta-analysis also suggest that single-case experimental designs can be used to explore the effectiveness of different forms of rehabilitation. This finding is important because evaluations of treatments for patients with specific impairments may only be possible using single-case designs (e.g. Coltheart and Byng 1989). Using single-case designs can also provide an efficient way to explore the effectiveness of alternative forms of treatment (Robertson 1994).

Interpreting restoration effects

In performing any type of review, it is difficult to decide how to aggregate findings across studies. Although quantitative aggregation does not occur in qualitative studies, these studies do aggregate findings when discussing the consistency of findings, summarizing results, categorizing studies, and so on. The current meta-analysis took three steps to guard against the possibility that we had masked effective treatments through inappropriate aggregation. First, we tested for homogeneity of effect size estimates by calculating Q statistics. Particularly effective treatment programs would have been detected as programs that deviated significantly from the mean effectiveness for that measure. Second, we assessed treatment effectiveness at several different levels of measurement so as to increase our chances of detecting specific improvements. Finally, we examined individually all studies that had a control condition.

Comparison with other reviews

At about the same time as the current meta-analysis was being performed, two other studies reviewed the effectiveness of treatments for individuals with cognitive impairments after acquired brain injury (see Carney et al. 1999; Cicerone et al. 2000). These two reviews differed in their scope and method of review from the meta-analysis because they used qualitative review procedures, and attempted to generate recommendations for clinical practice. Despite these differences, there were significant commonalties across the three reviews. Importantly, and consistent with the meta-analysis, the review by Carney and her colleagues concluded that treatment efficacy was stronger for compensatory than for restoration-based studies (see chapter 24). Further, if one focuses only on studies that were examined by both the Cicerone and meta-analytic reviews (n = 12), the two reviews were similar in their interpretation, although the Cicerone review was more positive about the possibility of remediating attention through training than this meta-analysis.

Analysis and treatment of naturalistic action

This section reviews work on naturalistic action as well as attempts to remediate its impairment following acquired brain injury. Naturalistic actions refer to goal-directed activities that require the production of several actions in a particular order so as to achieve a specific goal. Routine naturalistic actions refer to actions familiar to the participant prior to their performance (e.g., preparing coffee or tea, making a sandwich). Novel naturalistic actions refer to actions that cannot be performed by the participant prior to instruction (e.g., transferring from a wheelchair, preparing an unfamiliar recipe). Investigating impairments of naturalistic action and their remediation is clinically important because individuals with traumatic brain injury and stroke are frequently impaired when performing naturalistic actions (Buxbaum et al. 1998; Schwartz et al. 1999; Schwartz et al. 1998) and because many activities of daily living (e.g., food preparation, toileting, wheelchair transfer) require naturalistic action performance.

Investigations of purposeful action suggest that several cognitive processes are involved. For example, it appears that the psychological processes involved in the performance of single and multi-step actions overlap because patients with apraxia, a particular type of purposeful action impairment, are also impaired in their ability to perform functionally important everyday activities (Foundas *et al.* 1995). Attention also appears to be needed to learn novel actions and to produce routine actions. Reason (1984) investigated the relation between attention and skilled action production. In this study, 63 undergraduates were instructed to record in their diary whenever their actions deviated from their intended goal, and to answer a series of standard questions as soon as possible after the occurrence of an action slip. Analysis of these data showed that action slips occurred during the execution of a familiar action that required little attention to perform. This action was replaced by another action that tended to be performed in the same location, and required similar movements, although it frequently had a different purpose. Most action slips occurred at a time when participants reported they were preoccupied by some thought or distracted by an external event, and hence not paying attention to the task being performed.

A study involving 47 right-brain damaged stroke patients showed that performance on a neuropsychological test of sustained attention administered at two months post stroke predicted the functional status of these patients at two years on tests that included performance of everyday actions (Robertson *et al.* 1997). This result is also consistent with a recent study showing that attention test scores predicted the number of errors stroke individuals made while learning to perform novel naturalistic actions (Green *et al.* 2003). Tasks used in this study, such as making a Caesar drink, required about seven steps to complete, and were unfamiliar to participants prior to study.

One influential model of action hypothesizes that control over actions is mediated by two systems that select actions for input into a third system, the motor system that coordinates components of action to ensure their execution at precisely specified times (Cooper and Shallice 2000; Norman and Shallice 1986). According to this model, routine actions are controlled relatively automatically by the Contention Scheduling System. In novel situations or in situations that require the inhibition of alternative actions, however, actions are under attention or conscious control and are guided by a Supervisory Attentional System. The notion that conceptual aspects of naturalistic actions are performed by different neural and cognitive processes than those responsible for implementing actions is also consistent with representational models of apraxia formulated by Heilman, Roy, and others (Rothi *et al.* 1997; Roy and Square 1985). Empirical evidence also supports the separation of processes controlling the coordination of motor responses from the processes that conceptualize action because studies have shown that some brain-damaged individuals have impaired conceptual knowledge about actions, but intact motor performance, whereas others show the opposite pattern of performance (Bozeat *et al.* 2002; Heilman *et al.* 1982; Ochipa *et al.* 1992; Watson *et al.* 1986).

Treatment of naturalistic action deficits

The separation of conceptual and motor aspects of naturalistic action raises the possibility that different types of treatment are more effective in remediating motor versus conceptual naturalistic action deficits. Although one cannot be definitive, data reviewed in this chapter suggest that improving performance on functionally important activities that are controlled by consciously accessible components of attention (Reason 1984) may proceed more effectively if one focuses on the treatment of the impaired activity directly. In contrast, motor cortical deficits and perhaps involuntary aspects of attention may be treated more effectively by interventions that aim to reduce cognitive impairment through the restoration of the underlying neural and associated cognitive processes.

In recent research, our lab has investigated alternative training strategies to improve learning of novel naturalistic actions. An initial study (Curran *et al.* 2001; Curran 2002) evaluated whether it was possible to increase the rate at which individuals with mild cognitive impairment following stroke could learn novel naturalistic action sequences (e.g., make a pinhole camera). After a screening procedure to identify action sequences that were unfamiliar to a given participant in the study, the participant was taught six novel actions; half under each of two training conditions. In the demonstration with verbal description study training condition (DVD), the action sequence was demonstrated by the trainer and verbally described at the same time. In the other study condition, the demonstration only condition (DND), the action sequence was demonstrated by the trainer but no verbal description was provided. After the study trial was completed, the objects and tools required to perform the action were laid out, and the participant was instructed to try and perform the action sequence. Alternate study then test trials continued until the participant performed the action without error or for a maximum of six trials.

We hypothesized that providing verbal descriptions of actions as they were demonstrated would facilitate learning of the action by enabling stroke patients to develop a more accurate conceptual representation of the novel actions. Neurorehabilitationists often encourage patients to use verbal descriptions of planned actions to help them guide their behaviour (Luria 1963). Consistent with this hypothesis, results showed that stroke individuals made fewer errors and took fewer trials to learn novel actions in the DVD compared to the DND condition. The effect size of the difference between the two training conditions was large (effect size = 1.4).

A follow-up study showed that this result needed to be qualified because we found that stroke patients with more severe attentional/cognitive impairments did not benefit from the DVD condition, and in some cases took more trials to learn novel naturalistic actions in the DVD compared to the DND condition (Green et al. 2003). We are currently investigating this result further. Our current hypothesis is that this result was obtained because encoding novel naturalistic actions requires controlled processing and hence needs cognitive resources. Patients with limited cognitive resources have difficulty integrating verbal and visual-spatial information into a more complete memory representation, and thereby do not learn actions more quickly in the DVD than the DND condition.

In a divided attention experimental paradigm, we have compared the accuracy of novel naturalistic action performance originally viewed under full or divided attention conditions by college undergraduates (Park and Barbuto 2004; Park et al. 2004). Results showed that regardless of the nature of the secondary task, novel naturalistic action performance accuracy was higher in the full than in the divided attention condition, suggesting that encoding of naturalistic actions required controlled processing. Baddeley's (2000) new working memory model makes a similar point. The new model resembles the original three component model of working memory, but it also contains an episodic buffer that is hypothesized to integrate information from different modalities into coherent episodes. According to this model, the episodic buffer would be recruited to bind visuospatial and verbal information into an integrated memory representation in the DVD condition, a process that requires controlled processing.

A case study of two patients with Action Disorganization Syndrome (ADS) has shown that verbal descriptions may or may not help individuals perform naturalistic actions (Forde and Humphreys 2002). ADS is a neurological syndrome in which purposeful action performance is disorganized with frequent errors. Patients with ADS make large numbers of errors performing routine actions (e.g., making a cup of instant coffee). Errors include omitting necessary actions, repeating actions unnecessarily, and selecting the wrong object to perform a particular action. This particular study investigated two individuals who were equally impaired on routine action production, although a series of studies with these two individuals established that different cognitive and neural processes appeared to be responsible for their deficits. In a subsequent phase of the study the investigators showed that one patient was better able to complete routine naturalistic actions when presented with one verbal command describing the action to be performed relative to a no cueing condition.

In contrast, there was no difference in performance between these two conditions for the other ADS individual.

Concluding comments

The findings from the meta-analysis showed weak support for the hypothesis that attention can be restored through treatment because the effect sizes were relatively small and non-significant in studies with control conditions. Moreover, no study included in the meta-analysis actually investigated whether there was a significant change in activation of the damaged brain region after treatment. As noted previously, such a finding would provide support for the restoration hypothesis (Liepert *et al.* 2000). Taken together, there is no strong support for the notion that attention impairments can be remediated by restoring the underlying neural processes either at a behavioral or a neural level.

Although the meta-analysis findings fail to support the restoration of attention hypothesis, it would be premature to conclude that attention cannot be restored. Robertson and Murre (1999) have proposed that restoration may be possible only for individuals with mild to moderate brain lesions. This hypothesis remains viable and could not be evaluated in the meta-analysis. In fact, the finding that 11 of the 12 pre-post with control effect size measures assessing restoration were positive (although non-significant), may reflect restoration for the few participants with smaller brain lesions. This possibility needs to be investigated in future studies.

In contrast, there is good evidence to support the hypothesis that the performance of individuals with cognitive impairments on functionally important activities can be improved through training. We have recently investigated the cognitive processes underlying naturalistic action and have attempted to identify ways of remediating impaired naturalistic action after acquired brain injury. Our research showed that stroke patients with mild attentional impairments learned new naturalistic action sequences more quickly when they were verbally described as they were demonstrated. In contrast, patients with more severe impairments either did not benefit or were more impaired in the verbal description condition. This finding is important clinically because healthcare professionals working with acquired brain injury patients frequently describe actions as they demonstrate them.

The findings reviewed in this chapter suggest that cognitive rehabilitation should be based on a clear understanding of the underlying deficits and a clear statement of the goals of treatment. We call this a *deficit-based approach to treatment*. As the WHO ICF model of rehabilitation reminds us, treatment interventions can occur at several different levels. Findings reviewed in this chapter suggest that interventions need to be designed so as to respect the specific deficits of the individual being treated. For example, if the goal of treatment is to remediate learned non-use of a hemiparetic limb, restoration treatments may be appropriate. In contrast, our meta-analysis findings support the idea that compensatory approaches can lead to large improvements when the goal of treatment is to improve performance on tasks requiring attention. Our finding that verbal descriptions have differential effects on mild versus severely impaired stroke patients further supports the deficit-based approach to treatment.

In summary, despite its relative youth, the field of cognitive neurorehabilitation has made substantial progress in the past thirty years or so, and its future appears bright. New approaches to treatment are emerging that build on our increased understanding of basic cognitive and neural processes. Equally important, increasingly rigorous studies are critically evaluating whether these treatments are effective. This healthy interaction of theoretical analysis, better understanding of underlying cognitive and neural process, and careful evaluation of efficacy will yield a new generation of treatments for individuals with cognitive impairment.

9 Can disabilities resulting from attentional impairments be treated effectively?

McKay Moore Sohlberg

Abstract

The chronic, pervasive disabilities resulting from attention impairments has rendered this cognitive domain a rehabilitation priority. Individuals along the entire spectrum, from mild to severe brain injury, report long term dysfunction caused by persistent attention impairments (Brooks and McKinlay 1987; Mateer, Sohlberg and Crinean 1987). Subjective client complaints include reduced speed of processing, decreased ability to maintain attention, and distractibility, in addition to impairments in the working memory processes that are responsible for temporary maintenance and mental manipulation of information (Cicerone 2002; Mateer and Mapou 1996). This chapter examines the literature for evidence on the effectiveness of therapies for reducing the level of disability caused by such changes in attention.

Introduction

The question, 'Can disabilities resulting from attentional impairments be effectively treated?' requires understanding the concept of disability. The multiple modifications to the *International Classification of Functioning, Disability and Health* (ICF) by the World Health Organization (WHO) underscores the difficulty of confining disability to a single definition. The WHO has wrestled for decades with how to classify functional states associated with health conditions. They recognize the importance of language to describe changes in neuropsychological functioning (impairment) in addition to describing what an individual is able to and actually does perform with and without assistance in their natural environment. All aspects of community, social and civic life are considered potential sources of disability. (For information about current WHO classification scheme please see www3.who.int/icf/icftemplate.cfm and Chapter 4 in this volume.

Some researchers object to parsing disability from impairment and encourage a framework that views them simultaneously (Ylvisaker and Feeney 1998). Regardless of one's framework, attending to the effects of changes in cognitive function on people's ability to perform their everyday tasks is a universal concern to researchers and practitioners in the field of cognitive rehabilitation. What is not easily agreed upon, is what constitutes 'evidence' of changes in disability. This chapter begins with a discussion of the complexity inherent when trying to define and evaluate evidence of clinical effectiveness.

This discussion is followed by a review of the wide spectrum of attention intervention approaches and the corresponding evidence that they can reduce disability. The chapter concludes with recommendations for strengthening the link between research and practice in order to facilitate evidence-based attention treatment.

The challenge of evidence-based practice

In the last decade, the leaderships of clinical and research organizations concerned with addressing the needs of people with acquired cognitive disorders have joined the movement within healthcare to establish empirically-based practice guidelines. The U.S. National Institutes of Health (NIH Consensus Panel 1999; American Congress of Medicine (Cicerone *et al.* 2000) and the American Speech-Language-Hearing Association (Ylvisaker *et al.* 2002) have each committed resources toward developing evidence-based guidelines that causally link treatment protocols to expected clinical outcomes (Robey 2001). Increasingly, it has become important to temper the initial enthusiasm for having well-designed clinical studies dictate clinical practice with a balanced examination of the relationship between clinical research and clinical practice.

Proponents of evidence-based medicine (EBM) have traditionally advocated a hierarchy of evidence (Tonelli 2001). Table 9.1 illustrates a graded sequence of evidence. In cognitive rehabilitation, like other medical fields, Class 1 studies or well-designed radomized controlled trials (RCT) instill the highest confidence in the evidence (Robey 2001). However, hierarchies lump and grade evidence based on the assumption that each class of 'evidence is sufficiently similar to the others to allow for a universal judgment' (Tonelli 2001, p. 1437). Ylvisaker and colleagues (2002) underscore the risks from singular consideration of evidence from RCT when studying the diverse brain injury population. They note a client may (1) resemble those in the clinical trials who did not benefit from the intervention, (2) resemble those who were excluded from the study, (3) display important co-morbidity factors that influence response to treatment, or (4) not have the resources to receive a particular intervention. It is essential to consider all types of evidence, empirical and experiential, in clinical decision-making, as no single type of evidence is sufficient (Tonelli 2001).

Two excellent clinicians familiar with the research evidence and skilled in critical appraisal of the literature may disagree on the implementation of attention therapy (Rubenfield 2001; Ylvisaker *et al.* 2002). Interpretation of evidence is not a straightforward process. One reason is that evidence does not affect a clinician's practice unless it changes his or her beliefs and beliefs are in part influenced by a practitioner's existing convictions before encountering new evidence. The wide variety of experience with subgroups of people with brain injury by the many different specialties involved in cognitive

Table 9.1 Example of hierarchy of research evidence (Cicerone *et al.* 2000)

Type of evidence	Description
Class I	Well designed, prospective, randomized controlled trials
Class II	Prospective, nonrandomized cohort studies; retrospective, non randomized case-control studies; or clinical series with well-designed controls that permit between-subject comparisons of treatment conditions such as multiple baseline across subjects.
Class III	Clinical series without concurrent controls, or studies with results from 1 or more single cases that used appropriate single-subject methods, such as multiple baseline across interventions with adequate quantification and analysis of results.

rehabilitation results in divergent practice philosophies. Beliefs are also influenced by the degree to which a study is without flaw. New knowledge is discounted when it is unexpected, unless it is compelling in quality (Rubenfield 2001, p. 1445). Due to the heterogeneous population and complex issues related to brain injury recovery, compelling evidence in the field of cognitive rehabilitation is difficult to achieve. The quality of treatment studies is affected by the numerous research challenges.

'Scientific' clinical decision making is further prone to inconsistency due to the influence of patient values on this process. What constitutes a meaningful clinical outcome is in part a social judgment (Montgomery and Turkstra 2003). For example, regardless of the evidence supporting the effectiveness of direct attention training, a client who is not troubled by his difficulties sustaining attention and holding on to information should not be encouraged to undergo this treatment. A different client, however, who feels devastated by her inability to adequately hold on to information that she reads and hears and who is motivated to work on her impairments may be a good candidate for a diagnostic trial of attention training.

How then can we move forward in the quest to use evidence in our clinical decisions? To bridge the research and practice gap, it is important to acknowledge the value of well-designed research in addition to other forms of knowledge by considering the following:

1. Different sources of evidence including research outcomes, practitioner beliefs and values and client belief and values; and
2. The context of clinical treatment including possible influences of individual client characteristics as well as system resources and logistics.

This means that occasionally a client may be treated in the absence of strong research evidence if it can be established that the evidence does not apply (Ylvisaker *et al.* 2002). In this review of the research relevant to attention interventions designed to reduce disability, we will attempt to be mindful of the complicated nature of what constitutes 'evidence' and the myriad of factors that influence clinical outcomes.

Effects of attention intervention in reducing disability

Based on an extensive review of the literature for the Academy of Neurologic Communication Disorders and Sciences Evidence-Based Practice Guidelines (ANCDS EBPG) Traumatic Brain Injury subcommittee, attention interventions are classified into six distinct approaches:

1. direct training of attention processes;
2. specific skills training;
3. training metacognitive strategies specific for managing attention deficits;
4. training the use of external aids to compensate for attention deficits;
5. environmental modification/task accommodation; and
6. collaboration-focused approaches.

This classification scheme is admittedly simplistic and serves only as a method to organize and report results from a broad research base. The hope is that an examination of current intervention options, even those that are at present underspecified and loosely conceptualized, will help clinicians and their clients make optimal treatment decisions as well as help to advance our research questions.

Parceling out information about therapeutic techniques designed to address specific problems with attention is somewhat artificial due to the interdependence of attention, memory and executive functions.

Their close functional association and shared neurocircuitry accounts for the interdependence. Similarly, cognition overlaps with other domains including emotional, behavioral, and physical functioning (Sohlberg and Mateer 2001). The blurred distinction between attention and other cognitive areas and cognition and emotion, makes it important to examine intervention outcomes from multiple perspectives.

The six approaches to attention intervention are supported by differing amounts of research evidence. The direct process training, specific skills training and metacognitive strategy approaches have been subject to some experimental scrutiny, thus providing an initial research-base examining their efficacy. The use of external aids and environmental manipulations are part of mainstream clinical practice, but the efficacy of these approaches has been investigated less rigorously than the direct training of attention. The collaboration-focused approach is based on case reports and draws principal theoretical support from fields outside of cognitive rehabilitation. Although each approach will be described separately, they are often used in combination. For example, the simultaneous implementation of an external aid and direct training of attention processes is a common practice.

What follows is a description of each these approaches to attention intervention, with examples (where possible) from the literature showing evidence or lack of evidence in reducing disability. As discussed in the previous section, clinicians and researchers will want to weigh this information in conjunction with their own rehabilitation experiences and maintain cognizance of relevant values and system characteristics in order to make informed clinical decisions when treating or studying attention impairments.

Direct training of attention processes to reduce disability

Attention training is based on the notion that the repeated stimulation of attentional systems via hierarchical attention exercises will facilitate improvements in attentional functioning (Cicerone 2000; Sohlberg *et al.* 2001). The aspects of attention that are addressed vary widely among interventions, but regardless of their theoretical framework, most include functions related to sustaining attention over time (vigilance), capacity for information, shifting attention, speed of processing and screening out distractions. Intervention practices within this framework also differ by whether the exercises are matched to a client's specific attention abilities or are provided in a standard program to all clients. The frequency and duration in which the drill-oriented therapy is administered also varies considerably in the research reports (see Chapter 8 in this volume for a more complete discussion of this intervention).

The predominant outcome measures used in the attention training studies are impairment-based, neuropsychological test scores that do not easily translate into clinically meaningful improvement. Even if these test indices should prove to be ecologically valid in predicting improvements in independence or community reintegration, clinician judgment and client/family input would be required to determine if the cost-benefit ratio was acceptable. In other words, we must evaluate whether the magnitude of improvement in client functioning warrants the time and energy required on the part of the client and clinician. This post-hoc information is not provided in efficacy studies. Similarly, there is little attempt to measure maintenance of effects over time in attention training studies.

While the use of disability-related markers is sparse, there is an encouraging research trend to develop and use outcome measures which capture real world functioning. A review of the attention training literature conducted by the ANCDS EBPG Traumatic Brain Injury subcommittee (Sohlberg *et al.* 2003) revealed four different disability-related outcome markers to measure the effects of attention process training. The first marker was the use of descriptive reports about changes in subject functioning. A number of studies anecdotally report improvements in daily living skills, changes in vocational or independent living status that the researchers suggest are associated with treatment (Cicerone 2002; Sohlberg and Mateer 1987; Sohlberg *et al.* 2000). An obvious drawback is the lack of objectivity and control with the outcome measure. A second, somewhat more objective disability-related tool is the use of standardized rating scales for measuaring functional outcomes. The use of this outcome measure has yielded mixed results. The *Functional Independence Measure* (Granger and Hamilton 1987), a scale used to rate the level of assistance required to perform various activities of daily living, was used with a subset of one study (Novack *et al.* 1996) with no significant change in results reported following attention treatments. Similarly, Sohlberg *et al.* (2000) did not find significant changes on the Attention Questionnaire and the Dysexecutive Questionnaire (Wilson *et al.* 1996) following attention process training. Cicerone (2002), however, reported a significant reduction in the experience of attentional difficulties following attention training combined with strategy training on their self-report measure, a modified version of the Attention Rating and Monitoring Scale (ARMS) (Cicerone 2002).

Direct observation of attentional skills during a functional task was the third disability-related marker. It holds appeal due to its ecological validity; however, it is difficult to design the tasks that capture changes in attention that are treated by the attention training. Ponsford and Kinsella (1988) observed distractibility during a work related task; however they reported difficulties with ceiling effects using this measure.

A fourth, infrequently used marker that is systematic and based on authentic data is the use of *ethnographic reporting* or structured interviews. This approach attempts to capture and code the perceptions of subjects and/or caregivers regarding changes in attention ability thought to be associated with treatment. Only one study reported improvements using this measurement approach that were associated with changes on standardized attention tests (Sohlberg *et al.* 2000).

Interestingly, Sohlberg and colleagues noted that while neuropsychological tests and standardized questionnaires provide a quantitative index of level of impact resulting from an attention impairment, they do not provide information on the nature of the impact. In their report, they include an appendix with excerpts from interviews showing that people who did not endorse changes on questionnaires, spontaneously gave examples of improved attention during an interview. For example, clients that did not show improved performance ratings on an attention questionnaire, made statements such as 'I can drive while listening to the radio' or 'I can watch a whole movie' when asked if they had noted anything different in their day to day functioning. The reported everyday attention improvements were consistent with increased performance on corresponding attentional tests. The authors suggested that in order to investigate the impact of intervention, clients with brain injury may need to be asked about specific activities with relevance to their lives. Their report underscores the need to develop techniques that produce authentic data in order to assess changes in disability.

As stated, the predominant indicator of efficacy in studies evaluating attention training is impairment-based changes in neuropsychological scores. There are three published comprehensive reviews of the attention literature (Cicerone *et al.* 2000; Park and Ingles 2001; Sohlberg *et al.* 2003). Cicerone and colleagues reported the findings of a subcommittee of the American Congress of Rehabilitation Medicine (ACRM) in which they analyzed thirteen studies assigned to the category of remediation of attention deficits. In their meta-analysis, Park and Ingles (2000) coded and analyzed 26 studies as direct retraining studies. To measure outcomes, all of the studies in these reports employed some aspect of impairment-level testing via standardized assessment. Only three of these studies incorporated disability level information in their assessments (Novack *et al.* 1996; Ponsford and Kinsella 1988; Sohlberg and Mateer 1987).

There are two Class II studies evaluating attention training that were published during or after the year 2000 which included disability-related markers. A description of these two recent studies serves to illustrate the intervention and associated evidence relevant to implementing attention training.

Sohlberg *et al.* (2000) published an efficacy study of 14 post-acute clients with mild-severe brain injuries, who exhibited impaired attention abilities as determined by neuropsychological evaluation. Intervention consisted of attention training exercises from a commercially available attention training program administered three times per week in 60 minute sessions. The exercises were selected for each subject based on the results of their particular neuropsychological profile. These same subjects also received a single 60 minute session each week devoted to brain injury education for the same number of weeks as the attention drill work.

Outcomes for the two intervention programs (attention training and brain injury education) were measured and compared using both impairment- and disability-based measures. Impairment level measures were obtained using a battery of neuropsychological tests selected to assess different attention networks (vigilance, orienting, working memory, and executive attention). Disability-related measures were obtained using standardized questionnaires and structured interviews to assess subjects' perceptions of their neuropsychological and psychosocial performance in daily life. Results showed significantly improved scores on measures of working memory and executive attention that were correlated with self reports of improved attention in everyday settings. In contrast, brain injury education was associated with self reports of improved psychosocial function.

Cicerone (2002) evaluated the effectiveness of an intervention designed to address attention deficits following mild traumatic brain injury. Treatment participants consisted of a convenience sample of patients referred to a postacute brain injury rehabilitation program based on a diagnosis of mild traumatic brain injury (MTBI). Using a prospective, case comparison design, four subjects received attention remediation and four served as a control group based on their inability to receive treatment. The subjects were matched closely for age, gender, education, and months post injury, with all at least three months post injury.

Similar to the Sohlberg *et al.* (2000) study, the authors employed hierarchically organized attention remediation tasks targeting complex attention skills via working memory tasks that were tailored to match the specific attentional profiles of the individual clients. However, the focus was on using the attentional tasks as a method for training the use of metacognitive strategies such as verbal mediation, rehearsal, anticipation of task demands, self-pacing and self-monitoring rather than on improving attention. The intervention emphasized the conscious and deliberate use of such strategies to increase the participants' ability to allocate their attention resources and control the pacing of task performance. Hence, although there was repetitive administration of attention exercises, strategy training was a primary emphasis. The schedule of treatment was one hour per week for 11–27 weeks.

Treatment outcomes included psychometric measures, self rating for perception of change on the ARMS and informal reports of changes in status for vocational and social roles. Impairment-based measures compared pre and post-treatment scores on a number of attention tests with the performance of the no-treatment control group. Results showed that three of the four participants improved significantly on the attention tests, while none in the control group did so. More importantly, the treatment group also improved significantly on their self-report of a greater reduction of attention difficulties in comparison to no change in the control group. The author anecdotally reported that all of the treatment group participants returned to previous vocational and social roles while none of the comparison group participants did so during the same period. Change was attributed to improved strategy use rather than improved underlying attentional processing, although there was no attempt to separate out these factors.

Summary

It is not possible to compare the findings from different studies directly due to tremendous variability in the subjects (e.g., level of severity and time post onset), the treatment (e.g., type and selection of exercises and dosage), research methodology and outcome measurement. While attention training studies emphasize neuropsychological test performance, more recent studies are beginning to incorporate disability-related markers. Studies reporting positive outcomes following direct attention tend to share the following features:

1. individualized attention exercises;
2. treatment sessions that were 1 hour (versus 2 hours) in duration;
3. at least weekly treatment sessions;
4. outcome measures that included a range of different measures sensitive to attention and working memory; and
5. outcome measures that included disability-based measures using client self-report (Sohlberg *et al.* 2003).

Specific skills training to reduce disability

Treatment aimed at assisting individuals to learn or relearn skills of functional importance to them is another clinical option for addressing attention impairments. Evidence of the success of this approach is seen when performance on the target skill improves concurrent with training. Of relevance to this chapter is the teaching of skills that are hypothesized to depend upon attention, which some people may argue is inclusive of all functional activities. In their meta-analysis of attention rehabilitation, Park and Ingles (2000) analyzed four studies which addressed attention either by training a specific skill such as driving (e.g., Kewman *et al.* 1985), or by training attention skills intended to transfer to a specific related functional activity such as practice on video tasks to address driving-related perceptual deficits (e.g., Carter *et al.* 1988; Sivak *et al.* 1984; Wilson and Robertson 1992). This meta-analysis suggested that specific skills training significantly improved performance of the targeted tasks requiring attention.

There are many examples of Class II and Class III studies documenting the ability of people with brain injury to learn a variety of skills efficiently . Studies have shown that systematic training and practice results in learning driving (Kewman *et al.* 1985), academic skills (Glang *et al.* 1992) and vocational tasks (von Cramon and Mathes-von Cramon 1994) by people with attention impairments. The common element among all such studies is the use of deliberate instructional training methodologies grounded in learning and cognitive theories. They clearly define the relevant skills and subskills, carefully select training examples, build in methods for systematic corrections and provide sufficient practice (Sohlberg and Mateer 2001). Direct observation of performance on the trained skill is the disability-related outcome measure for this type of intervention. Unlike the process-oriented training, there is not an expectation for specific skills training to generalize to nontrained tasks, hence the measurement issues are less complex.

Metacognitive training for attention impairments

Metacognitive training reflects a blend of therapy approaches that includes cognitive, behavioral, or combined cognitive-behavioral techniques. The techniques may emphasize behavioral methods to train specific attention or goal-completion skills, or methods to help individuals achieve greater internalization of strategies for controlling and monitoring their attention (Cicerone *et al.* 2002; Sohlberg and Mateer 2001). For example, verbal self instruction (e.g., Meichenbaum and Goodman 1971) has been used with increasing frequency in brain injury rehabilitation to address a variety of cognitive issues, most commonly executive function deficits (Cicerone *et al.* 2000).

This author identified four reports of the use of metacognitive strategy-based training specifically designed to address attentional impairments following acquired brain injury (Butler and Copeland 2002; Fasotti *et al.* 2000; Webster and Scott 1983; Wilson and Robertson 1992). In an early Class III study by Webster and Scott (1983), a patient with a traumatic brain injury and resulting difficulties with attention was taught to subvocalize self-instructional statements. These statements prepared him to listen and ask for repetition if his attention had strayed (e.g., 'I must focus on what is being said, not on other thoughts which want to intrude.'). Results suggested improved attention on story recall measures and in functional activities in his home environment.

Fasotti and colleagues (2000) evaluated a strategy they termed Time Pressure Management (TPM), designed to compensate for 'information overload' and 'mental slowness' (p. 48). Similar to Webster and Scott (1983), they evaluated the effectiveness of a self instructional strategy. The strategy was comprised of four self-guiding steps:

1. identify if there are two or more things to be done at the same time for which there is not enough time (recognition of time pressure);
2. make a plan for what to do before the actual task begins (prevention of time pressure);
3. make an emergency plan in the event of overwhelming time pressure (dealing with time pressure), and
4. use the plans (encouragement of self-monitoring) (1983, p. 53).

The strategy was initially modeled by the examiner, followed by the patient instructing him- or herself out loud while writing and implementing the four strategy steps. The strategy was first used to remember the contents of videotaped short stories. Gradually it was practiced under progressively more distracting and difficult conditions. A control group was given four generic concentration suggestions (e.g., 'do not get distracted by irrelevant sounds' and 'try to imagine things that are said').

The results of this Class I randomized study with pre-training, post-training and six month follow-up measures suggested that both the concentration treatment and the TPM was effective in increasing the amount of material remembered. Although the TPM produced greater gains, the effects did not reach significance: however, this approach appeared to generalize to other measures of speed and memory which did not occur with the concentration treatment.

Goal setting was the metacognitive strategy evaluated in a Class III study by Wilson and Robertson (1992) to reduce attentional slips during reading in a person with brain injury. They used a behavioral shaping, goal-setting strategy to increase the length of time that the subject could concentrate during reading. They had the client practice reading a novel for the minimum periods sustainable without an attention slip and then take a break. They gradually increased the duration of the reading period. Conditions of distraction and more difficult text reading were also implemented. Results showed a significant decrease in the frequency of attention slips. The authors hypothesize that the training helped the client reduce capacity-occupying thoughts about concentration failures which in turn freed up some of his limited capacity during reading performance.

Butler and Copeland (2002) evaluated the use of metacognitive strategy training in combination with direct attention training in a young population (ages 6 to 22 years) with acquired attention deficits due to central nervous system treatment (e.g., brain radiation) for cancer (Butler and Copeland 2002). This Class I study compared scores on attention and arithmetic tests administered to participants in the Cognitive Rehabilitation Program (CRP; attention exercises and training of metacognitive strategies) with those of a comparison group who received no treatment. The metacognitive strategies included:

1. task preparation strategies ('use of magic/special words', 'soup breath', 'game face', 'personal best', 'warm up my brain');

2. on task strategies ('talk to myself', 'mark my place', 'start at the top, one row at a time', 'look for shortcuts', 'time out/start over', 'look at the floor', 'ask for a hint'); and

3. post task strategies ('check your work', 'ask for feedback', 'reward yourself').

The CRP group improved significantly on all impairment-based measures of attention, in contrast to the comparison group who manifested no changes. However, there was no generalization to the one disability marker, an arithmetic achievement test. While the improvements in attentional processing measured by neuropsychological tests were notable, the authors discussed the need to measure the ecological validity of the CRP. In their second phase, they plan to measure academic productivity (number of problems attempted) in addition to success as they feel this will be a more sensitive measure of changes in disability.

Summary

The four studies reviewed above suggest that it is possible to teach people with attention impairments to use self-instructional and goal setting strategies; the subjects in each study were able to learn and implement the target techniques. The studies reported mixed results using a variety of disability-related outcome measures within two broad categories: anecdotal report and direct observation of a functional skill. Client self-report suggested improved concentration during sexual performance and vocational activities as a result of metacognitive training (Webster and Scott 1983). Improved amount of information recall was reported as a result of the TPM self instructional training, but it was not significantly superior to general concentration training (Fasotti et al. 2000). A significant reduction in attention slips during reading was reported as a result of goal-setting training (Wilson and Robertson 1992). No improvement was observed on an arithmetic test following metacognitive strategy training plus attention process training (Butler and Copeland 2002).

Interestingly, the three studies (Butler and Copeland 2002; Fasotti et al. 2002; Webster and Scott 1983) that used impairment-based measures in addition to their disability-related markers reported improvements on cognitive test scores. As with direct attention process training, the methodological issues related to measuring possible changes in everyday functioning are challenging. All of the researchers highlighted the need to develop functional measures that can capture possible changes or more definitively determine that there is not generalization beyond neuropsychological tests when implementing metacognitive strategy training.

External aids for attention impairments

There are a number of experimental and case reports suggesting that the use of external aids is effective in managing difficulties in memory and executive functions (Kim et al. 1999). Given the interrelatedness of attention, memory and executive processes, it stands to reason that the use of external aids (e.g., written reminder systems or task specific aids) may compensate for attention deficits as well as deficits in memory and executive functions (Sohlberg and Mateer 2001).

Several training protocols based on cognitive and instructional theory have been specifically developed for teaching individuals with memory and attentional impairments to utilize external aids (e.g., Donaghy and Williams 1998; Sohlberg et al. 1998). Two experimental reports were identified that evaluated the use of eternal aids for a population that included people with attention impairments (Wilson et al. 2001; Wright et al. 2001). Wright and colleagues compared two different styles of pocket computer memory aids using a Class II within subject design. The outcome measures included qualitative questionnaire and interview data as well as computer logs of actual use of the computer aids. The authors concluded that people with brain injury could effectively use a computer-based external aid and that they found them useful.

In a Class I trial, Wilson and colleagues (2001) provided people displaying a wide variety of cognitive difficulties (including attention impairments) with paging systems that reminded them to carry out self-selected functional tasks. They measured the subjects' task completion in response to the paging reminders. The results indicated a significant increase in the initiation of functional tasks (e.g., taking medication) that for some subjects continued beyond the removal of the paging systems.

The disability-related outcome measures that have been used to examine the effectiveness of external aids include direct observation of use of aids, and self and caregiver report (e.g., Evans *et al.* 2003; Sohlberg and Mateer 1989; Wilson *et al.* 2001; Wright *et al.* 2001). In general, reports of using external aids to assist people with attention and other cognitive impairments to perform a wide variety of functional tasks suggest that it is important to conduct a needs assessment of the learner and environment in order to match the external aid to the individual. Effective implementation of the aid is dependent upon systematic instruction, incorporating care providers, and monitoring the effects of using the aid (Donaghy *et al.* 1998; Sohlberg *et al.* 1998).

Accommodation/environmental management for attention impairments

Disability advocacy law has resulted in the adoption of accommodation practices in vocational and academic settings. There are countless types of accommodations that can be implemented to assist individuals with attentional deficits. Teachers, employers and family members can modify task instructions, task expectations, supports for completing a task, and/or the environment in which a task is to be completed. Experimental investigations of the effectiveness of this approach are sparse. Instead, the literature focuses on descriptions of the types of accommodations that may be useful to people with cognitive deficits. For example, Thompson and Kerns (1999) described a number of classroom accommodations for students with brain injuries. Examples of strategies specifically for attention deficits included allowing students to take breaks, clearing clutter from work space, using earplugs or a headset during independent work, seating students away from noises such as windows or clocks, and posting information or task expectations on cue cards.

The issues in relation to accommodations specific for an individual are similar to those for external aids. That is, it is important to conduct individualized needs assessments, collaborate with key people in the environment, and systematically evaluate the effects of the accommodation (Sohlberg *et al.* 1998).

Collaboration approaches for attention impairments

Drawing from other psychological fields, such as family systems therapy, is the adoption of a more ecological, contextual framework within which to deliver cognitive rehabilitation services. The clinical power inherent in collaborating and forming partnerships with families and care providers is well recognized (Sohlberg and Mateer 2001). A collaboration approach to intervention is applicable not for only for attentional issues, but also for other cognitive and behavioral challenges resulting from brain injury. This collaboration approach is exemplified by Ylvisaker and Feeney (1998) who use positive, highly contextualized everyday routines to support people with cognitive difficulties in completing their desired daily goals. Collaborative alliances are formed with 'everyday people' who are supported in their role as coaches to the injured person as they teach that person to set goals and formulate, implement, and monitor a plan.

Another collaborative approach described by Sohlberg *et al.* (2001) teaches 'everyday people' to be careful observers of the contexts in which attention difficulties occur and to notice what helps and does not help. Families learn to conduct structured observations in order to help them select relevant goals and monitor progress on issues of concern to them. For example, the researchers used this approach with an adult with attention impairments in which his own observations led to the development and implementation of a tracking system that helped him attend to and follow classroom lectures (Sohlberg *et al.* 2001). Case descriptions that employ a combination of caregiver report and researcher anecdotal reports comprise the evidence for this approach to managing attention impairments.

Summary

A survey of the cognitive rehabilitation literature reveals a variety of approaches for addressing attention impairments including: direct attention process training, specific skills training, metacognitive strategy training, use of external aids, accommodations/environmental modifications and collaboration approaches. This chapter has attempted to answer the question: Are these approaches effective in reducing disability? The answer to this question lies in each practitioner's interpretation of the evidence. The heterogeneity inherent in the ABI population coupled with the strengths and limitations unique to each setting and practitioner and the range of opinions regarding what constitutes meaningful change makes it difficult, perhaps impossible, to design studies with clean, unequivocal outcomes.

In terms of experimental evidence, the outcomes of direct attention process training and metacognitive strategy training are predominantly restricted to correlations between impairment-based changes and some disability-related markers such as direct observation of activities, and caregiver/self-report within the contexts of interview and/or standardized rating scales. The evidence for disability-related changes for specific skills training and external aids is predominantly direct observation of target tasks and caregiver/self report. Case descriptions with a reliance on self/caregiver reports and researcher anecdotal accounts comprise the bulk of evidence for studies examining accommodations or collaboration-oriented interventions. Table 9.2 describes the range of disability-related markers found in the attention literature.

Table 9.2 Disability-related outcome measures in the attention literature

Disability markers	Study examples
Standardized rating scales or self-report measures that can be quantified	Attention Rating and Monitoring Scale (ARMS) allows rating frequency of attention symptoms using five point scale (Cicerone 2002) Attention Questionnaire allows rating frequency of occurrence for attentional breakdowns in different types of attention (Sohlberg *et al.* 2000)
Direct observation of performance	Measuring performance on attention dependent tasks such as driving (e.g., Kewman *et al.* 1985), arithmetic skills (e.g., Butler and Copeland 2002; Glang, Singer, Cooley and Tish 1992), use of an external aid (e.g., Wilson) or decrease in attention slips (Wilson and Robertson 1992)
Structured interview	Use of ethnographic reporting where clients' responses to questions about possible changes in functioning are analyzed and changes are coded (e.g., Sohlberg *et al.* 2000)
Self or caregiver report	Report of improvement concurrent with therapy; such as improved functioning with use of an external aid (e.g., Donaghy and Williams 1998; Wilson *et al.* 2001) or a detailed case report describing changes following family collaboration meetings (e.g., Sohlberg *et al.* 2001)
Anecdotal reports	Experimenter description of differences in global functioning such as employment and independent living pre- and post-treatment (e.g., Cicerone 2002; Webster and Scott 1983)

What is the bottom line? While there is not sufficient evidence to recommend any single intervention for a particular client profile or setting, there is evidence that different types of attention interventions can reduce disabilities in a variety of people with attention impairments stemming from brain injury. Each clinician must weigh the evidence in accordance with his or her own experiences, population, and client values. For example, the decision to move a student with an attention impairment to a less distracting seat is an easy accommodation that may reduce a learning disability. Teaching the same student to use a metacognitive strategy to improve learning has a much greater resource cost but if the student is an appropriate candidate, this latter approach may potentially reduce the learning disability across a number of environments. Research can provide one source of evidence to assist with this decision, but will never suffice.

Ultimately, the strongest evidence is from patient-specific hypothesis testing (PSHT) (Ylvisaker *et al.* 2002). In this approach, clinicians identify the most effective intervention based on the literature and what is known about their client. They measure the potential desired effects of the intervention. It is the strongest evidence because it is customized to the individual. As clinicians, we bridge the gap between research and practice by entering a rational decision making process that requires us to

1. be well versed on the research investigating the different treatment options for attention;
2. use this information in conjunction with relevant client-specific information;
3. develop in conjunction with our clients meaningful indicators of whether a selected treatment is working and
4. administer and analyze the results of these indicators during the treatment process.

As researchers, we can strengthen the research to practice bridge by striving to develop methodologies for measuring meaningful change that can be associated with intervention.

Section 3

Memory disorders

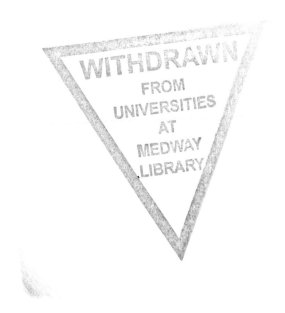

10 The neuroanatomy of memory

Hans J. Markowitsch

Abstract

The neuroanatomical correlates for memory encoding, consolidation, storage, and retrieval – and therefore for anterograde and retrograde forms of information processing – are discussed on the basis of time- and content-related subdivisions of memory. For content-based memory it is proposed that there are five long-term memory systems, each with its own neural circuitry. With respect to semantic and episodic memories (those two of the five memory systems which are of greatest importance for intellectual functioning), for encoding of information the interactive action of two circuits – the Papez and the basolateral limbic circuit – is proposed to be essential, with the first one acting more on the cognitive and the last one on the affective side. Memory storage of these two forms is assumed to require major cerebral cortical networks and for memory retrieval prefronto-temporal regions are assumed to trigger or activate the widespread cortical networks. It is proposed that both organic and psychogenic forms of retrograde amnesia act similarly in principle: in the organic forms the trigger structures for activating the storage nets are damaged, in the functional, psychogenic forms the stress hormone level is altered and influences those regions which have the highest number of stress hormone receptors – the amygdala and the hippocampus.

Introduction

The outstanding value of memory – compared to other cognitive functions – becomes especially apparent under pathological conditions. The loss of old and the inability to acquire new personal memories reduces the intellectual freedom of an individual drastically and affects his or her personality significantly. Without the 'glue' of memory, past and future lose their meaning and self-awareness is reduced or even lost. The old literature, dating back more than one century, provided case descriptions of patients with so-called global amnesia – preserved intelligence and short-term memory, together with permanent (anterograde) amnesia long-term and – also at that time – Hering (1870) (a physiologist known for his opponent-color theory or the Hering-Breuer reflex) stated that memory unites the countless single phenomena to a whole, and that without its binding power our consciousness would disintegrate into as many fragments as there are moments.

However, even at that time, scientists pointed to the fact that such patients may demonstrate rudimentary forms of long-term information processing (Markowitsch 1992). Furthermore, trying to simulate the amnesic syndrome in animals revealed more transitory effects and demonstrated that some kinds of information acquisition remained possible, while other kinds were impaired. This and various forms of learning, studied in non-brain damaged animals, led to the distinction between simple and complex forms of memory. For instance, into the forms of sensitisation, habituation, classical and operand conditioning, and concept formation (Gagné 1965). Furthermore, and this again principally only for human beings, it was emphasised that memory is embedded in other complex behavioural representations such as attention, thoughts, language, reasoning, and emotion. Memory processing consequently is quite difficult to localise, as cellular networks from the remotest neural periphery to the integration cortices participate in information processing.

Establishing the circuitry of normal memory functioning and tracing back possible relations between circumscribed or focal brain damage and different forms of memory impairment is of the utmost importance for memory diagnosis and rehabilitation in brain-damaged patients. Prerequisites for this endeavour lie in the application of knowledge coming from psychology.

In this overview the neuroanatomical correlates for memory encoding, consolidation, storage, and retrieval will be discussed on the basis of time- and content-related subdivisions of memory. Any discussion of brain–behaviour interrelations is dependent on the used or available methodology. The last century of brain research demonstrated numerous examples for this contingency. Kleist's (1934) painstaking analysis of the behavioural disturbances of thousands of gun or shrapnel lesioned veterans from the First World War let him to depict a quite detailed cortical map which contains for each of Brodmann's (1914) cytoarchitectonically defined areas one or several specific functions. Kleist's map probably comes closest to the old idea of establishing a *Landkartensystem* (geographical map-system) of the brain (Zülch 1976) (which had been looked for already by Gudden (1886), the personal physician of the mad Bavarian king Ludwig II). A contrasting view resulted from using electrophysiological techniques: John (1972; Bartlett and John 1973) and Pribram (1971) postulated holographic views of functional representation within the brain. While the results of the more recent functional imaging studies speak for an intermediate position, the debate of 'localisability' is a vivid one still (Brett, Johnsrude and Owen 2002; Goldman-Rakic 2000; Passingham, Stephan and Kötter 2002; Tyler and Malessa 2000).

It follows from all this research that it is not justifiable to equate the loss of a function after damage to a certain region with the control of this function by just this region in the normal brain (Chow 1967; Markowitsch 1984). The other extreme, that there is no specific brain locus for memory at all (Lashley 1950), is equally untenable.

On the psychological and psychiatric levels, Ebbinghaus (1885), Hering (1870), Ribot (1882) and other researchers from the nineteenth century laid the groundwork for a refined description of memory functions and actions. Diseases, resulting in memory disorders, in particular Korsakoff's disease (Korsakow 1890; Bonhoeffer 1901), but also various forms of senile and presenile dementia (Alzheimer 1907; Pick 1906) provided the bases for testing relations between memory divisions and their possible neural representations.

The present-day analysis of memory processes in the brain was helped by theoretical proposals on memory subdivisions which came from psychology (Tulving 1972, 1983, 2002). Tulving's ideas brought a framework for findings of memory preservation in amnesics (e.g., Warrington and Weiskrantz 1970) and induced a much more refined analysis of the so-called global amnesic syndrome. Even memory research in animals profited from this content-based splitting of memory functions (Mishkin and Petri 1984). Tulving's subdivisions will be used here, as his specifications seem to correspond closely to observations of selective memory loss in patients with certain forms of brain damage. Consequently, long-term memory is subdivided into episodic memory, semantic memory, perceptual memory, procedural memory, and priming (Figure 10.1). The episodic memory system is the only past-oriented memory system which makes mental time travel possible and thereby allows one to re-experience through autonoetic awareness (Markowitsch 2002), one's own previous experiences.

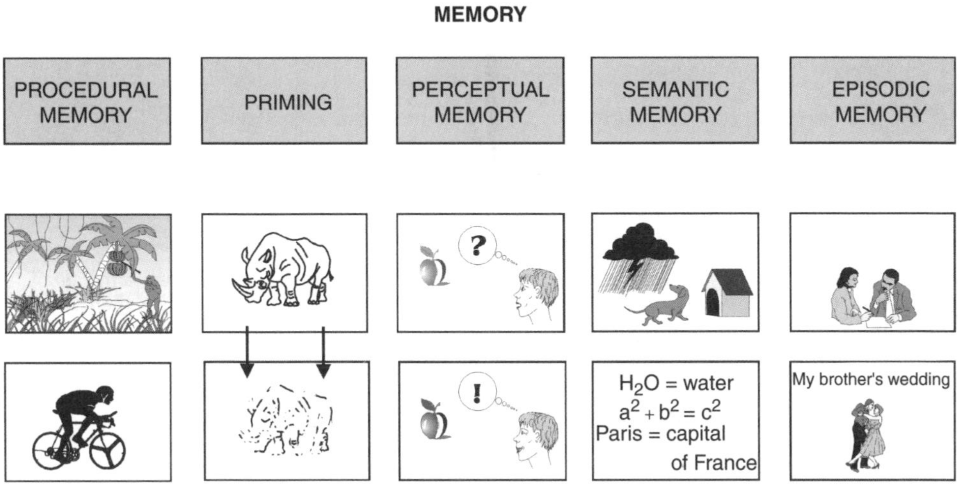

MEMORY

| PROCEDURAL MEMORY | PRIMING | PERCEPTUAL MEMORY | SEMANTIC MEMORY | EPISODIC MEMORY |

H_2O = water
$a^2 + b^2 = c^2$
Paris = capital of France

My brother's wedding

Figure 10.1 Five divisions of long-term memory (after Tulving and Markowitsch, in preparation).

Episodic memory has also been named event or autobiographical memory; it is usually affect-related. Semantic system refers to context-free facts, perceptual memory to the recognition of items, based, for example, on familiarity judgements. Procedural memory refers to various – perceptual, motor, cognitive – skills and priming to a higher likeliness of re-identifying a previously perceived stimulus (or, for conceptual priming, of identifying a stimulus from a previously perceived set or category of stimuli).

Aside from these long-term memory systems, short-term or working memory exists. Short-term memory is seen as the online holding of information for an initial time period after first confrontation with it (Cowan 2000), working memory refers to a multicomponent, active processing of information which also includes the transmission of already long-term stored information in a temporary buffer prior to retrieval, and which is composed of a controlling central executive system and a number of subsidiary slave systems (Baddeley 2002).

Brain damage, psychic shock conditions, or related interventions can either disturb the ability to form new memories – named 'anterograde amnesia' – or that of retrieving already stored memories – named 'retrograde amnesia' (Figure 10.2). Memory disorders, in fact, are a very frequent condition after various disease conditions (Table 10.1). From this fact it follows not only that information processing is controlled by a distributed network, but also that it is dependent on a large number of sensory, perceptual, attentive, emotional, and motivational processes, each with its own anatomical substrates.

Encoding of information

Information is usually transmitted via sensory organs. It then either may be encoded implicitly as primed information – activating mainly uni- and polymodal sensory cortex (Badgaiyan 2000; Naccache and Dehaene 2001; Schacter and Buckner 1998) – or as procedural memory – activating the basal ganglia, (pre-)motor cortical regions and possibly cerebellar structures (Eichenbaum and Cohen 2001; Knowlton *et al.* 1996). (Some authors question, however, a specific role of cerebellar structures in procedural memory.) Patients with basal ganglia degeneration such as those with Huntington's chorea and Parkinson's disease are particularly prone to procedural memory deficits (Heindel *et al.* 1989; Solveri *et al.* 1997).

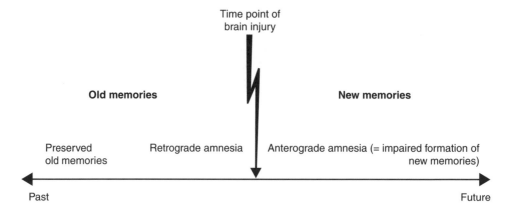

Figure 10.2 The 'Janus head of memory': Memory may be disturbed both with respect to future and past. With time point of brain injury also psychic stress and trauma situations are meant.

Table 10.1 Overview of patient groups in whom severe global amnesic disorders may be prominent

Etiology	Most common lesion sites
Intra-cranial tumors	Limbic thalamus (glioblastoma), medial temporal lobe (sphenoid wing meningioma), or posterior cingulate gyrus (lipoma)
Cerebral infarctions, ruptured aneurysms,	Bilateral lesions in hippocampus, aneurysm surgery medial temporal lobe and limbic nuclei of the thalamus (posterior cerebral artery) or in orbitofrontal cortex and basal forebrain (anterior communicating artery)
Viral infections (e.g., herpes simplex encephalitis)	Hippocampus and nearly all components of the limbic and paralimbic cortex
Closed head injury	Temporal pole, orbitofrontal cortex, fornix
Avitaminoses (e.g., B1 deficiency)	Limbic thalamus, mammillary bodies (as in Korsakoff's disease)
Neurotoxin exposure (e.g., trimethyltin intoxication)	Hippocampus
Temporal lobe epilepsy	Hippocampus and medial temporal lobe
Degenerative diseases of the CNS (e.g., Alzheimer's or Pick's diseases	Hippocampus, entorhinal cortex and amygdala
Anoxia or hypoxia (e.g., after a heart attack or drowning)	Hippocampus (CA1 sector)
Drugs such as anticholinergics, B-adrenergic blockers, benzodiazepines	Limbic system
Paraneoplastic limbic encephalitis	Limbic structure in medial temporal
Electroconvulsive therapy	Probably limbic system
Transient global amnesia	Usually limbic structures in medial temporal lobe when an etiology is found

In all the above-mentioned memory systems, the brain regions engaged in initial encoding correspond in principle to those relevant for later storage and also for later retrieval. This may also be true for perceptual memory which refers to the familarity with a stimulus, leading to its recognition at a later time (Yonelinas 2002). Perceptual memory probably largely engages uni- and polymodal cortical areas so, for the visual modality, regions within the occipital and temporal lobes. All of these memory systems function largely independent of limbic system structures and of conscious reflection. The two other memory systems, sketched in Figure 10.1, require staged encoding, starting with holding information on-line for later transmission and final consolidation ('engram formation') and storage.

Short-term and working memory

Short-term, or working memory, as described and defined in the Introduction, recruits prefrontal and (left) parietal structures, as was derived from results obtained from lesion work, evoked potential recordings and functional imaging studies (Belger *et al.* 1998; Goldman-Rakic *et al.* 2000; Jacobsen 1936; Markowitsch *et al.* 1999b). The online held information, which later becomes semantic or episodic memory, is then transferred to limbic system structures.

The bottleneck structures of the limbic system – semantic and episodic memory encoding

Semantic memory and even more so episodic memory require successful long-term storage time-limited representation in structures of the limbic system. While the fact-coding semantic memory system is oriented towards the presence (we only know the fact, but do not remember when we learnt it), the episodic memory system is past-oriented, allows mental time traveling and requires autonoetic consciousness (Tulving and Markowitsch 1998; Tulving 2002). Consequently, it is unlikely that it will exist in animals (Roberts 2002), in spite of various attempts to find episodic-like memory in them (e.g., Clayton and Dickinson 1998).

There is no definite time mark when the limbic system became regarded as essential for memory processing. Landmarks include the old results on Korsakoff's patients (Bonhoeffer 1901; Gamper 1929) and the description of patients with bilateral hippocampal damage and resulting amnesia (Bechterew 1900; Scoville and Milner 1957). Since then, components of the limbic system have been regarded as bottleneck structures through which information has to pass in order to become stored long-term (Brand and Markowitsch 2003). Bilateral damage to these structures lead to a kind of disconnection syndrome, resulting in anterograde amnesia for episodic and semantic information.

The major components of the limbic system can be subdivided into two interacting circuits: the medial (or Papez-) circuit centered around the hippocampus, and the basolateral limbic circuit (amygdaloid circuit). While Papez (1937) considered his proposed circuit (hippocampal formation → fornix → mammillary bodies → mammillothalic tract → anterior thalamus → thalamo-cortical peduncles → cingulate cortex → cingulum → hippocampal formation) as principally engaged in the analysis of emotions, subsequent work showed that it plays a critical role for the transfer of information into long-term memory. The basolateral circuit is more closely related to emotional processing, but is also relevant for encoding the emotional valence of experiences. It includes the amygdala, the mediodorsal nucleus of the thalamus and associated regions, largely situated in the basal forebrain and in its extensions to anterior insular and temporopolar cortical areas plus interconnecting fibers such as the ventral amygdalofugal pathway, the anterior thalamic peduncle and the diagonal band (Figure 10.3).

Though not all structures within the limbic system are of equal importance for memory processing – indeed a number of authors favour the hippocampal formation to the neglect of, for example, diencephalic regions – it can be said that amnesia of at least the severity as found in H.M. (a patient with

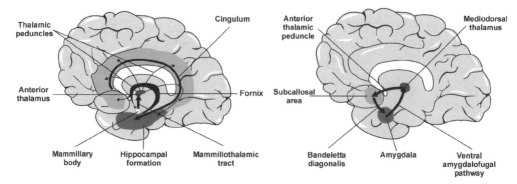

Figure 10.3 The medial (Papez) (left) and the basolateral limbic circuits (right). The Papez circuit is composed of the hippocampal formation, mammillary bodies, anterior thalamus and (conventionally) the cingulate cortex. These regions are interconnected via the (postcommissural) fornix, mammillothalamic tract, thalamo-cortical peduncles and the cingulum. The components of the basolateral limbic circuit are the amygdala, the thalamic mediodorsal nucleus and the subcallosal area (basal forebrain); here interconnections are the ventral amygdalofugal pathway, the inferior thalamic peduncle and the bandeletta diagonalis. The precommissural fornix in addition provides a bidirectional connection between the hippocampal formation and the basal forebrain. It is therefore one of those routes which interconnect both circuits. It is assumed that both circuits are relevant especially for encoding of information associated with the episodic and knowledge memory systems and that the medial circuit is more strongly engaged in the cognitive and the basolateral one in the affective side of information processing.

bilateral medial temporal lobe damage; Corkin 2002), can be found in patients with medial diencephalic damage (Markowitsch 1988; Markowitsch, von Cramon and Schuri 1993). Aside from cortical medial temporal regions, the amygdala has to be mentioned as modulating especially the phase of information consolidation (Paré 2003; McGaugh 2000, 2002). The amygdala is also centrally engaged in the Klüver-Bucy syndrome, characterized by hyperorality, hyperphagia, agnosia, amnesia, hypersexuality, tameness/placidity, and hypermetamorphosis (Klüver and Bucy 1937) and in a genetically based degenerative disease, named Urbach-Wiethe disease, which may lead to major disturbances in emotional memory encoding (Cahill *et al.* 1995; Markowitsch *et al.* 1994). It can be concluded that the amygdala provides the emotional flavour to episodes (Sarter and Markowitsch 1985).

The mammillary nuclei (Dusoir *et al.* 1990), the fornix (Calabrese *et al.* 1995), the retrosplenial cortex (Valenstein *et al.* 1987), the septum (Cramon and Markowitsch 2000; Cramon *et al.* 1993), and the basal forebrain (Damasio *et al.* 1985; Irle *et al.* 1992; Fujii *et al.* 2002) play major roles in memory encoding as well. (The brain damage in patients with 'basal forebrain amnesia' is most frequently caused by rupture of the anterior communicating artery.) More recently, results from functional imaging studies emphasized that prefrontal structures participate in encoding of semantic and episodic information (Kapur *et al.* 1994; Fletcher, Shallice and Dolan 1998).

These networks for information processing have been established on the basis of both patient data and data in normal subjects using functional imaging methods. Finally, recent research demonstrates that in part similar brain regions appear metabolically suppressed in patients with so-called non-organic, that is, psychiatric amnesias. For these, an increased release of stress hormones (which have their major receptors in hippocampal and amygdalar regions) is seen as the basis for what can be termed amnestic block syndrome and what can – in rare cases – result in an inability to acquire new episodic or semantic information long term (Markowitsch *et al.* 1999d).

Further consolidation and storage of information

Consolidation is a little understood, but probably very important phenomenon in the process of acquiring and storing information (McGaugh 2000). There are different views on the beginning and end of the consolidation phase. Sometimes, it is seen as directly succeeding the encoding phase, sometimes it is viewed as a process occurring after information has already been stored long-term. As both encoding and consolidation of episodic and semantic memories engage structures of the limbic system, they can be perceived as closely related.

Sometimes the amygdala is considered to be key structure in the process of memory consolidation (McGaugh 2002), as it is engaged in both emotional and memory processes and as at least episodic aspects of memory are strongly confounded by emotional coding. More generally, most of the limbic structures are engaged in processes of consolidation, especially in that way that every new retrieval of initially stored material re-activates and further associates, synchronises and binds it (Sara 2000).

The representation of the engram is related to that of the actual form or Gestalt of the engram – small, circumscribed or large, diffusely connected neuronal nets, morphological alterations of neurons, the genetic structure of neurons are examples. Genetic and biochemical processes may be common denominators (Kandel 1998). In recent years there is an increasing congruence that most of our memories are represented within widespread cerebral cortical networks. The expanded cortical association areas, with their large number of neurons and neuronal connections, are primary candidates for information representation. Especially for the episodic memory system, these may include and in part extend to structures of the 'expanded limbic system', as defined by Nauta (1979) (Figure 10.4). Evidence for the large cortical engagement in information storage comes primarily from patients with extensive neocortical damage – such as patients with degenerative brain damage: Alzheimer's patients, for example (Markowitsch *et al.* 2000a) – and from patients with anoxic or hypoxic conditions (Markowitsch *et al.* 1997).

There are, however, a few scientists who are of the opinion that most of our memories are represented outside our nervous system. Romijn (1997, 2002) considers a submanifest order of being as the principal storage place of memories. He is of the opinion that the whole universe in its spatial-temporal configuration would be permanently present in the submanifest order of being. Of this, a small portion would continuously materialise and thereby become available for psychic processing. Declarative memory would be found somewhere in the individual area of the submanifest order of being. Similar views are held by Sheldrake (1988) and Hameroff (1998). While the empirical evidence for such hypotheses is scarce, these authors even include assumptions from quantum mechanics and other modern physical theories in their ideas and interpret existing data in a such way that they fit their proposals.

Retrieval of information

While the traditional view of amnesia – in line with the term 'global amnesic syndrome' – assumed the existence of combined anterograde and retrograde amnesia (cf. also Mayes *et al.* 1997), more recently patients with selective retrograde amnesia have appeared in increasing numbers (Markowitsch 1995; Kroll *et al.* 1997). Patients with a progressively decaying cortical network (e.g., Alzheimer's disease or hypoxia) can be seen as the 'classical' ones, having (both anterograde and) retrograde amnesia. Furthermore, patients with transient global amnesia may be seen as classical, as there is both anterograde and retrograde amnesia, though this is limited to less than 24 hours (Markowitsch 1990).

'Non-classical' cases vary in loci and extents of brain damage and may in part reflect the influence of psychogenic (psychiatric) factors, there is a number of patients with in principal uniform brain damage.

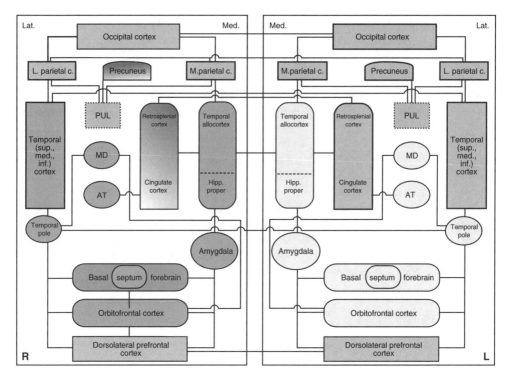

Figure 10.4 Sketch of the two cerebral hemispheres (R = right, L = left hemisphere; med. = medial, lat. = lateral) with some of those structures related to memory processing, in particular to the retrieval of stored information. It is assumed that limbic structures of the right hemisphere are much more strongly engaged in retrieving autobiographical information than those of the left hemisphere and that in principal the right hemisphere is heavily involved in retrieving episodic-autobiographical information while the left one mainly retrieves semantic material.

When the dominant deficit lies in retrograde autobiographical memory, these patients generally show a normal retrieval of knowledge and are able to learn new information long-term on a neutral level. The brain damage then is mainly in the right hemisphere with a focus in the infero-lateral prefrontal cortex and the anterior temporal cortex (excluding, however, the more posteriorly situated regions of the hippocampal formation) (Figure 10.5). Functional imaging studies confirm this view (Fink *et al.* 1996). Vice versa, when the brain damage is mainly left-hemispheric, the knowledge system is impaired while episodic memory is largely normal (Markowitsch *et al.* 1999a).

The frontotemporal cortex can be seen as a trigger region for retrieving that (episodic and semantic) information which is stored in widespread cortical areas. It can be assumed that especially the retrieval of episodic memories requires additional limbic activations (Figure 10.4). In fact, Markowitsch *et al.* (2003) and Piefke *et al.* (2003) found regions of Nauta's (1979) expanded limbic system as active during the retrieval of affect-laden autobiographical episodes. Piefke *et al.* (2003) furthermore found a hippocampal activation during the retrieval of episodes, encoded during the last five years, but not for episodes dating back 20 years.

Retrograde amnesia of the person's own biography always leads to the question of its possible psychogenic origin. As there are case examples of patients with retrograde amnesia who recover spontaneously after some time (Lucchelli *et al.* 1995), while for others there is no change apparent over years, the question of a psychogenic contribution becomes all the more virulent. Its importance

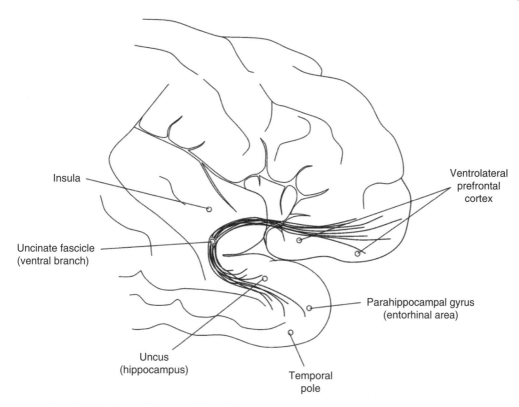

Figure 10.5 Sketch of the right anterior cerebral cortex with relevant structures and fibers engaged in triggering the retrieval of autobiographical episodes.

is further enhanced by the fact that there are numerous patients with various forms of dissociative amnesias (hysterias, psychogenic amnesia, psychogenic fugue, post traumatic stress disorder) (Markowitsch 2000a, 2001, 2002, 2003a, b).

Markowitsch *et al.* (1999d) propagated the existence of a mnestic block syndrome as a consequence of stress and trauma-related events and found corresponding changes in brain metabolism (Markowitsch 1999; Markowitsch *et al.* 1998) as well as an increase in brain metabolism to largely normal levels after cognitive recovery (Markowitsch *et al.* 2000b).

Conclusions

The last decade brought an enormous progress both on the experimental psychological and on the neuroscience side. On the psychological side, the divisions of memory in several systems lay the ground for respective work with patients. An astonishing convergence appeared between the formulations created by psychologists (Tulving 2002) and the findings of selective memory impairments in patients (Markowitsch 2000b) and of selective neural activations in functional imaging (Tulving *et al.* 1994; Cabeza *et al.* 2003).

Learning and memory engage a wide range of brain regions. There is, on the other hand, no equipotentiality in the nervous system for coding information. The principles of convergence and divergence of information transmission hold throughout the nervous system and there are both modality- and material-specific channels for information encoding, storage and even retrieval and there are bits of information which are rich in affect and consciously reflected (and consequently require wide neural nets), while others are processed only subliminally, may never gain conscious representation and may engage restricted nets.

The stages of information processing from encoding to retrieval engage various neural networks which differ in correspondence with the proposed memory systems. Furthermore, there is both for the anterograde (Markowitsch *et al.* 1999c) and the retrograde episodic memory site a principal correspondence between the functional and the organic level (Markowitsch 1996). Information is not represented statically in the brain – factors of attention, mood, the availability of internal associated cues, the hormonal level in the brain (e.g., glucocorticoids; Markowitsch *et al.* 1999d), and many additional factors influence, modify, and rearrange our knowledge. The phenomena of state-dependent learning and retrieval and of false memories are examples for the susceptibility and vulnerability of our memories. The concept of plasticity has gained considerable support and also the concept of life-long learning, proposed by the social sciences, demonstrates that information representation is much less hard-wired and rigid than assumed in the past.

Acknowledgements

Portions of my work included herein were supported by the Deutsche Forschungsgemeinschaft (DFG; Ma 795) and by the StiftungVolkswagenwerk.

11 The assessment of memory for memory rehabilitation

Veronica A. Bradley, Narinder Kapur and Jonathan Evans

Abstract

The assessment of memory as part of the process of memory rehabilitation is discussed in terms of practical considerations and a conceptual framework. The sources of evidence are described with particular reference to formal tests which may be useful in this context, and suggestions are made as to the value of certain tests or other assessment procedures in answering frequently-asked questions in the rehabilitation setting. Future developments in the field are considered.

Introduction: overview of memory assessment in clinical settings

Memory assessment in context

Memory difficulties are among the most commonly-reported and disruptive sequelae of acquired brain injury, and it is unlikely that any neuropsychological assessment for the purposes of rehabilitation would fail to include some assessment of memory. Since many rehabilitation techniques require the patient to learn to use compensatory strategies, it is important to identify strengths and weaknesses in memory, even if there is no complaint of memory disorder. In many cases, however, memory is the main focus of the assessment.

Memory assessment should ideally be carried out as close in time as is possible to the start of the rehabilitation programme, and should be planned, carried out and interpreted in the context of a wider assessment of the individual patient. Memory performance will be affected by other cognitive, emotional and behavioural functions, and will, in turn, affect performance on measures of these functions. Wilson (2002) argues persuasively for a broad theoretical base underpinning a holistic approach to cognitive rehabilitation. Assessment is an integral part of the rehabilitation process, and the need for a holistic approach is as important in assessment as it is in other parts of the process.

When feeding back results of the memory assessment to patients and their relatives, it is important that the results are communicated in a way that is meaningful. It is usually helpful:

- to use non-technical language
- to describe behaviours and abilities rather than tests and test scores, although descriptions of formal tasks can provide useful examples of the way in which memory can break down, and
- to highlight strengths as well as weaknesses.

Conceptual frameworks

The neuropsychologist requires conceptual frameworks when considering the selection of tests and other assessment procedures and interpreting memory performance. In the broadest sense, Wilson's (2002) provisional model of cognitive rehabilitation provides an important reminder of the relevance of models from other areas of psychology. However, more detailed models of cognitive functions are also needed. One such framework, based on the work of Tulving (e.g. Tulving 2002) and Markowitsch (e.g. Markowitsch 1998) is presented by Markowitsch in this volume (Chapter 10). In the interests of consistency, we have adopted this framework, which includes the following memory systems:

- *Episodic memory* – this generally refers to the encoding, storage and utilisation of personally-experienced events that can be related to specific spatial and temporal contexts.
- *Semantic memory* – this refers to an organized body of knowledge about words, concepts and culturally and educationally-acquired facts. It includes general knowledge, and covers a wide range of materials and modalities.
- *Working (short-term or attentional) memory* – this refers to a set of processes for holding and manipulating material in temporary store, over a period of seconds.

The above memory systems are routinely tested during neuropsychological assessment. The following memory systems are largely independent of conscious reflection. They are not routinely tested in the clinical assessment of memory but are nevertheless important in understanding the complexity of human memory and its breakdown.

- *Perceptual (perceptual identification) memory* – this refers to familiarity with a stimulus leading to its recognition at a later time. Impairment in this area may be demonstrated in assessing for agnosic disorders.
- *Procedural memory* – this is the ability to acquire new skills or to utilise previously-acquired skills, for example, the use of grammatical rules, or action skills such as riding a bicycle. Though not readily measured by standard psychometric tests, procedural memory is important in rehabilitation in that many densely amnesic patients are capable of procedural learning.
- *Priming* – information encoded implicitly influences performance on subsequent tasks. Experimental tasks such as stem completion demonstrate the priming process.

Also to be taken into account is:

- Emotional-motivational memory – this is not usually assessed directly but may be important in assessment and rehabilitation planning, since the amygdala, which is important in emotional learning, also has a modulatory influence on the strength of other forms of memory.

Additionally, the process of remembering can be broken down into stages, these being *encoding* or *registration, storage and consolidation,* and *retrieval.* Figure 11.1 shows factors that are important for lasting memory consolidation. These include stimulus and presentational characteristics as well as emotional and motivational factors.

Although anatomical localisation of deficits is not usually of primary importance in the rehabilitation setting, it may be important to link measurable deficits of memory with what is known about the likely anatomical or physiological effects of the patient's illness or injury. The brain areas associated with memory dysfunction are:

- medial temporal lobes
- the diencephalon and basal forebrain

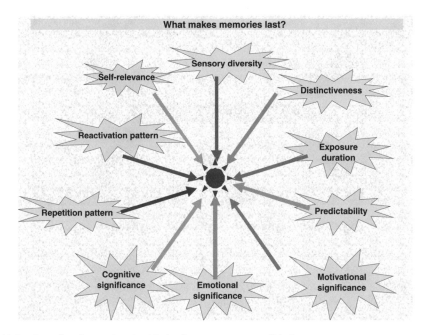

Figure 11.1 Encoding factors involved in lasting memory consolidation.

- frontal lobe neocortex
- temporal lobe neocortex.

Other areas of the brain subserve memory in its broadest sense. For further elaboration of the framework described in this section and the anatomical substrates of the systems and processes involved, see Chapter 10, this volume. For an alternative framework, Squire (1998) presents a taxonomy of long-term memory systems, together with the brain structures critical for each system.

Sources of evidence

Evidence is collected from a range of sources which are described below in some detail. Figure 11.2 summarises the different sources which contribute to a full assessment of memory.

The clinical interview

It is usually helpful to have a relative, friend or carer present at the interview, particularly when the patient's memory is moderately or severely impaired, as they may find it hard to recollect and recount examples of memory failure. We recommend starting the interview in a fairly unstructured way by asking the patient or family member to describe problem areas as they see them. This way, information is provided not just about the problems experienced, but also about which problems are perceived as most serious and disruptive. Note whether or not there is agreement between the patient and family member about the severity of a given problem. Once a spontaneous account has been given, the interviewer may wish to probe for frequently-occurring problems. It is also helpful to ask about aspects of memory which are felt not to have been affected, and to find out whether the patient's memory was considered to be good or bad premorbidly. The impact of reported memory problems on the patient's everyday life, and the demands made on their memory during their current

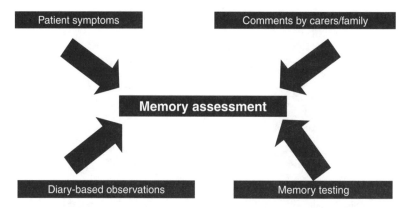

Figure 11.2 Contributions to memory assessment in memory rehabilitation.

routine should be clarified. If they have not returned to work, but hope to do so, how much does efficient performance at work depend on a good memory? Are employers sympathetic, and how much scope is there for using memory aids at work? To what extent have memory problems necessitated a change in the daily routine of the patient and their family? In some cases there may be questions about the relative contributions of organic and psychogenic factors. The neuropsychologist should look for signs of anxiety or depression which could be exacerbating the situation, and should be aware of the possibility of secondary gain which could lead to exaggerated accounts of symptoms as well as underperformance on formal tests.

Behavioural data: questionnaires and rating scales in the acute stages of recovery from brain injury

Assessment of patients during late coma or posttraumatic amnesia requires different instruments from those developed for post-acute use.

- The Galveston Orientation and Amnesia Test (GOAT) (Levin *et al.* 1979) is designed to assess post-traumatic amnesia (PTA) in the early stages of recovery following traumatic brain injury. It assesses orientation for time, place and person, and asks the patient to describe the last event they remember prior to the injury and the first event remembered post-injury. The test is usually administered repeatedly to monitor the patient's emergence from PTA.
- The Westmead Post-Traumatic Amnesia Scale (Shores *et al.* 1986) is another instrument devised for the measurement of post-traumatic amnesia. It omits some of the orientation questions included in the GOAT and does not include questions about the patient's last memory prior to injury and first memory subsequent to it. It does, however, include a recognition component that can be used if the patient cannot respond by recalling information. There is also a learning component; patients are tested on whether they remember pictures of objects from one session to the next. Like the GOAT, this test is usually administered repeatedly to monitor emergence from PTA.

Behavioural data: diaries, questionnaires and rating scales in the post-acute stages of recovery from brain injury

Diaries can be kept in a more or less formal way. The patient or family member may simply be asked to jot down in a standard diary, the memory failures of which they become aware. Alternatively, more detailed charts may be issued for completion so that the context of the memory failure, including whether or not there has been an attempt to use a memory aid, can be recorded.

In the case of questionnaires and rating scales, a thorough clinical interview may render their use unnecessary. However, some clinicians may prefer these more structured ways of collecting information, which can be particularly useful for ensuring the collection of standard data sets when admitting a patient to a rehabilitation unit in which different clinicians may carry out the initial interviews. Many such instruments are available (see Lezak 1995, for a review of most of these); some examples follow:

- The *Neurobehavioural Functioning Inventory*, devised by Kreutzer *et al.* (1999) includes a Memory/Attention Scale. There are two versions of the form, one for the patient and one for the family to complete. Responses to the items that make up the various scales are summed, and can be converted into standardised scores.
- The *Cognitive Symptoms Checklists*, developed by O'Hara *et al.* (1993) includes a memory checklist. Questions probe difficulties of various types, for example, those relating to safety or to money management. These checklists do not yield standardised scores, but are designed to form the basis of an in-depth interview in which rehabilitation goals will be agreed.
- The *Contextual Memory Test* (Toglia 1993) commences with a brief questionnaire designed to establish the patient's awareness of memory capacity. The patient is also asked to estimate how well s/he has performed after completing a test, and to describe strategies used. The questionnaire responses and estimates of success are examined in conjunction with performance measures on the recall tests in order to obtain an indication of the extent to which the patient's view of their memory is realistic.

Psychometric tests of memory: new learning and recall

Memory testing usually encompasses a range of task stimuli (e.g. verbal, figural, pictorial) a range of sensory and response modalities (e.g. auditory, visual) and a range of modes of response (e.g. recall, cued recall, recognition). Some tests will focus on retrograde (i.e. pre-illness) memory loss, while others will probe new learning and retention of material over delays of different lengths.

There are a number of factors to be taken into account when selecting appropriate tests. Many of these, such as construct validity, face validity and reliability, apply to selection of tests for use in a range of settings (see Kline 1993, for descriptions of test standardisation; Mayes and Warburg 1992, and Hickox and Sunderland 1992 for review of memory tests), and will not be discussed here. The neuropsychologist should always take into account the level of difficulty of tests in order to avoid floor and ceiling effects. In the rehabilitation setting, serial assessment will often be required and the existence of parallel forms is a bonus.

One further issue, which is particularly relevant to the use of formal tests in the rehabilitation setting, is that of ecological validity. Some tests have been developed with ecological validity in mind. However, traditional tests can be used flexibly in order to gain practically-applicable information, although test reliability and validity will be compromised when tests are used in this way and it is important that the neuropsychologist record in the patient's notes any departure from the standard testing protocol.

Lezak (1995) notes that there is a distinction to be made between *efficiency* (performance under non-optimal conditions) and *capacity* (performance under the optimal conditions usually required for standard administration of formal tests), and that this distinction is important for rehabilitation and vocational planning. It is helpful when planning rehabilitation to have an idea of the patient's efficiency as well as their capacity, and some of Lezak's suggestions in relation to establishing the latter can be reversed in order to establish the former. Thus, rather than testing in what Lezak terms a 'sterile' environment, the neuropsychologist may, for example, permit background noise during the assessment (by testing with the door open, or by arranging for a radio or tape to be playing in the background) or ask the patient to continue with the assessment even when they are fatiguing.

This kind of adjustment aimed at measuring the patient's mental efficiency may, to a certain extent, help to recreate 'real-life' situations, especially those which prevail in the workplace. Other modifications may give a more accurate indication of the patient's capacity. Sbordone (1996) suggests, inter alia:

- Simplification of test instructions.
- Repetition and clarification of test instructions.
- Practice and rehearsal.
- Rest breaks.
- Breaking up testing over several sessions.
- Use of external incentives and rewards.

Some of the tests which are commonly used or particularly appropriate for use in rehabilitation settings, and which are readily available to the clinician are described below. Table 1.1 summarises the main use of each test in terms of the aspect of memory measured, the method of testing and any special applications. This is by no means an exhaustive list and clinicians may prefer alternatives which will achieve similar ends.

The Wechsler Memory Scales

These are probably the best-known and most widely used batteries of memory tests. They have expanded in scope since the original scale was published in 1945. Revisions in 1987 and 1997/98 were welcome in bringing the tests up to date. The most recent revision, the WMS-III (Wechsler 1998a) is described here. The battery contains six primary subtests, used in calculating 'Index Scores' which are directly comparable with WAIS-III (Wechsler 1998b) IQ scores.

Two of these are tests of working memory (verbal and spatial). The WMS-III letter-number sequencing task is identical to the task of the same name in the WAIS-III; the WAIS-III also contains a digit span task. The 'Logical memory' test comprises two short stories which are read to the patient. Free recall is required immediately after presentation, after a re-reading of the second story and after a half-hour delay. In discussing the limitations of formal memory tests in the rehabilitation setting, Haut *et al.* (1992), specifically identified the absence of recognition measures as a weakness in the WMS-R. In the WMS-III, it is possible to examine recognition memory for the story. The other primary test of verbal memory is a paired associate learning task, again with recognition trial. In view of occasional ceiling effects with this subtest, an extended version with norms has been developed (Uttl *et al.* 2002). On the nonverbal side, a series of 24 photographs of faces is presented. Memory for these faces is tested through recognition; the patient is asked to pick out the target photographs from a set which includes distractors. In the 'Family pictures' subtest a family photograph and a series of scenes are presented. The patient is asked to recall who was in each scene, what they were doing, and their location in the picture. This new addition to the battery was designed as a visual analogue to the 'Logical memory' test, but it is not clear that it is entirely a test of visual memory as a certain amount of verbal encoding could improve performance. All of these tests include immediate and delayed recall components. Other optional subtests include a test of orientation, a word list learning task with a recognition trial and a non-verbal test of memory for designs. The battery is psychometrically quite complex, and a number of composite scores can be calculated in addition to the Index scores. Administration of the entire battery to neurologically-impaired patients is usually too demanding, but one advantage which this latest revision has over earlier versions is that norms for individual tests are available so that the clinician can select appropriate tests from the battery when time-constraints or lack of stamina on the patient's part preclude administration of the entire battery. One disadvantage of the current revision is the absence of a parallel form.

Table 11.1 Psychometric tests of memory

Test	Aspect of memory measured				Testing method			Special application				
	Episodic	Semantic	Working	Procedural	Recognition	Recall	Learning	Post-traumatic amnesia	Autobio-graphical memory	Prospective memory	Cognitive effort	Effect of context on memory
GOAT								●				
Westmead PTA Scale					●			●				
WAIS III Digit Span			●									
WAIS III Information		●				●						
WAIS III Vocabulary		●				●						
WAIS III/WMS III Letter-Number Sequencing			●			●						
WMS III Spatial Span			●			●						
WMS III Logical Memory	●				●	●						
WMS III Paired Associate Learning	●				●	●	●					
WMS III Family Pictures	●					●						
WMS III Faces	●				●							
AMIPB Design Learning	●					●	●					
AMIPB Figure Recall	●					●						

Continued

Table 11.1 Psychometric tests of memory—cont'd

Test	Aspect of memory measured				Testing method			Special application				
	Episodic	Semantic	Working	Procedural	Recognition	Recall	Learning	Post-traumatic amnesia	Autobio-graphical memory	Prospective memory	Cognitive effort	Effect of context on memory
AMIPB List Learning	•					•	•					
AMIPB Story Recall	•					•						
RBMT II/RBMT-E Appointment										•		
RBMT II/RBMT-E Belonging										•		
RBMT II/RBMT-E Faces	•				•							
RBMT II/RBMT-E Message	•									•		
RBMT II/RBMT-E Name	•					•						
RBMT II/RBMT-E Pictures	•				•							
RBMT II/RBMT-E Route	•					•						
RBMT II/RBMT-E Story	•					•						
Doors and People-Doors	•				•							
Doors and People-People	•					•						

Continued

Doors and People-Names

Doors and People-Shapes

Warrington RMT Faces

Warrington RMT Words

Camden Face Recognition

Camden Paired Associate Learning

Camden Pictorial Recognition

Camden Topographical Recognition

Camden Word Recognition

Rey Auditory Verbal Learning Test

California Verbal Learning Test

Hopkins Verbal Learning Test

Buschke Selective Reminding Test

Rey-Osterrieth Complex Figure

Table 11.1 Psychometric tests of memory—cont'd

Test	Aspect of memory measured				Testing method			Special application				
	Episodic	Semantic	Working	Procedural	Recognition	Recall	Learning	Post-traumatic amnesia	Autobiographical memory	Prospective memory	Cognitive effort	Effect of context on memory
Contextual Memory Test	•				•							•
Autobiographical Memory Interview	•	•				•			•			
Pyramids and Palm Trees		•			•							
Rey's Memorization of 15 items	•					•					•	
Tests of Neuropsychological Malingering			•		•						•	
Word Memory Test	•				•	•					•	
Test of Memory Malingering	•				•		•				•	

The Adult Memory and Information Processing Battery (AMIPB)

This battery (Coughlan and Hollows 1985) is an easy-to-administer set of four memory tests and two information processing tests, with two parallel forms.

Memory tests comprise story recall, word-list learning, figure recall and design learning. The design learning task is felt to be a particularly good measure of nonverbal memory since it is very difficult to encode any part of the design verbally. Both learning tests include a delayed recall trial following interference. The tests can be administered individually and norms are provided for each individual test. There is no overall memory quotient or composite score but this is not usually a disadvantage in the clinical neuropsychological setting, where the focus tends to be on relative strengths and weaknesses.

The Rivermead Behavioural Memory Test II (RBMT II)

The original Rivermead Behavioural Memory Test (Wilson *et al.* 1985) was devised specifically to meet the objection that many memory tests used in the clinical setting are adapted from laboratory-based tests and lack ecological validity. The authors updated the materials for publication of the revised version in 2003 (Wilson *et al.* 2003). The RBMT II contains a story recall test and picture and face recognition tests. (The faces in the latter test now reflect the multiracial nature of our society.) It also contains a number of subtests which are rather different from those contained in most other batteries, and which are felt to be closer to the everyday situations in which a patient might experience memory difficulties. In particular, a number of tests of prospective memory are included. The battery has the advantage of four parallel versions to allow for repeated assessments. It yields two scores, a screening score, based on a pass/fail grading of each item, and a more detailed profile score. The tests can be used with patients who have severe memory impairment, but are subject to ceiling effects if used to detect mild memory impairment. The authors have developed an extended version of the test, described below, to increase sensitivity to subtle deficit.

The Rivermead Behavioural Memory Test- Extended Version (RBMT-E)

This provides longer, and therefore more demanding, subtests. This has been achieved by combining parallel forms (Wilson *et al.* 1999). This version of the test, therefore, has two rather than four parallel forms. The authors have modified the test to avoid ceiling effects; this battery is less appropriate than the standard RBMT for patients with severe memory impairment.

Doors and People

This battery (Baddeley *et al.* 1994) was designed principally to provide an improved measure of visual episodic memory which would be acceptable to a wide range of subjects. It includes verbal recall and recognition tasks as well as non-verbal recall and recognition tests. Tests are relatively short and the battery is easy to administer. Norms are available for individual test scores and an overall score. Scaled scores are also provided for non-verbal–verbal and recall-recognition discrepancies.

The Recognition Memory Test (RMT)

The RMT (Warrington 1984) contains two subtests. The verbal test uses visually-presented words and the non-verbal test uses faces. Both are forced-choice recognition tests. A discrepancy score can be calculated to assist the evaluation of differences between scores on the tests. Each test contains

50 items, so they are less suitable than some of the shorter tests for patients who have very severe memory impairment or difficulty maintaining attention. However, there is also the possibility of a ceiling effect when the verbal test is used with very mildly-impaired patients. Forced choice recognition memory tests can be used to detect poor effort or malingering; of particular note in this context are scores which are below chance.

The Camden Memory Tests

This set (Warrington 1996) contains five tests, two verbal and three non-verbal, which are intended to be presented individually and not as a battery. They are all presented visually. Four are forced-choice recognition tests and do not require a spoken response. The fifth is a paired-associate learning test which requires a single word spoken response. These tests are shorter than the subtests of the Recognition Memory Test and include word and face recognition tests with similar formats. The least demanding is the 'Pictorial Recognition Memory Test', which is subject to ceiling effects when used with patients with mild or even moderate problems, but is extremely useful for patients who have severe memory impairments or limited stamina in the early days following neurological insult. As with the RMT above it may be helpful in detecting memory loss due to malingering.

The Rey Auditory Verbal Learning Test (RAVLT)

The RAVLT (Rey 1964) requires recall of an auditorily-presented 15-word list over five learning trials. Delayed recall is tested following an interference trial, and a recognition test is provided. A number of parallel forms have been developed since the initial publication of the test. A selection of these can be found in Lezak (1995). The test is not available from a commercial source; the clinician is free to design his/her own scoresheets for ease of administration. Normative data are provided by Spreen and Strauss (1998) and discussed by Lezak (1995).

The California Verbal Learning Test (CVLT)

Another word-list learning task (Delis *et al.* 1987, 2001), which differs from the RAVLT and AMIPB list learning tasks in that stimuli are semantically-related. In each list, items have been selected from a limited number of semantic categories and there are cued recall trials which request items within a given category. In the first version of the test, items which could make up shopping lists were used, with the aim of increasing the test's ecological validity: this aspect of the test has been abandoned in the second edition, in order to improve ease of understanding. Short and long-delay recall is required and there is a long-delay recognition trial. Norms are provided for a range of measures, such as vulnerability to interference and learning strategy. These measures can take time to calculate manually: however, computer-assisted scoring is an option. The first edition of the test did not have an alternative form, but one was developed and published by Delis *et al.* (1991). The second edition has two parallel forms, and this edition also includes a short form which roughly halves administration time.

The Hopkins Verbal Learning Test

A list-learning task (Brandt 1991), with a recognition trial, in which stimuli are semantically-related. It has the advantage of six parallel forms. The revised version (Benedict *et al.* 1998) includes a delayed recall trial: the recognition trial is therefore also delayed. The validity of the revised test has been investigated in relation to its discriminatory power in the diagnosis of dementia (Shapiro *et al.* 1999).

In the rehabilitation setting the test is more likely to be used in monitoring change over time than as a diagnostic tool.

The Buschke Selective Reminding Test (BSRT)

The BSRT (Buschke 1973; Buschke and Fuld 1974) also requires the patient to learn word lists, but the procedure differs from many other list learning tasks in that only words not recalled in a preceding trial are re-presented in the subsequent trial. There are a number of different versions of the test (see Spreen and Strauss 1998, for discussion). Parallel forms exist, but equal difficulty and reliability have not always been demonstrated for the adult versions.

The Rey-Osterreith Complex Figure (RCFT)

A test of immediate and delayed recall of a complex figure, this was devised by Rey in 1941 and standardised by Osterreith in 1944 (papers translated by Corwin and Bylsma 1993). Taylor (1979) contributed a parallel form and scoring criteria. Until 1995 the test was not available from a commercial source. Information detailed enough to permit the clinician to design their own stimuli and scoresheets are provided by Lezak (1995) and Spreen and Strauss (1998). A version is now commercially available (Meyers and Meyers 1995). This version includes a recognition trial.

The Memory Questionnaire included in the Contextual Memory Test

This was described earlier. The memory test itself (Toglia 1993) consists of two equivalent picture cards, each of which contain 20 line drawings around the theme of an everyday activity. The first card is presented for 90 seconds without explicit reference to the context (i.e. the unifying theme of the pictures). The patient is simply asked to memorise the line drawings and to recall them immediately after presentation and after an interval of 15 to 20 minutes. Raw scores are converted to standardised scores and compared with the control group appropriate for the patient's age. If the score is outside the normal range, or if poor strategy use (i.e. failure to recognise and make use of the theme of the pictures) is evident, then the second picture card is presented. On this occasion, the patient's attention is drawn to the theme at the time of presentation and during recall, when it forms the basis of cuing by the examiner. Optional cued recall and recognition trials are provided.

This test is designed for use in the rehabilitation rather than the diagnostic setting. It is intended to supplement other standard tests of memory by providing information about the extent to which the provision of contextual information can improve memory functioning and to assess the patient's awareness of their memory deficits.

Psychometric tests: Autobiographical memory

The Autobiographical Memory Interview (AMI)

As its title suggests, this takes the form of a structured interview (Kopelman *et al.* 1990). It encompasses two components. The first is what the authors call 'personal semantic' memory. It assesses patients' recall of facts about their earlier life. The second component relates to memory for 'autobiographical incidents', i.e. personally-experienced events. The interview probes the patients' recall of specific events in childhood and early adulthood, as well as memory for more recent personal events. A potential problem for a test of this type is the absence of any way of checking the accuracy of the patient's recall; even if a relative or carer is present they may not recall or be aware of certain incidents and events. As part of their validation procedure the authors checked the accuracy of recall with relatives of patients in their validation sample. They concluded that the tendency was for patients' responses to be accurate on about 90 per cent of occasions. Responses which are not obviously confabulatory (confabulatory responses[1] may be bizarre and illogical or may not be consistent with other information which the patient has given) are therefore scored as correct and, in theory therefore, the instrument can be used with patients who are not accompanied by a relative or carer. However, the question of reliability of answers needs to be kept in mind, as well as the possibility that autobiographical memory loss is present but is not tapped by the particular episodic memory items in the test.

An alternative procedure which can be used in assessing retrograde amnesia is described later in this chapter, p. 131.

Psychometric tests: Semantic memory

The Autobiographical Memory Interview (AMI)

This may, as described above, be useful in demonstrating deficits in personal semantic memory (Kopelman *et al.* 1990).

Pyramids and Palm Trees

Designed by Howard and Patterson (1992) this is a useful test of a patient's ability to access detailed semantic representations from words and pictures. It is a matching test which does not require a spoken response. The authors provide normative data from control groups, and a cut-off score. Although the test has been used extensively with clinical populations, norms from these populations are not included in the manual, since it is the pattern of performance, rather than the subject's absolute score, which is felt to be important in understanding semantic impairment.

The 'Information' and 'Vocabulary' subtests from the WAIS III (Wechsler 1998b) may also be helpful in this connection. The former gives an indication of the extent to which knowledge acquired premorbidly has been retained, while the latter may reveal a loss of knowledge of word meanings.

See p. 131 for further suggestions on the assessment of semantic memory.

Psychometric tests: Cognitive effort and malingering

Rey's Memorization of 15 Items

In this test (Rey 1964; full details in Lezak 1995), the need to remember 15 different items is stressed. In fact, the test consists of 5 sets of three items, which greatly reduces the memory load. There is some evidence that it possesses good specifiicity but lacks sensitivity, and is best used to detect blatant malingering strategies (Millis and Kler 1995). Kapur (unpublished) uses an adaptation of this test which contains only 12 items – forward and backward sequences of three letters and three numbers.

The Tests of Neuropsychological Malingering

Computerised forced-choice tests of three different types (Pritchard 1998). The 'memory' test is, in fact, a test of working memory, but it appears to the naive subject to be a memory test. A five-digit

---

[1]Confabulation can be elicited and documented by a structured interview procedure, e.g. Mercer *et al.* 1977) or by asking for recall of episodes in response to word cues, (Moscovitch & Melo1997).

number is presented for two seconds; the task is then to pick out the number from two five-digit numbers presented subsequently.

The Word Memory Test

Requires immediate and delayed recognition, followed by paired-associate and free recall of words initially presented in pairs (Green and Astner 1995; Green *et al.* 1996). The consistency of responses across trials and the response to different levels of difficulty are taken into account, and separate ability and validity measures can be obtained. Oral and computer-administered versions of the test are available.

The Test of Memory Malingering

Assesses two-choice recognition memory for a series of fifty pictures, with performance assessed over two learning trials and an optional retention trial (Tombaugh 1996, 1997).

Memory assessment in practice: rationale and selection of tests and assessment procedures

Most clinical investigations, including assessment of memory functioning in rehabilitation settings, are directly or indirectly intended to address issues relating to (a) diagnosis, severity and types of memory damage involved; (b) prognosis; and (c) possibilities for rehabilitation and monitoring change. One or more of the following questions will require an answer:

* What is going on?
* What is going to happen?
* What will help?
* Has memory changed?

In the following sections we will look at these questions in more detail and suggest tests and other assessment measures which may be useful in addressing them. The reader is referred to pp. 120–129 for test authors and additional detail for the tests shown below in bold print.

What's going on? Diagnosis and formulation

This question encompasses a number of subsidiary questions:

Is there memory dysfunction?

Everyday memory difficulties will usually be evident to the patient and to relatives or carers, and will be described in the clinical interview. Absence of reported memory symptoms in the presence of memory test deficits may be related to a number of factors, such as absence of demands on memory in everyday settings. It may, on occasion, reflect the presence of frontal lobe dysfunction. If there is a general complaint of memory impairment, but specific examples of memory failure are not volunteered, it may be helpful to ask the patient or relative to keep a diary record of memory failures. Questionnaires or rating scales, for example the Neurobehavioral Functioning Inventory may be helpful here. Presence of memory symptoms in the absence of memory test deficits may reflect the sensitivity of the tests used, or the presence of other factors such as heightened awareness of memory functioning due to anxiety. Behavioural observations may be made in situations in which the patient is given specific tasks to carry out as part of the assessment process.

Formal tests which are most sensitive to the presence of memory impairment in general are those requiring free recall (and in particular delayed free recall), such as the story recall tasks from the AMIPB or the WMS III, and the figure recall task or the visual reproduction subtest from the AMIPB and WMS-III respectively. Paired-associate learning tasks, such as that included in the WMS-III or the extended version of this task (Uttl *et al.* 2002) may also prove useful in addressing this question.

How severe is the memory dysfunction?

The Neurobehavioral Functioning Inventory yields scaled scores which can be compared to those of other patients of a similar age. However, as the authors explain there can be a number of reasons for high impairment scores. Severe impairment of memory is one of them, but high scores can also be explained by psychological distress or an attempt to exaggerate symptomatology. Conversely, minimal impairment scores do not necessarily imply mild memory deficit but may be associated with lack of awareness or denial.

It can be difficult for patients and their relatives to report the severity of memory deficits. What can be achieved day-to-day depends so much on the way in which memory problems are managed, and on subjective impressions which may be coloured by low mood or limited insight. Neuropsychometric tests are, however, well-suited to establishing severity of impairment. Scaled scores or centiles permit comparison with the patient's age-matched peers and with his/her premorbid level of functioning (note that the new Wechsler Test of Adult Reading, Psychological Corporation 2001, predicts WMS-III Index Scores as well as WAIS-III IQs). The WMS-III General Memory Index may be useful in grading patients with the global amnesic syndrome, but individual subtest scores or indices, which provide more detailed information about current strengths and weaknesses, are often more useful in rehabilitation settings.

The WMS-III and AMIPB have high ceilings and are appropriate for use with a range of patients, including those with subtle memory impairment. They tend to be less valuable if they are used with patients who have very severe impairments of memory. For these patients, use of tests such as the Rivermead Behavioural Memory Test II, Doors and People or the Camden Memory Tests will avoid floor effects.

Which memory domains and systems are affected?

Information relating to material-specific and system-specific systems may be obtained by specific questioning and observations. Verbal memory symptoms may be evident in memory lapses for phone messages, the content of a conversation, or what has been read. Non-verbal memory symptoms can be elicited by asking about memory for faces, including whether these are recognised as familiar, memory for direction and memory for location.

Problems with long-term episodic memory may be elicited by questions about specific events, such as holidays. Working memory difficulties may underlie complaints of being unable to keep track of conversation. Semantic memory impairment may give rise to word-finding difficulty, or failures of comprehension. Loss of motor knowledge may be probed by asking about dressing and other established perceptual-motor skills.

In the case of formal tests, verbal memory deficits may be elicited by tests that include memory for stories and word lists. Tests of this type are included in the WMS-III, the AMIPB and the Rivermead Tests.

The Camden Tests and the Recognition Memory Test contain verbal recognition tests; the Camden and the WMS-III contain verbal paired-associate learning tests.

Nonverbal memory impairment can be elicited by the AMIPB test of figure recall, the 'Faces Recognition' and 'Visual Reproduction' subtests of the WMS-III, and the visual recognition subtests of the Camden and Recognition Memory Tests listed above. Long-term episodic memory, when retrograde loss is suspected, can be assessed using the Autobiographical Memory Interview. The 'Crovitz' procedure (Crovitz and Schiffman 1974; see MacKinnon and Squire 1989, for an example of the use of the technique with amnesic patients) in which memories of autobiographical incidents are retrieved in response to specific cue words, is often used in experimental settings, but the clinician needs to gather their own set of normative data.

Semantic memory impairment may be examined using Pyramids and Palm Trees - a test of semantic access. The 'Vocabulary' subtest of the WAIS III demonstrates explicit knowledge of word meanings. General knowledge is readily assessable using the 'Information' subtest of the same battery. It is advisable to have details of the patient's educational history when interpreting test results: these tests are education-related. Verbal semantic breakdown may also show up on naming tests (most research supports the view that, if a patient no longer has a store of semantic information about a visually-presented object, they will be unable to name it). Performance on a range of non-memory tests which require previously-learned knowledge and skills, including gesture and comprehension of social situations, may be compromised in some cases of semantic breakdown.

Digit span tests provide a measure of auditory working memory, or immediate attention span, while the block-tapping subtest of the WMS-III assesses some aspects of non-verbal working memory. Implicit memory may be demonstrated by stem completion or by constructing tests that involve repeated identification of fragmented figures over successive trials. Examples of this type of test are described by Wiggins and Brandt (1988), who found similar tests to be useful in the detection of simulated memory impairment.

What is the aetiology of the memory dysfunction?

It is frequently the case that the underlying disease process or nature of the injury to the brain is established by the time the patient is assessed for rehabilitation. However, there may be a need to delineate the relative contributions of psychological and neurological factors. Questions probing the nature of the patient's difficulties will be asked in the clinical interview. A psychogenic contribution to memory problems should be considered when the following are reported:

- loss of personal identity and personal semantic memories
- disproportionate and dense autobiographical experiential amnesia
- inability to recognize family members
- memory symptoms related to absent-mindedness
- concentration perceived to be more impaired than memory
- significant variability in memory difficulties
- the patient complains of major memory impairment, yet enjoys reading and can retain what is read or enjoys and can readily follow films
- the patient has severe loss of memory for skills/habits in the absence of evidence of major pathology.

When formal testing is carried out, the neuropsychologist will look for inconsistency between the patient's day-to-day functioning and performance on memory tests; the latter may show profound impairment, yet the patient is able to answer questions about certain recent events, or to cope independently at home.

In general, recognition memory tests invoke less anxiety than recall tests, and this factor may be assessed by taking advantage of this observation. A number of tests of symptom validity are reviewed by Lezak (1995) and Spreen and Strauss (1998). These tests involve tasks which are presented as demanding, but are in fact quite easy for the patient who is not severely impaired to carry out. Recent standardised tests include the Word Memory Test, the Test of Memory Malingering and the Test of Neuropsychological Malingering. Performance on forced-choice recognition tests, such as the RMT or Camden tests described above, can be revealing in that the malingerer may score well below chance. Similarly, the forward digit span, a test of short-term memory, may be unexpectedly short. Rey's Memorization of 15 Items is quick and easy to administer and has been widely used but, as mentioned earlier, there is evidence to suggest that this test lacks sensitivity (Millis and Kler 1995).

A number of experimental techniques may also be worth considering, for example the 'coin in the hand' test in which the patient simply selects, on a large number of trials, the hand in which they have seen a coin grasped (Kapur 1994).

What are the cognitive mechanisms underlying memory dysfunction?

The role of encoding, storage and retrieval factors may be difficult to gauge from a clinical interview or behavioural observations. Some reported memory symptoms, such as forgetting what one has come into a room to collect, are suggestive of attentional loss rather than impairment of memory per se. Repeatedly confusing names of family members or confusing the day of the week with the month may reflect mild dysphasic difficulties.

Using formal tests, patterns of performance can be invaluable in establishing underlying cognitive mechanisms. In general, poor performance on immediate recall with good retention over a delay suggests problems at the encoding stage, while the reverse pattern may indicate a storage deficit. When retrieval mechanisms are compromised, this may be evident in a marked contrast between performance on recall and recognition memory tests. Recognition memory tests are usually less demanding for the general population, but this is reflected in the norms of standardised tests. Some learning tasks, such as the list learning, story recall and verbal paired associate tasks of the WAIS-III and the California Verbal Learning Test provide scaled scores for the learning slope so that learning efficiency can be gauged. The California Verbal Learning Test provides a range of measures of different learning characteristics (such as primacy and recency effects, semantic clustering) and contrast measures which help to distinguish storage from retrieval deficits. The Buschke Selective Reminding Test purports to provide measures of different memory processes, although there is some evidence that the numerous scores which can be derived are highly intercorrelated and may be assessing similar constructs (see Spreen and Strauss 1998, for discussion). Nevertheless, this is an accessible, and a popular test, particularly in the United States. The Meyers and Meyers (1995) version of the Rey Complex Figure Test yields different profiles which may help to distinguish disrupted encoding, storage or retrieval processes.

What's going to happen? Prognosis and prediction

What is the likely level of recovery of memory at a later time?

Many of the questions that patients and their relatives or carers will wish to ask the neuropsychologist relate to the extent to which cognitive impairments may be expected to recover and within what timescale. The severity of post-traumatic amnesia, assessed either retrospectively or concurrently, is a measure which is frequently used in making judgments about long-term prognosis. It is an imperfect measure, especially when made retrospectively, as it may in many cases be confounded by post-injury events such as sedation, pain control and the after-effects of surgery.

Concurrent measures of post-traumatic amnesia are the Galveston Orientation and Amnesia Test and the Westmead Post-Traumatic Amnesia Scale. The 'Information and Orientation' subtest of the WMS-III is shorter, and therefore easier to administer in the early stages, but has been developed for use in a range of conditions and is less sensitive as the patient improves.

In making predictions about eventual level of recovery and the time frame within which recovery is likely to occur, the clinician will need to consider a range of factors, including the patient's age, premorbid ability levels and lifestyle, time post-trauma and so on.

How will the memory problems affect functioning in everyday settings?

Other frequently-asked questions relate to the impact which impairments are likely to have on day-to-day life. The *International Classification of Illness, Disease and Health* (WHO 1980) distinguishes between *impairment*, which, in this context, is quantified through the use of formal psychometric tests, and *disability,* which is the impact of these impairments on the performance of everyday activities. The classification has now been revised (WHO 2001): the new classification describes the effects of impairment of body structure and functions in terms of 'activity limitation' and 'participation restrictions'. One of the roles of the neuropsychologist, when feeding back information following formal assessment, is to express information about impairment in these terms.

Observations of memory performance in occupational therapy settings that mimic domestic, social or work settings may be useful in helping to predict adjustment to everyday situations outside the clinical environment.

How helpful are psychometric tests of memory in predicting the extent to which measurable impairments give rise to disability? Much has been made of the dearth of tests in which good ecological validity (e.g. Johnstone and Callaghan 1996; Larrabee and Crook 1996) and content validity (e.g. Johnstone and Frank 1995; Dodrill 1997, 1999; but see Bell and Roper 1998, for an opposing view) have been demonstrated. As noted in above, there are tests, such as the Rivermead Behavioural Memory Tests, which have been shown to have good ecological validity. It is also important to bear in mind that predictions about everyday performance are made by experienced clinicians on the basis of information from a range of sources. Demands made on the patient in their everyday life, relatives' reports, the patient's mood state, insight into cognitive status and behaviour during assessment, and the nature of errors made during formal assessment should be taken into account along with formal test results.

What will help? Recommendations for rehabilitation

The clinical interview is important in establishing premorbid skills and abilities, the patient's aspirations, previous use of memory aids, insight into memory loss and motivation to improve. The extent to which the patient is supported by relatives or carers is also relevant. The Contextual Memory Test questionnaire is particularly useful in establishing the patient's awareness of memory problems, while the relevant Cognitive Symptoms Checklist is helpful in identifying areas of concern and agreeing rehabilitation goals.

In the case of cognitive deficits, a range of cognitive functions should be sampled – impairments of attention, language and so on can affect performance on memory tasks and influence coping strategies. If a patient has mild to moderate memory impairment, in the context of good executive function and minimal additional cognitive deficit, this bodes well for many forms of memory intervention, especially those which involve concentration and new learning on the part of the patient. Global indices of memory impairment that fall in the amnesic range are more compatible with interventions that involve changes in environment and appropriate counselling of relatives and care-staff. Depending upon the cognitive mechanisms underlying memory impairment, strategies to improve or compensate for particular deficits can be devised (Skeel and Edwards 2001). For example, where there is a deficit in encoding, intervention may focus on attentional control or the use of mnemonic strategies at the encoding stage. Where retrieval deficits have been demonstrated, cuing systems may be utilised, while spared processing systems may be used to compensate for modality-specific memory impairment.

Has memory changed? Monitoring and evaluation

Measures such as the GOAT and the Westmead Battery are often helpful in monitoring recovery from acute memory loss associated with severe traumatic brain injury or subarachnoid haemorrhage. Subjective memory ratings, diary-based recording of memory lapses, or those obtained from electronic monitoring of events, such as opening pill bottles, may be helpful in asssessing the effectiveness of intervention strategies. Examples of questions which can usefully be included in monitoring an intervention (in this case the introduction of an electronic pager), are provided by Wilson *et al.* (2001).

When monitoring change over time using formal tests, it is preferable to select tests which have parallel forms. The AMIPB and the RBMT-E have two parallel form, while the RBMT II has four, and the Hopkins Verbal Learning Test six forms. Some of the computerised batteries that are used in trials of drugs developed for the treatment of dementia have parallel forms and are suitable for use in sequential assessment. Examples are CAMCOG (the cognitive section of the Cambridge Mental Disorders of the Elderly Examination – CAMDEX, Roth *et al.* 1986), and the system developed by Wesnes and colleagues, the validity of which has been investigated with a small group of brain-injured patients Keith *et al.* (1998). There is evidence that practice effects vary from test to test. Wilson *et al.* (2000) found that digit span, doors recognition memory (from the Doors and People Tests), and word list recall showed little change with repeated testing, whereas verbal fluency did show practice effects. Behavioural measures and questionnaires have minimal practice effects, and can thus be given much more frequently.

Future developments in memory assessment

The issue of the ecological validity of neuropsychological tests is, as previously mentioned, particularly important in the rehabilitation setting. It is envisaged that there will be more tests of proven ecological validity available by the end of the decade. Tests which take particular advantage of computer technology are already in development. In particular, the use of virtual reality techniques may be important in developing ecologically valid tests.

Advances in communication technology may change methods of test delivery. In the future some tests may be administered through the Internet, or by means of a videophone.

There is a need for memory tests specifically designed to monitor the effects of therapeutic intervention. These tests will have matched parallel forms and data on practice effects.

Finally, the development of functional brain imaging is already having an impact on neuropsychological research. Upright MRI scanners in which the patient can sit rather than lie are already in existence (Nakada and Tasaka 2001), and memory testing that is combined with functional brain imaging may shed light on compensatory mechanisms underlying memory test performance.

12 Can memory impairment be effectively treated?

Elizabeth L. Glisky

Abstract

This chapter reviews evidence for the effectiveness of memory rehabilitation approaches that have focused on the treatment of memory impairment. Interventions targeting impairment have usually involved either the use of repetitive practice or the teaching of mnemonic strategies. Although patients with memory disorders have learned new information using these methods, generalization to materials and situations beyond the training context has seldom been found, and so there is little evidence that impairment has been reduced. Nevertheless, in the context of disability-focused treatments, there is some evidence that a general mnemonic skill can be acquired after considerable practice of functionally-relevant specific behaviors. Similarly, strategy training may be more effective when focused on real-world problems. These findings, along with recent discoveries of neuroplasticity in the adult human brain suggest that further research directed at reducing impairment may be warranted. Such research should focus on people with relatively mild memory disorders and limited damage to brain regions important for memory and should target functionally useful tasks.

Introduction

In recent years, there has been almost uniform agreement that the most effective way to provide rehabilitation for individuals with memory disorders is to focus on reducing the disabilities caused by memory dysfunction thereby enhancing functioning in everyday life (Glisky and Schacter 1989; Wilson 1997, 2002). Earlier attempts at remediation that relied on repetitive practice of meaningless materials provided few if any benefits for memory and little reason to believe that such methods could relieve the underlying memory impairment and have any practical consequences. Recent findings suggesting that the human brain is much more plastic than previously thought, however, have renewed interest in the possibility that impairments in memory may be treatable in some cases (Ogden 2000). In this chapter, I will take a look at some old findings in light of new evidence and suggest that there may be some merit in reconsidering, at least in a research context, whether and under what conditions treating memory impairment may be an appropriate goal for rehabilitation.

Impairment vs. disability

According to the definition provided by the World Health Organization (1980), impairment refers to damage to a physical or mental structure, whereas disability refers to reduction or loss of a functional activity in daily life that occurs as a result of the impairment (see Chapter 4). Interventions that focus on memory impairment attempt to alter the internal neurobiological or cognitive state of the individual, with the expectation that such change will have general benefits for memory in a range of situations in everyday life and thus reduce disability. For this kind of treatment to be judged successful, memory benefits must generalize beyond the specific materials and context of training. Interventions that focus on disability, on the other hand, intervene directly at the behavioral level without any expectation or necessity for internal change and without any assumptions that improvements will generalize. Such interventions are judged successful if the specific functional disability is alleviated. This chapter reviews interventions that have focused on memory impairment, evaluates the extent to which they have been able to achieve generalizable benefits, and considers how they might be modified to increase the probability of attaining long-term generalized improvements in memory functioning.

Repetitive practice

Focus on impairment

The method that has been used most often to treat memory impairment is repetitive practice and exercise. In most cases, patients are asked to sit in front of computers for long periods of time (although paper and pencil methods are also used), playing a variety of memory games that require them to remember all kinds of useless pieces of information, including random words, digits, line drawings, nonsense objects, and locations on the computer screen. Only occasionally are people asked to remember anything of importance. Clearly the goal of such interventions is to stimulate or activate the damaged cognitive and neural processes that are involved in memory so as to restore their function and re-enable memory. Numerous studies (Benedict, Brandt, and Bergey 1993; Berg, Koning-Haanstra, and Deelman 1991; Godfrey and Knight 1985; Middleton, Lambert, and Seggar 1991) have tested this possibility, requiring memory-impaired patients to complete up to 32 hours of practice in the laboratory, often followed by supplemental exercises at home, and the results are clear: there is no evidence that repetitive practice of such meaningless material results in restoration of memory function or provides any generalizable benefits whatsoever. Although the specific materials practiced may be learned, memory in any general sense is not improved.

Focus on disability

Domain-specific learning

Despite the consistent failure to find any *general* benefits of repetitive practice, it is nevertheless clear that practice is essential for memory-impaired individuals to learn new information. So, for example, the studies that have demonstrated the acquisition of domain-specific learning in amnesic patients have all incorporated many hours of practice (for review, see Glisky and Glisky 2002). However, the benefits of practice, in most cases, are highly specific; there is typically little generalization to new information and contexts. These findings thus suggest that the underlying impairment has not been reduced, but rather that despite the impairment new learning can still occur.

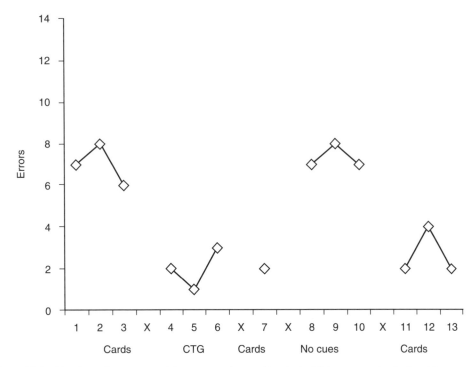

Figure 12.1 Number of errors per trial on a complex cooking task. CTG = computer task guidance. Reproduced from Kirsch *et al.* (1988) with permission of the author.

Learning a general mnemonic skill

There have, however, been a small number of demonstrations of generalizable improvements in memory obtained from studies that focused on treating disability rather than impairment. For example, in 1988, Kirsch and colleagues reported a single case study in which they used a computer to present cues to a severely amnesic anoxic patient to guide him interactively through the steps of a cookie-baking task. They employed a variation of an ABA design in which instructions were presented on rolodex cards during baseline and by an interactive computer task guidance system (CTG) during the intervention. The finding of interest, illustrated in Figure 12.1, was that the gains achieved during CTG were substantially retained after the computer was withdrawn and the instruction reverted to the rolodex cards. It was clear that the patient had not learned the cooking task itself because when all cues were withdrawn, performance reverted to baseline levels, but when cards were reintroduced, once again the patient was able to perform as he had with the CTG. Kirsch *et al.* suggested that the patient had learned a general mnemonic skill during the CTG trials – how to interact with a cuing system – and this skill had generalized from the computer to the card cuing system.

A similar outcome was reported in a case study of a patient with Korsakoff's syndrome by Heinrichs and colleagues (Heinrichs *et al.* 1992). In this study, the patient was taught her daily schedule of 12 activities and the times of those activities, using the method of vanishing cues (Glisky, Schacter, and Tulving 1986). As can be seen in Figure 12.2, after 17 training trials (trials 11–27), the patient had learned all of her daily activities although she was able to recall correctly only about half of the scheduled times for those activities. This level of performance was maintained across an additional 16 control trials, during which time no further training was offered (indicated by the second X in

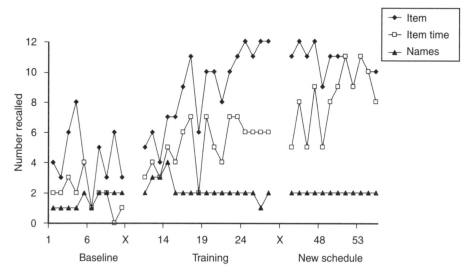

Figure 12.2 Number of daily scheduled activities and times recalled at baseline, during training, and without training following a change in the schedule. Adapted and reproduced from Heinrichs *et al.* (1992) with permission of Lawrence Erlbaum Associates.

Figure 12.2). Importantly, when her schedule was changed, she was quickly able to learn the new schedule without any additional training (trials 44–55). Heinrichs *et al.* observed that the patient appeared to have developed some kind of self-cuing skills as a result of the training and was subsequently able to apply them to a new, similar situation. Although memory had not improved in any general sense (note the lack of learning of the names of fellow patients, which were untrained), it still appeared that generalization to a similar task had occurred.

Finally, a recent study by Wilson and colleagues (Wilson, Evans, Emslie, and Malinek 1997; see also Wilson, Emslie, Quirk, and Evans 2001) showed that, following 12 weeks of practice using a simple paging system, NeuroPage, to cue daily activities, a mixed group of memory-impaired patients were able to carry out 85 per cent of those activities (compared to only 37 per cent at baseline) and continued to do so (74 per cent success rate) even after the pager was removed. This finding again suggests that many of these patients may have learned a generalizable mnemonic skill – how to use cues in their environment to remind them of their daily activities.

These three studies, in contrast to the earlier studies using repetitive practice, demonstrate that, at least under some conditions, a general mnemonic skill can be learned, suggesting perhaps that some aspects of memory impairment were reduced. What then might those conditions be? In these latter studies, training was focused on reducing disability, and people were engaged in practicing specific behaviors that were important and relevant to their daily lives. Practice was continued for quite a long period of time in both the Heinrichs *et al.* study – 55 trials over 6 months – and the Wilson *et al.* study – 12 weeks with daily practice. Importantly, the patients appeared to learn more than the specific activities practiced, suggesting that they had incidentally acquired a more general skill with potential application to other situations in everyday life.

Mechanisms of change

Although one might debate whether memory impairment was diminished in the foregoing studies, the findings are consistent with results of recent studies of sensory and motor impairments that have been treated successfully following extensive amounts of practice. For example, Nudo and colleagues

(Nudo, Barbay, and Kleim 2000) have found that practice of motor movements is not effective if it merely engages simple repetitive movements. Rather, such exercises are beneficial only if they involve the learning of a functional skill. Also, outcomes are often quite specific, benefiting only a narrow range of functions that bear a close relation to the one trained. Examination of the brain regions affected by such practice indicates increased activation and changes in the anatomy and physiology of regions of motor cortex adjacent to areas of damage, suggesting that impairment was directly impacted. Plasticity has also been demonstrated in numerous animal studies. In particular, several studies have reported that enriched environments stimulate dendritic growth and synaptic connectivity in normal rats (Kolb 1995) and enhance recovery of cognitive deficits in injured animals (see Hamm, Temple, Buck, Deford, and Floyd 2000). Although the functional consequences of enriched environments have been inconsistent in animals and unstudied in humans, the animal studies nevertheless provide further evidence that enriching experiences may produce neural changes that might promote recovery (Kolb and Gibb 1999). Finally, there have been reports of neurogenesis in the adult human hippocampus, a region of the brain known to be important for memory (Eriksson *et al.* 1998); in animals, the growth of new neurons in this region has been linked to the learning of hippocampally dependent memory tasks (Gould, Beylin, Tanapat, Reeves, and Shors 1999).

Together these studies suggest that the adult human is capable of new learning after brain injury, if given extensive practice on functionally meaningful activities. This learning should be reflected in cognitive and neural changes that are quite specific and permit generalization only to highly similar activities requiring the same acquired skill. How the new learning and skill are represented in the brain is, at this time, still uncertain. One possibility is that the learning of new factual information may be represented neocortically, reflecting intact semantic memory. Consistent with this possibility are studies reported by Vargha-Khadem and colleagues (1997) showing that children with hippocampal loss early in life and a persistent dense amnesia for the episodes in their lives, are nevertheless able to acquire considerable amounts of semantic knowledge in school (presumably as a result of lots of practice). In these cases, however, the episodic memory deficit was not diminished. Whether neuroplastic changes can be induced in the hippocampus by extensive practice and whether such changes will reduce the episodic memory impairment remains to be determined. The use of functional neuroimaging in rehabilitation studies should, in the near future, help to provide answers to these questions.

The goal of rehabilitation is always to achieve a meaningful clinical outcome. Repetitive practice can achieve such an outcome if it is focused on information or tasks relevant to everyday functioning. Whether treatment targets the underlying impairment or focuses on relieving disability may be of little concern to the practising clinician, as long as real-world goals are attained. Nevertheless, it is still important both theoretically and clinically to understand the mechanisms of change. Discovering what brain regions are associated with positive outcomes will help us understand how new learning occurs in brain-injured individuals, what we can expect from our interventions, and how we can adapt our procedures to facilitate those outcomes.

Mnemonic strategies

Focus on impairment or disability

Another common intervention that has been used to treat memory impairment is the teaching of mnemonic strategies. A variety of different strategies have been attempted with varying degrees of success (for reviews, see Butters, Soety, and Glisky 1998; Glisky and Glisky 2002). Probably the most frequently used method has been visual imagery (for review, see Richardson 1995), but verbally-based organizational and elaboration strategies have also been employed. Early rehabilitation studies often tried to use strategies to teach people unrelated word lists or paired associates – things with little real-world value. These were clear attempts to treat impairment, the assumption being that if a strategy was learned it could be applied broadly to a range of materials. Later studies were focused on teaching patients information with more relevance in everyday life, such as the names of people in their immediate living or work environments. These interventions were focused on alleviating disability and there was no expectation that the strategies would generalize beyond the training context.

Generalization to real-world contexts

The findings with respect to mnemonic strategies have been mixed. As with practice and exercise, people can learn specific pieces of information using strategies, but evidence of generalization to new materials and contexts is weak. When generalization is observed, it is restricted to closely related tasks and materials. In most cases, people do not use the strategies spontaneously outside the training context, suggesting that a generalizable skill has not been acquired. There have, however, been a couple of exceptions to these negative findings. Kaschel and colleagues (2002) reported that a group of mildly-impaired patients of mixed etiology did show transfer to relevant everyday memory situations (i.e., stories, appointments) after 30 sessions of imagery training, but these were for the most part quite similar to the training tasks. Similarly, Berg, Koning-Haanstra and Deelman (1991) reported transfer to a group of strategy-dependent tasks following 18 hours of organizational strategy training (plus homework). In both studies, effects were maintained across a 3–4 month interval. In a later four-year follow-up study, however, Berg and colleagues (Milders, Berg, and Deelman 1995) reported no advantage for the strategy-trained group, and suggested that perhaps a refresher course in the intervening years might have encouraged long-term maintenance.

Strategies appear to be particularly useful for learning arbitrary associations such as name-face pairs that lack meaningful associative relations or obvious links to prior knowledge. In these cases, strategies likely provide an associative structure, helping people to link unrelated things together and connect them to other information in the knowledge system. Like practice and exercise, however, strategies also seem most effective when applied in real-world contexts; little seems to be gained from teaching strategies isolated from their functional application. Kaschel *et al.* (2002), for example, trained people to form images of everyday actions like changing a light bulb and then practiced transfer to a range of everyday tasks. Berg *et al.* (1991) also worked with common problems of daily life, and in both studies, patients themselves identified the particular problems to be included in training. The relevance of strategy-training in patients' lives is likely an important contributor to its success.

Who is most likely to benefit?

Finally, numerous studies have demonstrated that strategies benefit only people with mild to moderate impairments. Individuals with severe memory disorders often cannot learn the strategies or apply them effectively (Gade 1994; Kaschel *et al.* 2002; Richardson 1995; Wilson 1987). Even those with mild impairments, who can learn the strategies, often tend not to apply them in other contexts, and so strategy training applied to functionally useless materials is not beneficial. Nevertheless, strategies may be used very effectively to help people acquire new information that is relevant in their daily lives.

The evidence with respect to mnemonic strategies is much like that obtained from the studies of repetitive practice, although perhaps somewhat more positive: Strategies can be effective to help memory-impaired individuals learn new knowledge and skills relevant in their daily lives, but in many cases they tend not to be maintained over time or applied beyond the context of training. Patients with mild disorders are most likely to benefit and may show transfer to related situations if training is continued over long periods of time and strategies are learned in the context of real-world problems.

Whether this constitutes a reduction of the memory impairment per se or an alleviation of a disability really cannot be determined at this time without more knowledge of the brain regions affected by the intervention.

Mechanisms of change

It is noteworthy, however, that only mildly-impaired patients benefit from strategies or show any indication of generalization. These patients have some residual memory function and likely only limited damage to the neural structures important for memory. In particular, they may have relatively small lesions in the medial temporal lobes, which are important for the acquisition and retention of the strategies, and relatively intact frontal lobes, which are necessary for the construction and initiation of strategies. Patients with frontal deficits, although they may be able to learn strategies, may not initiate them spontaneously, and so will fail to show generalization. Strategy training should therefore be most beneficial to those with relatively preserved frontal function and limited damage to medial temporal lobe structures. To the extent that the frontal lobes, through the use of strategic encoding processes, can associate the elements of a new experience together and relate them to similar information in the knowledge system, the information delivered to the medial temporal lobe memory system is likely to be well-integrated and meaningful, placing less of a burden on the binding processes of the hippocampus and surrounding brain regions. This highly organized packet of information may then be more easily processed by medial temporal lobe structures that are only partially functional. Thus, to the extent that patients are able to use mnemonic strategies, the efficiency of the damaged cognitive and neural structures involved in memory should be improved, thereby reducing memory impairment.

Conclusions

Evidence for successful treatment of memory impairment is weak and probably, at this time, should not be the focus of clinical intervention. Nevertheless, further research into treatment of memory impairment seems warranted, given the suggestive findings outlined above, and the new evidence for plasticity in the adult human brain. Research should focus on treatments for people with relatively mild memory disorders and limited damage to regions of the brain that are important for memory. This segment of the brain-injured population is significant in number and may be underserved by disability-focused interventions, many of which may be too simplistic for people functioning at a relatively high level. Further, because of their more limited damage, those individuals with mild impairments should be optimal candidates for interventions that are focused on achieving neural changes. To the extent that some neurons in the memory regions continue to function, it may be possible to stimulate further growth and connectivity through extensive amounts of practice.

It is also important to conduct training in the context of functionally useful tasks. All of the evidence from rehabilitation studies in the sensory and motor domains as well as in the cognitive domain suggests that practice of meaningless tasks or information is not beneficial. Further, to the extent that training focuses on important real-world tasks, and includes attempts to achieve generalization to a broader range of tasks or contexts, the goals of impairment- and disability-driven interventions are not inconsistent. It seems likely, however, that if generalizable improvements are to be achieved, interventions will have to continue for months rather than for just a few hours. It may also be important to start interventions soon after injury in order to stimulate surviving neurons or promote the growth of new ones. Further studies are still needed, however, to assess the optimal timing for interventions.

Finally, we might consider providing more stimulating environments for our patients during rehabilitation to see whether we can encourage neuronal growth. Exactly how to structure these environments is uncertain at this time, but environments that enable the practice of functionally meaningful tasks and activities would seem to be a good place to start (Ogden 2000). We might also try to construct tasks that require the hippocampus in order to explore whether the practice of such tasks might stimulate the growth of new neurons in this brain region. There is reasonable consensus among cognitive neuroscientists that the function of the hippocampus is to bind various aspects of an experience together, linking the focal content of an experience with its spatiotemporal context. Although to my knowledge no interventions of this sort have been attempted, it should be possible to create tasks that require such linking (perhaps using analogs of the tasks used in animals) and have people practice them over extended periods of time.

We now have the neuroimaging tools to monitor the effects of our interventions at the level of the brain and to determine whether pre-morbid function has been at least partly restored or whether compensation or reorganization of function has occurred. Activations in perilesional regions would suggest that tasks were being accomplished in much the same way and by the same or similar neural circuits as prior to injury and that impairment was likely reduced. On the other hand, activations in regions remote from the lesion would be consistent with a reorganization of function in new neural circuits.

Acknowledgement

Preparation of this chapter was supported by Grant RO1 AG14792 from the National Institute on Aging.

13 The effective treatment of memory-related disabilities

Barbara A Wilson

Abstract

Everyday problems (i.e. disabilities) arising from organic memory impairment are the most handicapping for people with organic memory impairment and for their families. It is these problems that should be targeted in rehabilitation. Although there is little evidence that rehabilitation can restore lost memory functioning, there is considerable evidence that disabilities can be treated. Evidence is presented from a randomized control trial in which people were randomly allocated to a pager or to a waiting list. At a later stage, those with the pager were then monitored without the pager and those on the waiting list were given a pager. Significant improvements in remembering everyday targets only occurred once the pager had been received. It is also possible to improve the learning ability of memory impaired people through a teaching technique known as errorless learning. Again, evidence is provided from several studies showing the benefits of errorless over errorful (or trial-and-error) learning. One of the reasons why memory rehabilitation is successful in the treatment of disabilities is that it encompasses a wide range of theoretical approaches. No one model, theory, or framework is sufficient to address the many and complex problems of people requiring cognitive rehabilitation.

Introduction

Memory disabilities are those everyday problems that arise from a memory deficit or impairment. While an assessment of memory might identify a particular problem with one aspect of memory, say poor delayed recall of verbal material, this does not tell us how disabling this impairment will be in real life for the individual concerned. It might not be too bad for someone who does not need to remember verbal reports and instructions and who is surrounded by people who habitually remind that person when it is time to do something. For someone who is expected to respond rapidly to constantly changing information, however, such an impairment could be devastating. Attempts to restore lost memory functioning, i.e. attempts to treat the basic underlying memory impairment appear to have always been unsuccessful (see, for example, Glisky and Schacter 1986; Wilson 1995). This issue is further addressed by Glisky in Chapter 12 of this volume. In contrast, there is ample evidence to suggest that the related disabilities can be treated effectively. It is, of course, the everyday problems or disabilities that are most handicapping for memory impaired people, who are most concerned with such things as remembering appointments, conversations, where they are going later in the day or who came to visit yesterday. They are not particularly concerned with or indeed affected by scores on a particular test or the knowledge of the size of the hippocampal lesion.

Rehabilitation is usually defined in functional or practical terms. Take the definition of McLellan (1991), for example, who wrote:

> Rehabilitation is a process whereby people who are disabled by injury or disease work together with professional staff, relatives and members of the wider community to achieve their optimum physical, psychological, social and vocational well being.
>
> McLellan (1991, p. 785)

The point of rehabilitation, then, is to enable people with disabilities to function as adequately as possible in their own most appropriate environments. The purpose of rehabilitation is not simply to improve performance on tests: therefore changes in test scores should never be taken as an indicator of rehabilitation success.

Although successful rehabilitation can be judged by the reduction of a disability, that same rehabilitation may have no effect on underlying impairments. Of course, it would be highly desirable to restore or retrain basic memory functions, but attempts to do this remain woefully inadequate. It is possible that our rapidly expanding knowledge of the brain and how it works may result in new treatments that can restore lost memory functioning, i.e. can treat the impairments. With new pharmacological agents, new technology, neural transplants and genetic engineering, who knows what is possible in the future – particularly if these new developments are combined with good rehabilitation practice? However, even if such developments do occur, their effectiveness must be judged in terms of how well they alleviate the problems of brain injured people in their everyday lives. This chapter argues that it is possible, even in the current state of play, to alleviate some of those everyday problems, and evidence will be presented to show that memory disabilities can be treated successfully.

Studies to determine if a paging system can reduce everyday memory and planning problems

A pilot study

In the early 1990s Larry Treadgold, an engineer, and Neil Hersch, a neuropsychologist, began working on some software to run a paging system to help Larry's son, who had survived a severe head injury and was trying to return to college. This became known as 'Neuropage', a system using radio-paging technology to send reminders of things to do at predetermined times (Hersch and Treadgold 1994). On Neuropage messages can be regular repeat ones such as 'take your tablets', or one-off messages such as 'Beryl's party in half an hour'. People can receive one message a week or more than 100 during the day. It is an extremely flexible system that is easy to use and suitable for a wide range of individuals. I saw the system in use in California in 1994 and agreed to evaluate it in the United Kingdom. In Table 13.1 we list the reasons why some people find external memory aids such as this difficult to use.

Table 13.1 Problems with external memory aids

People with memory problems
• Forget to use them
• May have difficulty programming them
• May use them in an unsystematic or disorganised way
• May be embarrassed by them

Two single case studies to show the system could improve independence and reduce costs to health and social services

In 1998, Evans, Emslie and Wilson reported the case of a 50-year old woman, R.P., who had sustained a stroke seven years earlier. The pager enabled R.P. to carry out everyday tasks that had previously required prompting from her husband. For example, she wanted help with watering plants, washing underwear, taking medication and attending a clinic as a voluntary helper. Once given the pager, she was immediately able to carry out these tasks independently. Furthermore, before having the pager, R.P. used to spend one week every three months in respite care to give her family a break. Since she had the pager the family never felt the need for respite care. This saved several thousand pounds a year.

In 1999, Wilson, Emslie, Quirk and Evans reported the case of a young man, George, who learned to live independently with the help of the paging system. George had sustained a very severe head injury several years earlier, and took part in the randomised control study described below. At this time he was living with his parents. Almost four months after this study, George's parents contacted the NeuroPage research team to ask about availability of the pager on a longer term basis. We were able to provide George with a pager and monitor him over a three month period. At this time he was living in his own flat with 24-hour a day care provided by social services. He received an average of 14 messages per day with a maximum of 20 on any one day. Not only did George gradually cut down the number of messages he received each day, but he was soon able to cut down on the amount of care he received. By the end of the three month period George had 12-hour a day care instead of 24 hours: a considerable saving for social services. Details of cost savings are provided in Wilson and Evans (2002). Once again, we were treating the disabilities and not the underlying impairment.

A randomised control study

Once the pilot study was completed, my colleagues and I were ready to embark on a randomised control trial to persuade potential purchasers of the paging service that NeuroPage was an effective way of reducing the everyday problems of people with acquired brain injury. We had also obtained funding to do this from Anglia and Oxford NHS Research and Development Initiative. We accepted referrals from throughout the United Kingdom: anyone with memory and/or planning problems of any age provided they could read a test message on the screen of the pager. Once entered into the trial, we allocated people randomly to one of two groups. Those in group A were to receive a pager immediately following the baseline period while those in group B were to go on a waiting list prior to receiving the pager. We decided to use this crossover design so that all people were able to benefit from the pager at some time during the study. Most people were referred by occupational therapists or clinical psychologists and most had sustained a head injury or a stroke, although we had a few people with other conditions, such as a developmental learning difficulty or Korsakoff's Syndrome.

Following the referral, clients were interviewed, usually with a family member, therapist or other carer to determine which reminders they would find helpful. Next they were assessed to ensure they could read and could learn to press the button on the pager when the alarm sounded. They were also given a brief, neuropsychological test battery to establish memory, executive and attention functions.

During the two week baseline period target behaviours were recorded as described above. Those in group A then received their pagers, while group B waited for a further seven weeks before pagers were distributed. After this time, people in group A returned their pagers and those in group B were now allocated a pager. People were assessed on the achievement of target behaviours at three time periods: at baseline, at weeks 6 and 7 post baseline (i.e. the last two weeks on the pager for group A and the last two weeks of the waiting list for group B) and at weeks 13 and 14 post baseline (i.e. the final two weeks of the study). More than 80 per cent of the 143 people who completed all 16 weeks of the study

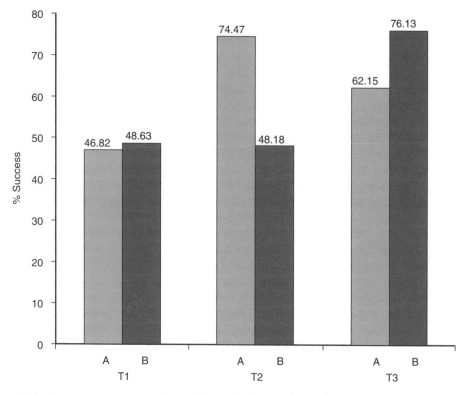

Figure 13.1 Percentage success rate for participants in Group A (pager first) and Group B (pager later) at Time 1 (baseline) and Time 2 (weeks 8 and 9) and 6.

(from 209 initially referred and from 173 who completed the baseline phase) were significantly more successful in carrying out everyday activities such as self care, self-medication and keeping appointments when using the pager in comparison with the baseline period. For most of those we were able to monitor seven weeks after removal of the pager (i.e. those in group A), improvement remained well above baseline levels.

To summarise the actual group figures, achievment of targets did not differ between the two groups during baseline (group A achieved 46.82 per cent and group B achieved 48.63 per cent of targets). When assessed at time two, group A (who had the pagers first) achieved 74.47 per cent of targets while group B (who were still waiting for a pager) achieved 48.18 per cent (i.e. no different from baseline). Group A returned their pagers and at the end of the study had dropped back a little way: they were now achieving 62.15 per cent but were still significantly better than baseline. Group B, meanwhile, had risen to a success rate of 76.13 per cent. This was significantly better than at times 1 and 2. The evidence, then, strongly supported the findings from the pilot study that NeuroPage reduces the everyday memory and planning problems of people with brain injury (Wilson, Emslie, Quirk and Evans 2001). These results can be seen in Figure 13.1.

From research to clinical practice

The successful research studies encouraged the local health authority (Lifespan National Health Service Trust, which has since become Fenland and East Cambridgeshire Trust), to set up a clinical NeuroPage service for people throughout the United Kingdom. We have recently surveyed the first 40 people referred to this service (Wilson, Scott, Evans and Emslie 2003). The age range of this group was 14–81 years with a mean age of 38.25 years. The mean time post injury was 4.56 years with a range of three months to 15.33 years. The majority of clients were men (only 8 women were in the group). The most frequent diagnosis was traumatic brain injury (13 people) and stroke (7 people), although a number of different diagnostic groups were represented, including neurofibromatosis (1) and multiple sclerosis (1). The number of messages sent out per week ranged from 2 to 147, with many of these being daily repeat messages (e.g. 'take medication'). The number of different messages sent each week ranged from 2 to 33. By far the most frequent messages were those relating to medication – 514 messages sent out each week reminding people to take their medication. Reminders about orientation, such as telling clients the day and the time, were next with 380 messages sent each week. The third most frequent messages related to food, e.g. 'prepare dinner' or 'eat your lunch': 193 'food' messages were sent each week. Among the least frequent messages were those about finances (e.g. 'pay electricity bill'), transport (e.g. 'arrange taxi for tomorrow') and NeuroPage (e.g. 'call NeuroPage with messages'). Respectively there were 4, 8 and 11 of these messages sent each week. The majority (77.5 per cent) i.e. 31 of the 40 clients found the pager successful. This compares well with the randomised control study (Wilson *et al.* 2001) in which 71 per cent of clients referred completed all stages of the study and 80 per cent of these clients showed an improvement in achieving their everyday targets. Once again, the nature of the messages show that memory disabilities are being targeted and, on the whole, successfully overcome.

Studies to help memory impaired people learn more efficiently

Background to errorless learning studies

In 1963, Terrace described his work with pigeons using a technique he called 'Errorless Learning', or learning without making mistakes. He taught pigeons to discriminate a red key from a green key (apparently a hard discrimination to make for pigeons). Having trained the pigeons to peck reliably to one colour, he introduced a different colour when the birds were in a position where it was difficult to peck. Thus Terrace gradually faded in one colour in such a way that the pigeons learned the task while making no, or very few errors en route. The principle was soon taken up by people working with children (and later adults) with developmental learning difficulties. Sidman and Stoddard (1967), for example, taught learning disabled children to discriminate circles from ellipses, and Walsh and Lamberts (1979) used errorless learning principles to teach children to read. Errorless learning is used to this day in the teaching of intellectually handicapped children. As both this group and people with memory problems share a difficulty in new learning, it would make sense to see if this method worked in memory rehabilitation.

Another theoretical impetus stimulating the use of errorless learning in cognitive rehabilitation came from studies of implicit memory and implicit learning in cognitive psychology and neuropsychology. It has been established for many years that people with the amnesic syndrome can learn some things normally or nearly normally: these are tasks where conscious recollection of the information to be remembered is not required. Learning is demonstrated through implicit means – in other words conscious recollection is not required. Accuracy at tracking a visual stimulus on a screen, for example, typically improves with practice, even in people with severe memory deficits who may not even remember having done the task earlier. Glisky and Schacter (1986) attempted to use the intact implicit learning abilities of people with amnesia to teach them new skills. Although they were sucessful in certain cases, learning typically required more effort than one normally expects in implicit learning tasks.

In some cases anomalies are seen in implicit learning studies. When assessing amnesic patients on a perceptual priming (fragmented pictures) task, one may see the usual overall improvement (the fragments are identified progressively earlier over trials) together with a few examples of no improvement over trials. If a fragmented picture of a monkey is called a 'cat' on trial one, it may be called a 'cat' on trial after trial despite the amnesic person seeing the correct answer later in the sequence in every trial. These anomalies led Alan Baddeley and I to consider whether errors injected into a system that has a very impoverished episodic memory may be difficult or impossible to eliminate? In order to benefit from our mistakes we need to remember them. As implicit memory is not good at error elimination, it may be that we should avoid errors for people with poor explicit and episodic memory. We went on to ask the question, 'Do amnesic people learn better if prevented from making mistakes during the learning process?'

For our first study (Baddeley and Wilson 1994) we saw three groups of people: those with a severe memory deficit as defined by zero delayed recall of a prose passage; young control subjects and older control subjects. We administered a stem completion task under two conditions: namely errorless and errorful learning. In the errorless condition people were prevented from making mistakes: they were given a stem and told the correct answer immediately. In the errorful condition they were forced to make mistakes: they were given a stem and asked to guess what the word might be before being told the correct answer. Conditions and words were counterbalanced. After three learning trials participants were tested by being given the two letter stems and asked for the correct word. Errorless learning was superior to errorful learning for all subjects but, in the case of the people with amnesia, every one of them showed better performance under the errorless learning condition.

The probability of learning under errorful and errorless conditions can be seen in Figure 13.2a and 13.2b.

As a result of these findings, I changed my clinical behaviour immediately, and now I never ask memory impaired people to guess unless I am giving them a test which requires guessing. Instead I say, 'Only tell me if you are sure.' It was interesting to note that when I explained to relatives what the experiment was about, several of them said, 'Oh, yes, I know what you mean', and gave me examples of intuitive errorless learning. For example, the wife of one man who had sustained encephalitis said:

> When he first came out of hospital, he tried to help in the kitchen but he couldn't remember where the bowls went and where the spoons went. I thought he'll work it out but he never did. Eventually, I went through things with him. I said the bowls go there and showed him, and the spoons go there and showed him and then he learned.

Obviously, the answer to our question was, 'Yes, amnesic people do learn better if prevented from making mistakes during the learning process.' This, however, was not enough. I did not want to teach people stem completion tasks. It was necessary to demonstrate that errorless learning could also be applied to real life tasks.

Some clinical studies

The first published studies that applied errorless learning principles to the rehabilitation of memory impaired people would appear to be those of Wilson, Baddeley, Evans and Shiel (1994). We reported several single case studies of people with non-progressive brain damage, including a man who had survived encephalitis, a stroke patient, a man with Korsakoff's Syndrome and a man with head injury who was still in post traumatic amnesia. In each case we taught two tasks, one in an errorful way and one in an errorless way. The tasks were matched as far as possible for difficulty and number of subcomponents. Tasks included recognition of objects (for a man with agnosia and amnesia), names of famous people, entering messages into an electronic organiser and orientation items. In each case errorless learning was superior to errorful learning. We were encouraged as we had shown this effect with people of different diagnostic groups and at different times post insult.

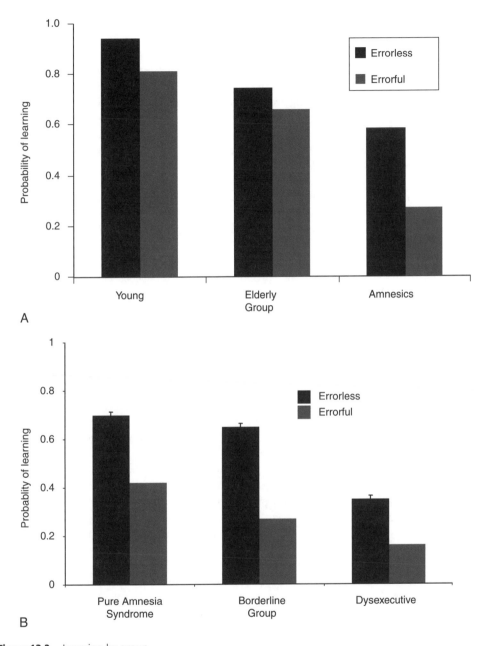

Figure 13.2 Learning by group.

Since then, errorless learning has been used by others. Wilson and Evans (1996), Squires *et al.* (1997) and Evans *et al.* (2000) have used it to teach a variety of tasks to people with non progressive brain damage; and Clare *et al.* in a series of studies have used errorless learning, in combination with other strategies for improving learning, with people with Alzheimer's disease. This last group of studies will be described next.

Errorless learning to help people with Alzheimer's disease

Clare and colleagues published their first paper on this topic in 1999 (Clare, Wilson, Breen and Hodges). This was a report of a man who had been diagnosed with dementia of the Alzheimer type six years earlier. He was seen at a memory clinic and invited to take part in a study investigating whether errorless learning was effective in helping people with AD learn or relearn information. The man, V.J., agreed to take part. Following an assessment and a discussion with V.J. and his sister with whom he lived, it was decided to address a particular concern of V.J.'s, namely difficulty remembering the names of people at a social club he attended each week. Armed with a Polaroid camera, Linda Clare went with V.J. to his club and photographed 14 of V.J.'s friends. He was then seen at home each week for several months. During baseline measures, it was clear that V.J. could recall reliably three names of the people shown him in the photographs. These names were retained in the set so that V.J. would always experience some success. The remaining 11 names were taught one at a time, one for each week, using a combination of errorless learning, spaced retrieval and vanishing cues. The procedure involved presenting one photograph and saying, 'This is (e.g. Gloria). Can you think of a way to remember her?' Gloria was described as, 'Gloria with the gleaming smile.' Other descriptors were used for other names/people. The name was then presented using vanishing cues, so, for example, 'Gloria'; Glori _'; Glor _ _' etc. V.J. was required to complete the missing letters each time. Once V.J. was able to write the entire name, a spaced retrieval method was employed in which he was asked to recall the name at gradually increasing intervals. The over riding principle was to ensure no (or very few) errors were made during learning. The correct name was written on the back of each photograph and V.J. was told never to guess and only say the name if he was sure. If he was not sure he was asked to look at the name on the back. Following each weekly session, V.J.'s sister spent a few minutes a day practising the name. In addition, V.J. attended the club each week so he could practise there.

Once all 11 names had been learned, Linda Clare went to the club with V.J. and took the photographs. He was required to look at a photograph, find the correct person and introduce this person by name to Linda. This was the generalisation stage and V.J.'s only error was with a woman who had dyed her hair and changed her hairstyle since the photograph was taken.

Mean recall scores for the 11 names were 20 per cent correct over the baseline sessions; 98 per cent correct following intervention and 100 per cent correct at the three month, six month and nine month follow up. Furthermore, V.J. was very pleased with his relearning, saying that he had thought he would never learn anything new again and now he could greet everyone at the club by name. V.J. was able to maintain this new learning with short daily practices despite the fact that his disease was progressing.

In 2001, Clare *et al.* published a three year follow up of V.J. After the nine month follow-up period, V.J. and his sister were asked to stop the daily practice sessions and the photographs were removed. His only practice, therefore, was during his weekly visits to the club. He was regularly assessed on the set of faces, including the three he had always known without any training, but was given no feedback on whether or not these were correct. V.J. was monitored for a further two years. His performance remained stable for the first year and then showed a modest decline over the second year, although it remained well above baseline levels. Potentially, this is a highly important clinical finding. If people with AD can be taught practically useful everyday information and hold on to this information in the face of neuro-logical and neuropsychological decline, it could reduce the stress on carers and postpone admission to long term care.

It is not only names that respond to this treatment even though it is probably true to say that names respond consistently to errorless learning. In 2000, a small group study from the same team (Clare *et al.* 2000), demonstrated that other problems, including remembering to use a memory board and reducing the number of repetitive questions, also responded to an errorless learning treatment strategy.

Once more, there is evidence that it is possible to reduce the disabilities associated with organic memory impairment.

For an interesting review of errorful and errorless learning, the reader is referred to Fillingham, Hodgson, Sage and Lambon Ralph (2003).

Rehabilitation should have a broad theoretical base

For a number of years rehabilitation practitioners have argued that there are several theoretical or methodological contributors to rehabilitation (Gianutsos 1989; Wilson 1987; McMillan and Greenwood 1993). It is certainly not a pure discipline, and those who argue that one model is sufficient (e.g. Coltheart 1991; Seron *et al.* 1991; Mitchum and Berndt 1995) fail to realise that not only do most people requiring cognitive rehabilitation have multiple cognitive deficits, they frequently have other non-cognitive problems such as anxiety and depression that may impact on cognitive functioning and also require treatment in their own right. Recently, I published a paper entitled, 'Towards a comprehensive model of cognitive rehabilitation' (Wilson 2002) and argued that no one model, theory or framework is sufficient to address the complex problems faced by people with cognitive problems resulting from brain injury. We should recognise the contributions made by theories of learning, behaviour, emotion, recovery, plasticity, assessment and others. One of the big changes in rehabilitation over the past 20 years or so has been the recognition that dealing with the emotional consequences of brain injury is an integral part of cognitive rehabilitation (Prigatano 1995, 1999; Williams, Evans and Wilson 2003). Thus we need to know about models of emotion and consider whether the emotional difficulties are due to biological, psychosocial or psychodynamic factors (Gainotti 1993). Another big step forward is the recognition that rehabilitation is a partnership between patients/clients, their families and rehabilitation staff. We have to understand such frameworks as goal setting and goal planning in order to negotiate the goals and ensure the smooth running of this partnership. Assessment for rehabilitation is of crucial importance, but it is not only assessment of cognitive functioning that matters. We must also assess the functional consequences of the impairments: how the problems manifest themselves in real life, the areas in which the families want help, and whether the cognitive problems are exacerbated by anxiety. We can turn to behavioural assessment models and theories here. The list is endless but the point remains that we need to draw on a variety of theoretical bases, models and frameworks if we are to achieve good clinical practice and ensure effective treatment of memory disabilities.

Section 4

Spoken language disorders

14 Language: cognitive models and functional anatomy

David Howard

Abstract

The first section of this chapter introduces cognitive neuropsychological models of single word processing. Box and arrow models can indicate the functional architecture of the language system but provide only a first level of description; they need to be supplemented by detailed descriptions of how the modules operate. They are however very useful clinically in guiding a description of different levels of impairment, and identifying intact language abilities. This approach is then compared with a number of competing theoretical perspectives.

The second section considers how language is represented in the brain. The classical Wernicke-Lichtheim model, although widely represented in textbooks, is inadequate. Evidence from lesion studies of people with brain damage is considered together with their limitations. Functional imaging has revealed a large network of areas in the brain that are involved in language processing in normal people. Although functional imaging studies have brought substantial progress in our understanding of language representation in the brain, much is still unclear about the nature of processing taking place, how it is implemented at a neural level and the interactions between different regions during language tasks.

A cognitive neuropsychological model of language

The progress of the last 20 years has shown that the nature of the impairments of people with disorders of language is best understood in terms of a model of normal language processing. How people with aphasia use language in real life communication and the ways they employ language to establish their identity in a social world are beyond such models; real life limitations will, of course, in part at least reflect the underlying linguistic impairments. Models of language are useful in interpreting the results of language assessment, and, it can be argued, in designing therapy that should be based on both a knowledge of impaired processes and the intact language processing resources. As Basso and Marangolo (2000, p. 228), put it:

> The most important contribution of cognitive neuropsychology to aphasia therapy lies in the massive reduction of the theoretically-motivated choices left open to the therapist. Clearly articulated and detailed hypotheses about representations and processing of cognitive functions allow rejection of all those strategies for treatment that are not theoretically justified. The more detailed

the cognitive model, the narrower the spectrum of rationally motivated treatments; whereas the less fine-grained the cognitive model, the greater the number of theoretically justifiable therapeutic interventions.

At a single word level, all the current information processing models used in understanding disorders of language can be seen as developments of Morton's (1969) 'logogen model'. The central component in this model is a lexicon in which each known word is represented. Each lexical item (word) can be seen as a 'demon' that seeks evidence (or activation) that it is the required word; once a logogen – representing a lexical item – reaches its threshold, having accumulated enough evidence in accordance with its specification, it 'fires' making a response available at the next level. For an item in the input lexicons (with separate lexicons for spoken and written words), that can be a specification of the word's meaning or its output phonology. For an item in the output lexicons, it would be a specification of the word's phonology or orthography (spelling pattern).

These information processing models of normal processing identify a sequence of stages in different tasks such as spoken language comprehension, spoken language production, reading aloud and repetition. A simple model of spoken word comprehension is shown in Figure 14.1.

The processes specified in the model each transcode one level of representation into another. Retrieving the meaning of a spoken word requires sequential retrieval of information at a number of levels – auditory, phonemic, lexical and semantic. In the case of spoken word comprehension, there are tests that only require access to information at that level. Non-word minimal pair judgments require access only to a phonemic representation (one that specifies in pre-lexical form the segments, or, perhaps, the features of a heard word). Auditory lexical decision (deciding if a spoken string is a real word or not) can be done on the basis of lexical activation alone. It could also be done on the basis of retrieval of word meaning at a semantic level, but this is not necessary. So there are, for example,

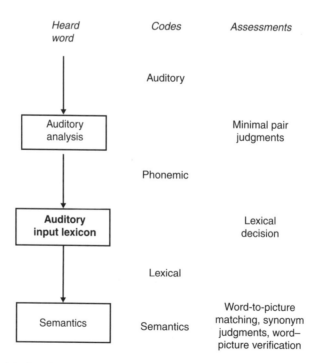

Figure 14.1 A model of spoken word comprehension.

patients who can do lexical decision accurately for words that they cannot understand (e.g. Franklin, Howard, and Patterson 1994). Word comprehension tasks, such as word-to-picture matching or synonym judgments, rely on retrieval of semantics.

The importance of such models to the assessment and treatment of people with aphasia is that data shows that different components can be selectively impaired. An implication of this is that processing at different levels is largely independent from processing at other levels. So, for example, access to a word form at the level of the auditory input lexicon may be impaired when both auditory analysis (as assessed by minimal pair judgments) and semantics (as assessed by good written word comprehension) are intact. The system for spoken word comprehension, nevertheless, comprises a sequence of stages; as a result normal operation at one stage necessarily requires input from earlier stages. The result is that one would expect to find knock-on effects. A person with impaired auditory analysis will, therefore, also perform poorly in tasks tapping lexical access and spoken word comprehension. A person with an impairment at a lexical level will have normal minimal pair judgments, but have difficulties in spoken word comprehension; and a person with difficulties in access to semantics will have poor understanding of spoken words, but good performance in minimal pair judgments and lexical decision.

Table 14.1 shows the performance of three patients on tasks tapping different levels in auditory comprehension; all of the patients have better comprehension of written words than spoken words, showing that they must have impairment at some level in spoken word comprehension. It shows precisely the pattern the model in Figure 14.1 suggests.

Figure 14.2 elaborates the model to add the components necessary for spoken word production. Again this is a sequence of stages. A semantic representation accesses a representation of the word's phonological form. Phonological assembly then converts this into a form suitable for driving articulation. The critical claim here is that the processes of word production are largely independent of those necessary for word comprehension, although the central semantic component is common to production and comprehension. This captures the frequent observations that people with aphasia can have difficulties in spoken word comprehension without difficulties in spoken word production (as in 'pure word deafness') e.g. Auerbach, Allard, Naeser, Alexander, and Albert 1982), and that, conversely, word retrieval can be impaired without difficulties in word comprehension (as, for example in 'lexical anomia') (e.g. Howard 1995). In contrast, profound difficulties at a semantic level affect both word comprehension and production as in some people with aphasia (Hillis, Rapp, Romani, and Caramazza, 1990; Howard and Orchard-Lisle 1984) as well as people with semantic dementia (Garrard and Hodges 2000; Hodges, Patterson, Oxbury, and Funnell 1992).

Figure 14.2 also includes additional routines to accommodate word repetition. The sublexical mapping from auditory input to spoken output is needed to account for people's ability to repeat non-words that have no lexical representation. The direct connection from the input lexicon to the output lexicon permits repetition of real words without semantic mediation (McCarthy and Warrington 1984).

Evidence used in identifying the levels of breakdown in word production come from three different types of source. First, the variables that affect word retrieval accuracy, such as word imageability (or concreteness), frequency and length. Imageability effects suggest difficulties at a semantic level, or in

Table 14.1 Performance of three people with aphasia on three tasks tapping different levels in spoken word comprehension. (Per cent correct; impaired scores are in italics)

Task	TON	MK	DRB
Minimal pairs	67	94	91
Lexical decision	69	67	97
Synonym judgements	67	74	78

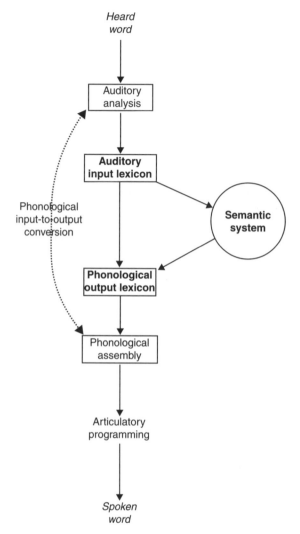

Figure 14.2 A model for spoken word comprehension and production and repetition (based on Whitworth, Webster and Howard in press).

the input to or output from semantics. Poorer performance with longer words indicates an impairment in post-lexical processes of phonological assembly or articulation. Frequency effects are more complex; in semantic dementia, for example, the semantics of less frequently used words is more severely affected (Lambon Ralph, Graham, Ellis, and Hodges 1998). Word frequency can also affect the mapping from semantics to the phonological lexicon or damage to lexical representations (e.g. Howard 1995). The second source of evidence used is the nature of errors produced. In general semantically related errors are consistent with either impairment to semantics (Hillis *et al.* 1990; Howard and Orchard-Lisle 1984) or difficulties in access to the output lexicon (Caramazza and Hillis 1990). Phonologically related errors are most probably due to either impairment of lexical phonological representations or in phonological assembly (Nickels 1997). Unrelated non-words (neologisms) may reflect difficulties in lexical retrieval (Butterworth 1979) or severe impairments in post-lexical phonological assembly. The third kind of evidence is performance in other tasks that share processing components. For instance, an impairment in phonological assembly should be evident in spoken picture naming, in word and non-word repetition and in word and non-word reading (Caplan, Vanier and Baker 1986). Similarly, a central impairment in semantics will result in difficulties in spoken and written word comprehension and spoken and written word production (Hillis *et al.* 1990). Converging evidence from all three sources can be used to identify the level or level(s) of impairment contributing to the processing difficulties of a person with aphasia.

The routines needed for written word comprehension and production as well as reading aloud and writing to dictation are added in Figure 14.3. The result is a diagram of considerable complexity; yet this model in this form deals only with single word comprehension and production. It requires elaboration to accommodate the procedures needed for sentence comprehension and production.

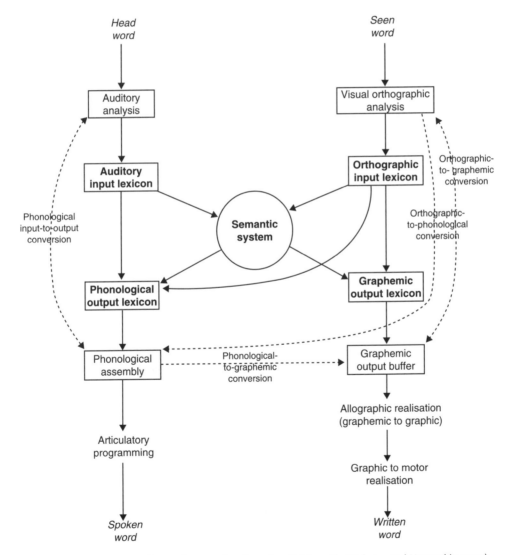

Figure 14.3 A model of single word processing (based on Whitworth, Webster and Howard in press).

Some critics have expressed disquiet about the complexity of these models. But language is complex, and the complexity of the model is necessary. As Coltheart *et al.* (2001) put it, 'All the complexities of the model are motivated. If any box or arrow were deleted from it, the result would be a system that would fail in at least one language-processing task at which humans succeed' (p. 211).

Closely related models have been used to explore and explain a variety of patterns of impairment in single word processing that occur in people with aphasia, for example by Morton and Patterson (1980), Patterson and Shewell (1987), Ellis and Young (1988), and Hillis and Caramazza (1995) amongst many others. In this diagrammatic form these models are a considerable aid to diagnosis and analysis of aphasic disorders, yet they are clearly a simplification. Each of the boxes – that is modules – carries out processing and will necessarily have internal structure. For instance, Levelt, Roelofs and Meyer (1999) advance a detailed model of phonological encoding that details a number of sub-processes involved in phonological assembly including spell out of the phoneme sequence, assignment of stress patterns and articulatory programming that has received some support in understanding the detailed patterns found in people with aphasia who make phonological errors in production (e.g. Howard and Smith 2002; Nickels and Howard 2000).

Worries that using models of this kind to analyse language in aphasia would result in the proliferation of modules proposed in an ad hoc way to account for individual patterns of performance (e.g. Seidenberg 1988) have proved unfounded. The model in this form has proved remarkably durable. In fact the pressure has been towards simplification; for instance, Hillis and Caramazza (1995) have argued that the 'direct routes' from the auditory input lexicon and the orthographic input lexicon to the phonological output lexicon may be unnecessary. They argue that the summation of information from a lexical route via semantics and a sublexical route is sufficient to account for the existing data.

Competing models

Two kinds of important criticisms can be made of the cognitive neuropsychological model described in the previous section. The first is that they postulate more levels of processing and representation than are necessary. By Occam's razor, a simpler model that can accommodate the same data would be preferable. The second criticism is that, by not being explicit about the detailed operation of the component processes, it has too much power. A model that is explicit about the forms of processing can make specific quantitative predictions about performance.

One proposal for simplification is to combine the input and output lexicons, leaving one lexicon used for both spoken word production and spoken word recognition, and another for written word recognition and production as proposed by Allport and Funnell (1981, see Figure 14.4A). Selective deficits in production or comprehension can then be accounted for by impairment to connections specific to the task. Some evidence in favour of this proposal comes from Behrmann and Bub's (1992) finding with one patient that words impaired for reading were also difficult to write to dictation. One difficulty faced by this model is that it has difficulty in accounting for word production deficits that appear to be due to a specifically *lexical* impairment, with no comprehension difficulties for the same words (e.g. Howard 1995). A second difficulty comes with people who make semantic errors in single word repetition – sometimes called 'deep dysphasia' (Howard and Franklin 1988). When 'woman' is repeated as 'lady', it is clear that the semantics corresponding to the stimulus has been accessed; this necessarily requires that the lexical entry for *woman* has been correctly accessed. The difficulty is to explain why access to this lexical entry fails to result in correct spoken word production.

Martin and Saffran (1992) and Martin, Dell, Saffran, and Schwartz (1994) developed an interactive activation model in which bidirectional links support both word comprehension and production.

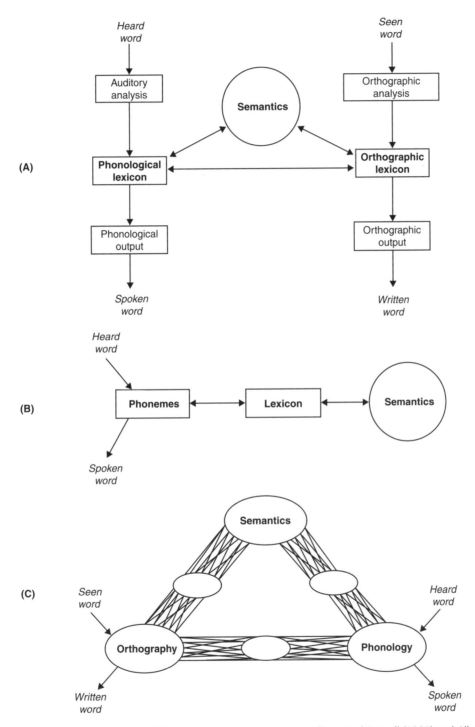

Figure 14.4 Competing models: **(A)** Two lexicon model, based on Allport and Funnell (1981) and Allport (1985). **(B)** Interactive activation model with a single lexicon and a common network for comprehension and production, based on Martin et al. (1994). **(C)** The triangle model, with distributed representations joined by bidirectional connections via hidden units, based on Seidenberg and McClelland (1989) Plaut et al. (1996) and Patterson and Lambon Ralph (1999).

They used a computational version of this model to account for the pattern of errors in both repetition and naming of a person with aphasia, N.C. Strikingly they were able to show that a model with a single phonological lexicon could account for semantic errors in repetition. However, a number of difficulties with this model became apparent, leading Dell *et al.* (1997) to abandon it in this form as a model of word comprehension, confining its scope to accounting for patterns of errors in naming. These difficulties included: (i) the finding that, even in its unlesioned form the model made 37 per cent errors in word comprehension (Nickels and Howard 1995) (ii) it failed to account for the relationship between naming and repetition in people with aphasia other than NC (Dell *et al.* 1997), (iii) it could not account for normal people's ability to repeat non-words (Nickels and Howard 1995). Its ability to account for the patterns of naming errors found in people with aphasia has also been seriously challenged (Ruml and Caramazza 2000; Ruml, Caramazza, Shelton, and Chialant 2000).

A more radical computational model – the triangle model (see Figure 14.4C) – has been advanced by McClelland, Plaut, Seidenberg and Patterson (Patterson and Lambon Ralph 1999; Plaut, McClelland, Seidenberg, and Patterson 1996; Seidenberg and McClelland 1989). This has only three components: semantics, phonology, and orthography. Each of these domains is linked by bidirectional connections with hidden units. There is no lexical representation; the same network is used for both real word and non-word processing. Knowledge about individual words is distributed across the connection strengths of the units connecting each level; these connection strengths are acquired during a learning process. This model is, to some extent, motivated by a wish to develop a model that is neurologically plausible, with multiply connected, distributed representations. In addition to the rejection of any localised representation, the triangle model has a single phonological domain and a single orthographic domain serving both input and output. Early explorations of the direct mapping from orthography to phonology (i.e. reading aloud) shows that a single computational system is able to account for the basic findings in single syllable word reading from normal people and people with a variety of kinds of acquired dyslexia, although this is only successful with a particular local representation of graphemes and phonemes in the phonological and orthographic domains (Plaut *et al.* 1996). Further promising results are reported in Plaut and Shallice's (1993) implementation of the mapping from orthography to phonology via semantics, that they use to model deep dyslexia – a reading disorder characterised by semantic errors in single word reading.

These results are promising, but they only involve simulations within limited domains, using only feed-forward mappings. As Plaut *et al.* (1996) emphasise, the behaviour of a computational model is difficult to predict in advance. Simulations are required. As a result it is premature to evaluate whether the full interactive triangle model has the potential to account for the range of associations and dissociations in performance found in people with aphasia.

Language in the brain

Interest in how and where language is represented in the brain goes back to before Broca's famous paper in 1861. A flurry of work in the latter half of the nineteenth century that attempted to link sites of lesions in people with aphasia with their patterns of language performance resulted in the Wernicke-Lichtheim model of language (see Figure 14.5) (Howard 1997; Lichtheim 1885). This has three principle components, all located in the left hemisphere. Broca's area in the left inferior frontal gyrus is responsible for spoken language production, controlling the actions of the articulatory motor cortex, which lies just posterior to it. Wernicke's area lies just behind the primary auditory cortex and is used for language comprehension. This is linked to Broca's area by the arcuate fasciculus that is necessary for repetition. Wernicke's area also modulates spoken language production; damage to either Wernicke's area or the arcuate fasciculus results in fluent but paraphasic speech. Semantic representations are not

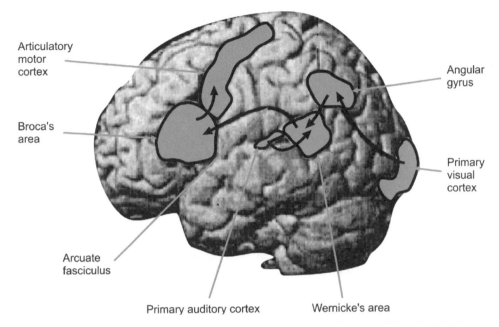

Articulatory
motor
cortex

Broca's
area

Arcuate
fasciculus

Primary auditory cortex

Wernicke's area

Angular
gyrus

Primary
visual
cortex

Figure 14.5 Areas of the brain involved in language processing according to the Wernicke-Lichtheim model; based on Geschwind (1979).

localised, but consist of associations between different types of sensory features localised in different parts of the cortex. To this set of regions, Déjerine (1891) added the angular gyrus, necessary for both written word recognition and for writing. In reading aloud, visual input to the primary visual cortex connects to the angular gyrus that then projects to Wernicke's area. This in turn connects via the arcuate fasciculus to Broca's area that drives the reading response (Bub, Arguin, and Lecours 1993).

This model was built on a very limited corpus of data from people with quite careful post-mortems but often very poorly described aphasia (Caplan 1987). Although a variety of kinds of data inconsistent with this model were available from very early on (see e.g. Mohr 1976), and it was subjected to trenchant criticism from several quarters (e.g. Freud 1891; Head 1926; Marie 1906), it has shown remarkable longevity. It is still rare to find a textbook that does not present this as the correct view about language localisation. It has been, as Mohr (1976) notes, almost immune to falsification.

The cognitive neuropsychological model described in the preceding section says nothing about how the modules involved might be represented in the brain. Each of the information processing modules might, in principle, be distributed across cortical regions or localised. The occurrence of selective deficits after localised brain damage does, however, suggest that parts of the brain are specialised for processing of individual functions.

Yet there is considerable similarity between the Wernicke-Lichtheim model and the cognitive neuropsychological models. Both specify modules for spoken word production and recognition, and visual word recognition and the connections between them. Yet the difference is that the intentions are radically different: the cognitive neuropsychological model is a model of information processing, whereas the Wernicke-Lichtheim model is a model of neurological organisation where psychological functions are directly equivalent to neural structures. As Wernicke (1874) put it 'the basic elementary hypothesis that can now hardly be challenged [is] that the central nerve endings are invested with the role of psychic elements' (p.143 in Eggert 1977 translation).

From the early 1970s, the development of *in vivo* structural imaging of lesions using CT and, later, MRI scans allowed a much richer database to be developed to assess the adequacy of this model, with much more careful description of the patients' language disorders. An obvious technique – sometimes called 'hotspotting' – was to take a set of people with aphasia, all showing a common symptom, and overlay the areas of their lesions. The area whose lesion is critical to producing the symptom should be in the area of overlap. The most successful use of this approach is by Dronkers (1996) who showed that a small region in the anterior insular cortex was affected by the lesion in all of 25 people with articulatory apraxia and none of a group of 19 people with left hemisphere lesions who did not have articulatory difficulties. Dronkers concluded that the anterior insula played a role in articulatory programming. Hillis *et al.* (2004), however, found results with acute studies that did not support this conclusion. They point out that the anterior insula is the typical region of lesion overlap for people with left middle cerebral artery stroke. In a study with people with acute language difficulties (in the first few days after stroke) they found that articulatory apraxia was associated with reduced cerebral blood flow in Broca's area.

The study by Dronkers (1996) is rather exceptional in producing clear (although controversial) results using the lesion overlap approach (see Howard 1997 for a review). There are a number of reasons for this. First, even if a particular region is critical for performing a particular function, we would not necessarily expect to find an area of lesion overlap. In addition to lesions of the critical area, any lesion elsewhere that disconnects it from its inputs or its outputs will have, functionally, the same effect. Second, it makes the assumption that only the areas that are structurally affected by a lesion will be non-functional. Recent metabolic scans have shown that areas of hypometabolism are typically much more extensive than structural lesions (Hillis *et al.* 2004). Third, it makes the assumption that the neural architecture of language functions will be universal; that is all people will localise different functions in the same way. The plausibility of this assumption is challenged by demonstrations of reorganisation and relocalisation of functions after brain damage (e.g. Jenkins and Merzenich 1992), and inconsistency between people in the areas where temporary electrical lesions of the exposed cortex during surgery result in effects on language functions (e.g. Ojemann 1991).

Recent work on the cortical representation of language has concentrated on using functional imaging, using PET or fMRI scans, to investigate the areas of the brain that receive increased blood flow while normal people are engaged in language tasks. This approach has a number of features. First, by using healthy subjects it circumvents potential problems of relocalisation or reorganisation as a result of a lesion, and, by seeking areas that are active across a group of subjects it can identify areas of common activation, discarding exceptional patterns as statistical noise. Second, it shows areas that are involved in a task; lesions in contrast may provide information only about the areas that are necessary (Price and Friston 2002).

While functional imaging can show the areas active when people perform a particular language task, drawing conclusions about the processing that those areas are doing is less straightforward. This is partly because there is substantial evidence of automatic processing of language. For example, on hearing a word a normal person will automatically activate its meaning, as well as probably its output phonology and its orthography. As a result, cunning experimental design is needed to isolate the areas responsible for different types of processing. Second, the interpretation of *increases* in cerebral blood flow is not simple. For example, consider the comparison of the areas activated during the hearing of real words and non-words. On one view, only real words can activate a lexical entry for auditory word recognition, so one might expect increased regional cerebral blood flow (rCBF) with real words compared to non-words in the region responsible for spoken word recognition. Another hypothesis is that real words will be quickly and efficiently recognised requiring little synaptic activity whereas the unsuccessful attempt to recognise the non-word will result in much greater processing effort. On this hypothesis, we would therefore expect to find greater rCBF for non-words than words in areas involved in auditory word recognition. Thirdly, functional imaging provides no information about the *sequence* in which activated areas become involved.[1] Interpretation of this is further limited by real anatomical uncertainty on how language related regions of the cortex are connected. For example there is still considerable uncertainty whether Broca's and Wernicke's areas are connected by the arcuate fasciculus (Passingham 1993). Fourth, it is unclear what we might expect to be localised. In particular, are different kinds of codes going to correspond to activations, or will we see activations corresponding to transcodings (cf. Fig. 14.1)? And, what kinds of representations will be broadly distributed (resulting perhaps in no localised changes in rCBF) and which will be localised in a consistent way across subjects?

Nevertheless there is now a considerable body of research work using these approaches to identify the language areas. The next part of this section provides a brief overview of some selected representative results of this effort; for a more detailed review see, for example, Price (2000).

In Figure 14.6A the black shaded area shows the regions that Mummery *et al.* (1999) found were significantly more activated by hearing words than by noise. This should identify the areas involved in phoneme perception, auditory lexical access, and also, perhaps, automatic activation of semantics. The activation extends across much of the superior temporal gyrus in both the left and right hemisphere, excluding the temporal pole. The right hemisphere activation is not expected in terms of the Wernicke-Lichtheim model, and, in the left hemisphere, the activation is more extensive than the model suggests. Nevertheless the bilateral activation is compatible with the observation that severe word sound deafness (a difficulty in phoneme perception) requires bilateral temporal lesions (Buchman, Garron, Trost-Cardamone, Wichter, and Schwartz 1986). The grey areas in Figure 14.6A show the areas that Giraud and Price (2001) showed were activated more by repeating heard words than by naming sounds. Both of these tasks involve spoken word production; the activations should, therefore represent phonological and lexical processing of heard words. This shows much less extensive activation, mainly limited to Wernicke's area bilaterally.

Figure 14.6B summarises three studies that look for areas active in speech production. The areas shaded in black show the regions that Price *et al.* (1996) found were significantly more active when repeating words than when listening; this should show the whole set of areas involved in phonological word form retrieval and generation of articulation. This includes large bilateral activations in the perisylvian regions, including Broca's and Wernicke's areas and their homologues in the right hemisphere, as well as articulatory sensorimotor cortex bilaterally, the supplementary motor area and the cingulate gyrus. The involvement of both Wernicke's and Broca's area was postulated by the Wernicke-Lichtheim model, although activation of their right hemisphere homologues was not anticipated. Lesion evidence suggests that these right hemisphere regions are not necessary for speech production – large perisylvian lesions in the right hemisphere rarely result in more than very subtle language impairments. In contrast, lesions extending over these areas on the left frequently result in global aphasia (Willmes and Poeck 1993). The areas shown in grey were those activated more by repeating words than listening to words and saying 'OK' (Giraud and Price 2001). This comparison, that should isolate areas involved in phonological word retrieval, shows activation bilaterally in superior temporal cortex, and in right articulatory sensorimotor cortex. There is also activation of the left anterior insular cortex – the area that Dronkers' (1996) lesion study identified as critical in causing articulatory apraxia – and in the left posterior inferior temporal lobe at the junction with the cerebellum, a region that Price (2000) showed was activated in common by a set of eight different tasks involving phonological word retrieval. The areas that Price identified in this conjunction are shown in white in Figure 14.6B; in addition to the activation in the posterior inferior temporal cortex there is another area of activation involving the left anterior insula and/or the frontal operculum.

---

[1] The recently developed technique of magneto-encephalography (MEG), although it provides poorer localisation information and is only sensitive to activation in areas near to the skull surface, provides very precise information about timing. Used in conjunction with functional imaging, MEG has considerable potential in unpacking processing sequences.

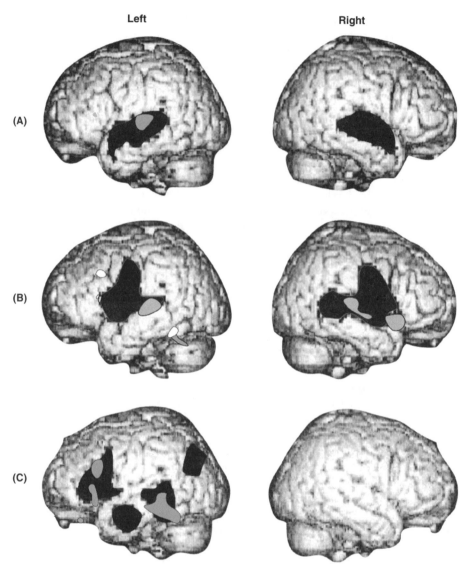

Left

Right

(A)

(B)

(C)

Figure 14.6 Areas of the brain active during single word processing language tasks: **(A)** Auditory word recognition; **(B)** Spoken word production; **(C)** Semantic processing. For a detailed description see text.

A careful study by Wise *et al.* (1999) sought to identify areas involved in phonological retrieval and articulation by comparing word repetition with listening. The areas more active in repetition than listening were articulatory sensorimotor cortex bilaterally, the rostral cerebellum, the anterior cingulate and the left posterior pallidum. Among these are some areas that, when damaged, result in long term difficulties in speech production such as the sensorimotor cortex, and the cerebellum. Other areas that, when damaged, result in short-lasting or more permanent impairments in speech production are not activated, such as Broca's area, the supplementary motor area and the anterior insula (this latter area was activated as much by listening as repetition). There are other areas that are activated – the posterior pallidum and the anterior cingulate – that, on the basis of lesion evidence, have no documented effects on speech production.

While these data show that a whole network of areas are involved in phonological retrieval and speech production, their roles are not yet clearly established from functional imaging studies. Interestingly, Broca's area is not consistently involved in speech production tasks; this casts serious doubt on its proposed role as a source of 'motor word images'. Broca's area is much more consistently activated in tasks involving the comprehension of syntactically complex sentences (Caplan, Alpert, and Waters 1999; Grodzinsky 2000); this accords with the observation that many – but not all – people with Broca's aphasia have difficulties in the comprehension of such sentences.

Wernicke (1874) and Allport (1985) argued that semantic representations, at least for concrete words, were distributed across different cortical regions as a set of sensory features associated with different sensory modalities. If this is true, functional activation studies may find it difficult to find any activations that are large enough to reach significance. The first studies by Petersen *et al.* (1988, 1989) associated semantic processing with the left dorso-lateral frontal cortex, but used a difficult task (noun-verb association) that, because it was difficult, required considerable executive functions. Vandenberghe *et al.* (1996) compared activations from associative semantic judgments on pictures or words, with the activations from size judgments on the same stimuli. They found that semantic judgment on words and pictures activated an extensive network in the left hemisphere, illustrated in black in Figure 14.6C. This includes, in addition to an activation in dorso-lateral frontal cortex, the anterior part of the middle temporal lobe, the posterior inferior temporal gyrus extending into the middle temporal gyrus, and the posterior parietal lobe. Once more it is not clear what these areas are doing. The frontal activation seems to occur only where active – and often difficult – semantic judgments are made, and may represent a decision-making, executive component (Roskies, Fiez, Balota, Raichle, and Petersen 2001). The activations in the inferior temporal gyrus are consonant with data from people with semantic dementia, who, as a result of atrophy in the inferolateral temporal lobe show progressive deterioration of semantics (Garrard and Hodges 2000; Hodges *et al.* 1992). The activation in the posterior parietal lobe is less easily interpreted, but may possibly relate to information about object location (Mummery, Patterson, Hodges, and Price 1998), action semantics (Devlin *et al.* 2002), or verbally learned knowledge (Noppeney and Price 2003).

The study by Noppenney and Price (2002) investigated the regions that were specifically concerned in semantic decisions on spoken words, using the judgment 'Is the sound described by the stimulus word usually loud?', using a number of other conditions to control for the activations attributable to input and output. Although the semantic judgment used in this study is very different from that used by Vandenberghe *et al.* (1996) the activations show considerable similarity with both the posterior inferior temporal and dorso-lateral frontal regions activated. Interestingly, in view of Wernicke's (1874) hypothesis that semantic representations are associative networks across sensory modalities, this semantic judgment about the auditory properties of words did not recruit activation in areas that seem likely to code words' auditory properties.

Many other lines of evidence support the importance of inferior temporal regions for semantic processing. For example, Wise *et al.* (1999) and d'Esposito *et al.* (1997) showed that the middle fusiform gyrus on the floor of the left temporal lobe was specifically activated by more imageable words. This result can be related directly to the finding that most people with acquired aphasia after stroke have specific difficulties with abstract words (e.g. Franklin 1989). Aphasia-causing stroke typically involves lesions involving the middle cerebral artery, leaving this area that is specifically involved in processing more imageable, concrete words intact.

But what are these inferior temporal regions doing? One possibility is that semantic representations are 'stored' here. Another is that they are involved in the *access* to semantic representations, which may, as Wernicke suggested, be widely distributed. There is some evidence for specialisation within the inferior temporal regions; for instance, the posterior areas on the left are activated more by tools and the temporal pole bilaterally is more activated by animals (Devlin *et al.* 2002).

Attempts to identify the regions responsible for visual word recognition have not yielded much agreement. Early proposals included medial extrastriate cortex in the occipital lobe (Petersen *et al.* 1988; Posner, Petersen, Fox and Raichle 1988) and posterior middle temporal gyrus (Howard *et al.* 1992), but neither is probably correct. One serious problem is that the patterns of activation when written words are presented depends greatly on word presentation duration and rate (Price *et al.* 1994). More recently, Cohen, Dehaene and their colleagues (Cohen *et al.* 2000, 2002; Dehaene, Le Clec'H, Poline, Le Bihan, and Cohen 2002) have argued that the visual word form area is in the fusiform gyrus in the left inferior temporal lobe. Moore and Price (1999) found that this area is activated as much by pictures as written words, and showed that the posterior part of the superior temporal gyrus extending into the parietal lobe was more active for word reading than picture naming. However, when regions more active for reading than for repetition are identified, controlling for the sensory input differences, the posterior part of the infero-lateral temporal cortex is identified (Price 2000).

Conclusion

In summary, functional imaging studies of normal function yield networks of areas involved in different language tasks. The areas involved include those postulated by the Wernicke-Lichtheim model, but are much more extensive. Basal language areas in the inferior temporal lobe are clearly involved in visual and semantic processing, as Nielsen (1946) had suggested. Homologous regions in the right hemisphere show much more extensive involvement than lesion studies had supposed. While considerable progress has been made in the last fifteen years in delineating the areas of the cortex involved in language functioning, the nature of the processing taking place in these regions is not yet clearly established.

15 Tried, tested and trusted?

Language assessment for rehabilitation

Lyndsey Nickels

Abstract

This chapter provides a critical review of clinical assessments used to evaluate acquired language impairments. It reviews assessments aimed at examining both language functions ('impairment'-based approaches), and language activities ('functional' measures). In particular it discusses the adequacy of these assessments as tools in the rehabilitation process. For example, do the assessments lead to a clear description of the language function? If they are to be used to measure treatment efficacy, do they have good test-retest reliability and are they sensitive to change? In addition, the question is raised as to whether there is any relationship between performance on measures of language function and degree of impairment in language activities. The chapter concludes that rehabilitation focused assessment should be hypothesis-driven and goal-focused, and that broad-ranging, comprehensive assessments are inappropriate.

Introduction and overview

This chapter is concerned with current practice in the assessment of acquired language impairments (aphasia). However, we must first determine the purpose of an assessment.

A broad definition might be that an assessment is a diagnostic tool, but what is it that we are trying to diagnose? This takes us to the heart of the debate regarding assessment of acquired language disorders. The diagnosis might be differential diagnosis of aphasia from, for example, dysarthria, dyspraxia or dementia. Alternatively, it might be of the 'type' of aphasia – assigning the individual with aphasia to a 'traditional' syndrome category such as Broca's, Wernicke's or Conduction aphasia. In another view, the role of assessment might be to diagnose the impact of aphasia on communication or quality of life. As we will see, the diversity of assessment for aphasia reflects the different perspectives regarding the aims of the diagnostic process.

Here, I suggest that the purpose of an assessment should be to enable formulation of a hypothesis regarding the areas of strength and weakness in functioning, in order to set appropriate goals for therapy (see also e.g. Byng, Kay, Edmundson and Scott 1990; Howard and Hatfield 1987), and to evaluate the outcome of the therapy process. While this may not be the only role for assessment, the adequacy of assessments as tools in the rehabilitation process is clearly critical for the aphasia therapist, and hence

Table 15.1 The scope of the aphasia therapist (Byng 1993, pp. 127–8)

As the aphasia therapist works towards recovery with a person with aphasia they...

- 'Delineate the uses of language made by the person with aphasia prior to becoming aphasic
- facilitate adjustment to the change in communication skills
- investigate the nature and effects of the language deficit with respect to the whole language system
- attempt to remediate the language deficit itself
- increase the use of all other potential means of communication to support, facilitate and compensate for the use of impaired language
- provide an opportunity to use newly acquired and emerging language skills, not just in a clinical environment, but in more normal communicative situations;
- attempt to change the communication skills of those around the person with aphasia to accommodate the aphasia.'

is the focus of this chapter. It is also important to note that I do not intend to imply that assessment is the only factor for setting goals for treatment. Assessment should be a part of a collaborative process of goal-setting, involving the individual with aphasia and their communicative partners as major players.

Before we can discuss further the adequacy of assessments in the rehabilitation process, we must first consider the scope of that process. As listed in Table 15.1, Byng (1993) argued that aphasia therapists cover a broad range of domains as they work towards recovery with a person with aphasia.

However, not only must the aphasia therapist have the skills to address these different areas, they also have a duty to document the efficacy of their rehabilitation, no matter which approach or combination of approaches is their focus. This requires appropriate assessment before rehabilitation begins, during the rehabilitation process and after rehabilitation (by the therapist) has ended. Howard and Hatfield (1987) note that measuring changes in aphasia requires testing that is

> *Reliable* enough to give consistent measures; that is *sensitive* enough to measure the improvement that the particular therapy involved is intended to produce; and that is *valid* so that it measures changes that are of real consequence in the patients' lives.
>
> (Howard and Hatfield 1987, p. 113)

Hence, reliability, sensitivity and validity will be three main themes running through this paper.

The review of assessments will broadly follow the World Health Organization (WHO 2001) *International Classification of Functioning, Disability and Health* (ICF) in its organisation (see chapter 4). First I shall discuss assessment of language functions (impairment-based approaches) and subsequently assessment of communication activities (functional measures) and quality of life/psychosocial issues. Because of the potential confusion between the WHO use of the term 'function' and the use of the term 'functional' within the rehabilitation community, I will for the most part avoid the use of the former term – instead primarily using 'language impairment' as a shorthand for 'impairment of language functions'. Table 15.2 gives examples of the WHO classification in the language domain.

Language functions: assessment of the language impairment

There are two main approaches to the assessment of the language impairment, which can be broadly described as the 'battery approach' and the 'hypothesis-testing approach'.

The battery approach can be caricatured as one where, whatever the presenting symptoms of aphasia are, you always do the same thing – an aphasia assessment battery. While the choice of battery may be modulated somewhat by severity or time post-onset, it is more likely to reflect the training, theoretical

Table 15.2 Examples of language functions and communication activities from the WHO-ICF classification

Language functions	
Reception of language	Spoken language Written language Sign language
Expression of language	Spoken language Written language Sign language
Integrative language functions	Mental functions that organize semantic and symbolic meaning, grammatical structure and ideas for the production of messages in spoken, written or other forms of language.
Communication activities	
Communicating – receiving	Spoken messages Non-verbal messages Written messages
Communicating – producing	Speaking Producing non-verbal messages Writing messages
Conversation and use of communication devices and techniques	**Conversation:** Starting, sustaining and ending an interchange of thoughts and ideas, carried out by means of spoken, written, sign or other forms of language, with one or more people one knows or who are strangers, in formal or casual settings. **Discussion:** Starting, sustaining and ending an examination of a matter, with arguments for or against, or debate carried out by means of spoken, written, sign or other forms of language, with one or more people one knows or who are strangers, in formal or casual settings **Using communication devices and techniques:** Using devices, techniques and other means for the purposes of communicating, such as calling a friend on the telephone.

perspective and country of origin of the clinician. An individual with aphasia is assessed using the whole of a particular test battery, usually resulting in an overall measure of severity and a profile across the subtests which may be compared to the non-aphasic population and/or the average aphasic, and may be used to assign the individual to an aphasia syndrome category. This approach is embodied in standardised aphasia assessments such as those listed in Table 15.3.

Table 15.3 Examples of (English) Language Batteries for the assessment of aphasia

Full assessments
Boston Diagnostic Aphasia Examination (BDAE, Goodglass and Kaplan 1983), Minnesota Test for Differential Diagnosis of Aphasia (MTDDA; Schuell 1965), Porch Index of Communicative Ability (PICA; Porch 1967, 1981), Western Aphasia Battery (WAB, Kertesz 1982),

Screening assessments
Aphasia Screening Test (AST; Whurr 1996), Frenchay Aphasia Screening Test (FAST; Enderby *et al.* 1987; Enderby and Crow 1996).

In contrast, the hypothesis-testing approach uses observations from interacting with the individual with aphasia (and/or others reports of the individual's language behaviour) to form a hypothesis regarding language processing. The hypothesis must be related to a particular theory of language processing (usually instantiated in a model, e.g. Kay, Lesser and Coltheart 1992) and will comprise predictions regarding which language functions are intact and which are impaired. This hypothesis may be very general (e.g. possible word-finding impairments, and intact comprehension) or more specific (e.g. a semantic impairment from observation of semantic errors in word production, see Table 15.4 for examples). On the basis of this hypothesis the clinician chooses the assessment that they believe initially will be the most informative to support/refute the hypothesis. This assessment may be a formal assessment, but may equally use informal assessment methods in the first instance (e.g. observing accuracy of answers to biographical questions). The results of assessment will then be used to revise the hypothesis, and cyclical testing will continue until such a point where a sufficiently clear picture is formed to provide a focus for therapy. Howard and Hatfield (1987) note that treatment-planning does not rely on demonstrating beyond all reasonable doubt what the underlying impairment is 'all that is required is a hypothesis sufficiently detailed to be able to motivate therapy. ... Treatment is then a test of the hypothesis' (p. 130). This is illustrated graphically in Figure 15.1.

The hypothesis testing approach to assessment is most commonly associated with the cognitive neuropsychological approach, and the assessment materials provided by the Psycholinguistic Assessments of Language Processing Ability in Aphasia (PALPA); Kay, Lesser and Coltheart 1992; but see also e.g. Pyramids and Palm Trees Test, Howard and Patterson 1992; Sentence Processing Resource Pack, Marshall *et al.* 1998). However, the majority of experienced clinicians have advanced hypothesis formation skills, often described as 'clinical intuition'. This term devalues what is in fact a highly sophisticated mechanism of observation of symptoms and matching to a stored internal database of previous cases (both observed and learned), in order to form a hypothesis about the likely impairment underlying the symptom, the skills that may be retained and what co-occurring impairments there may be. This sophisticated skill is often so automated that clinicians may be unable to articulate the steps leading to the formation of the hypothesis, but a hypothesis it is nonetheless. Moreover, many experienced clinicians using a battery approach will be able to predict the performance on some parts of the assessment battery, prior to administration – this is hypothesis formation on the basis of observed behaviour. It is also important to note that the hypothesis testing approach to aphasia assessment is not restricted to impairment level assessment – it can (and should) be used to guide choice of assessment at activity and participation levels too, this will be discussed further below.

Adequacy of standardised aphasia batteries I: identification of the impairment

There has been a great deal of debate regarding the adequacy of standardised aphasia batteries for the rehabilitation-focused assessment of aphasia (see, for example, Byng *et al.* 1990; David 1990; Goodglass 1990; Kay, Byng, Edmundson and Scott 1990; Kertesz 1988, 1990; Weniger 1990, Weniger and Sarno 1990). Byng *et al.* (1990) question whether 'the clinician's time is well spent in carrying out any of these assessments if they neither clarify what is wrong nor specify what treatment should be provided' (p. 67). However, as they note, assessment batteries (specifically, MTDDA, PICA, BDAE, WAB) were not designed primarily to elucidate the underlying nature of the language disorder: interpretation is in terms of diagnosis of a syndrome on the basis of the surface symptoms of the language impairment (but see Goodglass 1990, and BDAE third edition, Goodglass, Kaplan and Barresi 2001). It is widely acknowledged that individuals within these syndrome categories are not homogeneous, and hence the categories do not reveal the individual variations in the nature of the language impairment. The key difference between advocates of the two approaches appears to rest on the

Table 15.4 Examples of hypotheses, their source and ways of testing these hypotheses

Example of an initial hypothesis	Evidence on which hypothesis was based	Examples of means of testing hypothesis:	
		Formal	Informal
Word-finding impairment	Informal interview – 'empty speech' with circumlocutions, clear awareness of inability to retrieve correct lexical items and appropriate response to questions.	*Assessment of naming:* e.g. Boston Naming Test (Kaplan et al. 1983); Graded Naming test (Mckenna and Warrington, 1980)	*Biographical questions requiring specific responses* (and preferably where experimenter knows the answers from other sources): e.g. What's your son's occupation?; What suburb do you live in?
...with good comprehension		*Comprehension assessment:* e.g. Pyramids and Palm Trees (Howard and Patterson, 1992); Word-Picture matching subtests 47/48 from PALPA	*Biographical forced choice or yes/No questions with semantically related distractors:* e.g. Is your son an civil engineer or electrical engineer? Do you live in a house or a unit? Does your daughter live in Manchester? (When in fact she lives in Liverpool).
Semantic impairment	Informal interview – semantic errors in word production		

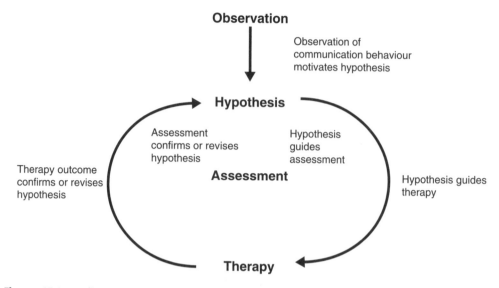

Figuere 15.1 A diagrammatic representation of the Hypothesis Testing approach to assessment and treatment of aphasia (Adapted from Cole, 1993).

perceived importance of these limitations in the syndrome classifications. Proponents of the battery testing approach, such as Kertesz (1988), suggest that they do not detract from the usefulness of syndromes in general, and in particular for planning therapy. In contrast, Byng *et al.*, as advocates of the hypothesis testing approach (e.g. Byng *et al.* 1990; Kay *et al.* 1992) argue that as the syndromes are heterogeneous, and also accuracy in assigning individuals to categories is often less than perfect, they tell one very little about underlying language impairment and hence are of little benefit for focusing treatment.

Goodglass (1990) argues that while syndrome classification is part of the role of standardised aphasia batteries, they also aim to provide the clinician with an overview of language skills (see also Goodglass *et al.* 2001). Indeed, at least in the UK and Australia, this is the more common goal for clinicians performing the assessments. However, an overview of language skills as assessed by performance on certain subtests is only of value when interpreted within a theoretical framework. The batteries do not provide this framework, although the data from them can, of course, be used to generate a hypothesis regarding language function within other theoretical frameworks. However, as surface symptoms are not reliable indicators of underlying language impairment, often, and at best, the assessment must lead to further testing. For example, the six item auditory comprehension of object names subtest on the BDAE may lead to an observation of impaired auditory comprehension, but the nature of this impairment remains obscure – only with further testing will it be possible to determine whether the impairment is one of semantic processing, or of impaired processing of auditory input, or non-language skills (e.g. acoustic processing, visual recognition) or task demands (e.g. memory, attention). Even if performance on this subtest is unimpaired, further testing would be required to determine if single word auditory comprehension was intact under more stringent conditions (e.g. with semantically related distractors, and for abstract words; it is of note that the third edition of the BDAE now incorporates semantically related distractors in the testing of auditory comprehension, and more stimuli: n = 17 for objects in the standard form). The critical question is whether having performed the battery provides sufficient additional information over and above informal observation and selective assessment to warrant the time taken to perform it. In my personal experience the answer was often 'no', although as a student with less developed observational skills and only emergent hypothesis testing skills, the overview provided would no doubt have been useful to me. Nevertheless, whether a screening battery or informal assessment also would be sufficient for this purpose is open to debate.

Hence, as a clinician converted to cognitive neuropsychology early in my career, I would join with Byng, Kay, Howard and others to argue that the hypothesis testing approach is the most efficient and clinically useful approach to assessing language impairment. It allows clear identification of the retained and impaired language functions with two primary limitations, the accuracy and degree of detail of current theories of language processing and the skill of the clinician at relating observations to theory to form hypotheses. However, it is important to note that neither the battery approach nor the hypothesis testing approach specifies what specific treatment, nor which treatment approach, is appropriate. Nevertheless, it is argued that a clearer understanding of the underlying nature of the language disorder better enables the clinician to determine which kind of treatment might be appropriate (for further discussion see, for example, Basso and Marongolo 2000; Caramazza 1989; Hillis 1993; Howard 2000; Howard and Hatfield 1987; Mitchum and Berndt 1995; Nickels 2002; Shallice 2000; Wilshire and Coslett 2000; Wilson and Patterson 1990).

Adequacy of standardised aphasia batteries II: measuring change

Performance on aphasia batteries is also commonly used to measure the evolution and change of aphasia for an individual over time (both with and without therapy). However, they have also been argued to be inadequate on these grounds (e.g. David 1990; Kay *et al.* 1990; Weniger 1990). As discussed earlier, one of the requirements of assessments for measuring effects of treatment is that they should show sensitivity to change. While over the battery as a whole there are large numbers of stimuli, within each subtest the numbers of items are generally (and necessarily) small. This means that improvement in a specific area (as a result, for example, of therapy targeted at that area) will not be represented in the overall score (nor will it be significant on its own because of the small number of stimuli). (Once again it is interesting to note that the revised third edition of the BDAE generally incorporates more stimuli per subtest).

In addition, aphasic individuals are generally variable in performance on particular stimuli from one testing session to another. For example, Howard, Patterson, Franklin *et al.* (1984) demonstrated that while the overall naming accuracy remained stable from session to session, naming performance on an item one day did not reliably predict performance a couple of days later. Moreover, in addition to the intrinsic variability arising from the language disturbance itself, extrinsic variability (from influences external to the aphasia) may cause variation – e.g. performance is worse in the afternoon (Marshall, Tompkins, and Phillips 1980). The smaller the numbers of items in an assessment, the harder it is to distinguish 'real' change from the 'noise' caused by variability. Hence, as Howard and Hatfield (1987) conclude 'standardised tests that measure a non-specific overall level of deficit cannot be expected to measure specific improvement – particularly when the unreliability of performance is taken into account' (p. 114).

In sum, standardised aphasia batteries are argued to be wholly inadequate for rehabilitation, they neither specify the impairment nor allow clear documentation of change over time (see also David 1990; Howard and Hatfield 1987; Kay *et al.* 1990; Weniger 1990). It is suggested that for rehabilitation, a hypothesis-testing approach to assessment of language impairment is most efficient. Identification of the language profile (impairments and retained skills) using reliable measures containing sufficient stimuli to enable confident and replicable diagnoses within a theoretical model of language processing. These same assessments can and should be used to evaluate change over time and the effects of therapy (incorporating appropriate methodological controls, see for example Howard and Hatfield 1987; Nickels 2002).

Communication activities and participation I: functional assessments of language use

No therapist would disagree with the statement that a therapy is of no use unless it has a benefit for the individual's life; not just for their performance on an assessment that bears little resemblance to any communicative act (e.g. lexical decision). While it is possible, of course, that improvement with no functional communicative benefit may have psychological benefits – e.g. reduced levels of depression, increased self-esteem – it is beyond the scope of this paper to discuss this further. In this section we will address assessments that attempt to measure language use in context.

It is less than clear where to draw the boundary between investigations of language impairment and functional measures of language use. Worrall (2000) notes that there has been confusion in the literature as to whether the functional approach extends to the impairment level. She suggests that, when used by speech-language pathologists, reference to this approach (and the term 'functional communication') does not include the domain of impairment. Crucial to this debate is the distinction and relationship between functional communication and pragmatics. Pragmatics is the linguistic field examining the system of rules that regulate the use of language in context (Bates 1976). Assessment techniques include pragmatic profiles, conversational analysis and discourse analysis, all of which may be considered to measure aspects of communicative behaviour. Hence, some authors argue that these are measures of functional communication at the activity level (e.g. Armstrong 1993; Ferguson 1994). However, these assessments do more than document the success or failure of language use in context, but rather systematically attempt to identify which aspects of this process differ from the norm. This is clearly parallel to the aims of the impairment-focused assessments (within the hypothesis-testing approach) described in the section above.

Worrall (2000) notes that while pragmatics is a field of linguistics that has been applied to disordered communication, the concept of functional communication stemmed from the medical rehabilitation setting. More recently the distinction between the approaches has often become blurred, with speech-language pathologists using the terms interchangeably, and some authors using pragmatic theory to develop functional communication assessments (e.g. Skinner *et al.* 1984; Holland 1980). However, this discussion will broadly distinguish between those functional communication assessments developed as measures of limitations in communication activities and participation (measures of disability and handicap) and those from a more linguistic/pragmatic perspective which also examine in more detail how and why these limitations might be occurring.

Assessments of functional language use

Assessments of limitations in language use are of two major types. Those of the first type are rating scales and observational inventories, examples of which are given in Table 15.5. The ASHA-FACS, for example, has both qualitative and quantitative scales for scoring an individual's ability to complete a variety of everyday activities across four domains: social communication (e.g. exchanges information on the telephone), communication of basic needs (e.g. responds in an emergency), reading, writing and number concepts (e.g. understands simple signs) and daily planning (e.g. follows a map). Murray and Chapey (2001) note that the ASHA-FACS is unusual amongst these assessments in that it has undergone extensive standardisation and has been demonstrated to have good reliability and validity.

The rating scales and inventories rely on the raters' assessment regarding performance in a given situation, without direct observation of that situation (at the time of rating or even at any time). In contrast, a second type of assessment involves direct observation of performance on test items and

Table 15.5 Examples of assessments of functional language use

Title	Abbreviation	Author(s)
1. Rating scales and observational inventories		
Functional Communication Profile	FCP	Sarno 1969
American Speech and Hearing Association Functional Assessment of Communication Skills	ASHA FACS	Frattali *et al*. 1995
Communicative Effectiveness Index	CETI	Lomas *et al*. 1989
La Trobe Communication Questionnaire	LCQ	Douglas, O'Flaherty and Snow 2000
2. Assessments requiring direct observation of performance		
Communicative Activities of Daily Living	CADL	Holland 1980
	CADL-2	Holland *et al*. 1998
Amsterdam-Nijmegen Everyday Language Test	ANELT	Blomert *et al*. 1994

scoring at the time (see Table 15.5 for examples). For example, in the ANELT scale A (ANELT-A: Understandability), ten scenarios of daily life situations are presented to the person with aphasia, who is asked to give a verbal response. One such scenario is: "You have just moved in next door to me. You would like to meet me. You ring my doorbell and say …". Responses are rated on a five-point scale, representing the content of the message, independent of the linguistic form of the utterances. ANELT-A rated by experts correlates highly with a rating by naive subjects and with the Aphasia Partner Questionnaire (a significant other is asked to indicate on a five-point scale to what extent he or she thinks the person with aphasia is able to verbally express what they intend in a number of everyday situations), and is thus argued to have strong 'ecological' validity (Blomert 1995). However, while these assessments are argued to be reliable, they have been criticised because they have (and give) a somewhat restricted view of how aphasic individuals might spontaneously interact in real-life situations: performance in a role-play/scenario based setting may not necessarily reflect performance of the same activity in real-life.

Murray and Chapey (2001) note that for many of these functional communication tools further research is required urgently to determine whether they have sensitivity to change over time (as well as general sensitivity, reliability and validity) (see also Worrall, McCooey, Davidson *et al*. 2002). For example, Lomas *et al*. (1989) compare 'recovering' (6–10 weeks post onset) and 'stable' (more than 65 weeks post onset) groups of people with aphasia on the CETI, on two assessments around 7 weeks apart. The CETI requires rating of communicative ability for 16 communication situations on a (visual analogue) scale from 'not at all able' to 'as able as before stroke', as rated by a significant other. Although the recovering group show a significant improvement while no significant change is shown by the stable group, it is of note that some (36 percent) of the stable group show variability of as great (or greater) magnitude than 54 percent of the recovering group. (Although some of these change scores are worsening of ratings, the point still holds that there can be a great deal of variability in the measure).

Moreover, Worrall (1992, 2000; Worrall *et al*. 2002; Davidson and Worrall 2000) suggests that it is naive to expect a single assessment to be appropriate to assess all individuals with aphasia, all cultures, all impairments, and all settings, and that clinicians should not rely on a single assessment of functional communication. In an attempt to go some way towards addressing this problem, the Everyday Communication Needs Assessment (Worrall 1992; Functional Communication Therapy planner, Worrall 1999) includes an interview to evaluate an individual's communicative needs, a questionnaire to assess social support and observations and ratings of interactions in the individual's natural environment.

This assessment goes some way towards the goal of functional communication assessment that both reflects what really happens (in the aphasic and non-aphasic population), what is really important (to the individual with aphasia and their communicative partners) and what can be acted upon for rehabilitation.

In a commentary on Frattali's (1992) discussion of the assessment of functional communication, Sacchett and Marshall (1992) also question the appropriateness and adequacy of a single measure of functional communication. However, they argue that an assessment that attempts to capture the whole of an individual's functional communication ability will inevitably be inadequate, just as was the case for the impairment-focused measures above. Such a measure will inevitably only briefly sample each communicative area, role or skill and as such have little sensitivity to change, especially when that change results from therapy focused on one particular functional need (e.g. telephone catalogue ordering, Hinckley, Patterson and Carr 2001). Instead they argue for assessment that focuses on specific areas motivated by prioritisation by the clinician, the individual with aphasia and their communicative partners. This assessment should aim to identify the reason for failure, prior to attempted rehabilitation. Moreover, the assessment should be detailed enough and sensitive enough to enable observation of change as a result of rehabilitation. Pound, Parr, Lindsay and Woolf (2000) discuss in detail evaluation of outcome, (particularly for therapies 'beyond' the impairment level; see also Pound 1998; Byng *et al.* 1998). They suggest that once the goals for therapy have been set, the problems that underlie those goals (which may be at the functional level or the impairment level, or indeed concern psychosocial/quality of life issues) are rated by the person with aphasia. These pre-therapy ratings are then compared with post-therapy ratings. This approach has the benefit of specific focused assessment that may be supplemented with more objective assessments in any particular domain. However, the (test-retest) reliability of the ratings is likely to be a problem, as is a possible placebo effect of therapy on the rating process.

Assessments of language use from a linguistic/pragmatic perspective

As noted earlier, assessments from a linguistic/pragmatic perspective include conversational analysis (e.g. Whitworth, Perkins and Lesser 1997; for discussion see Perkins, Crisp and Walshaw 1999) and discourse analysis (for discussion see Armstrong 2000; Togher 2001).

It is important to note at this point that there is also a confusion in the literature regarding the term 'discourse' – some authors use it simply to mean connected speech beyond the level of the sentence. Hence under this definition analyses of connected speech such as that of Berndt *et al.* (2000) would be included. Here, we are excluding these analyses, which are more clearly impairment-focused, and only including those 'discourse' measures that are clearly examining pragmatic aspects of connected speech. Admittedly it is a hard line to draw on occasions.

These assessments from a linguistic/pragmatic perspective would appear to be better suited to Sacchett and Marshall's model for functional assessment. Common to these approaches is the need first for a sample of communicative behaviour, which is then analysed with respect to any one of a number of aspects of communicative behaviour (e.g. turn-taking behaviour, conversational repair, discourse cohesion, content and efficiency of language). Hence, the focus of the analysis can be highly specific according to the hypothesis to be tested. However, these approaches can have methodological problems. For example, Armstrong (2002) asked 12 adult non brain-damaged participants to produce a recount of an illness they had experienced. The recounts were analysed using Halliday's (1994) analysis of clause complexes (units comprising two or more clauses; analysing length and semantic content). Armstrong found a great deal of variability between the speakers, not just quantitatively but also qualitatively, with greater stylistic variation than has been previously predicted to occur within a single discourse genre such as a recount. Hence, determining what is or is not a 'normal' pattern of discourse for an individual with aphasia is far from trivial.

There can also be problems with measuring change over time due to the variability in individuals across samples. While Boles and Bombard (1998) argue that 5–10 minute conversational samples can provide adequate, representative interactions (providing comparable measures to the longer samples from which they were derived), there was none the less a high degree of variation in each measure across samples. Indeed, Manochiopinig, Sheard and Reed (1992) suggest that assessments like these, which are based on the observation or analysis of a conversation, are unsuitable for the precise measurement of performance over time. Perkins *et al.* (1999) discuss this issue in detail, with reference to conversational analysis. Part of the problem is philosophical; discourse and conversation analysis are essentially qualitative approaches, and some authors argue that quantification is inappropriate. But yet, as Perkins *et al.* note, some quantification is possible, and necessary, for evaluation of change over time. In examining quantitative analysis of collaborative repair for eight individuals with aphasia, Perkins *et al.* found highly significant variation across four conversational samples. Clearly, this is problematic for measuring change over time (although Perkins *et al.* suggest that a measure of within-participant variability could be taken into account when interpreting change as a result of therapy. This measure could be determined by multiple pre-therapy baselines or perhaps from normative studies). In contrast, qualitative measures seemed more consistent – for all but one individual, key features of repair sequences were present in all four samples. Hence, Perkins *et al.* recommend use of qualitative measures from conversational analysis to investigate the outcome of treatment.

More recently Herbert *et al.* (2004) attempted to develop a practical and reliable conversational measure to quantify successes and failures in word retrieval and to evaluate the effects of therapy on word retrieval in conversation. They found that some measures were comparable across conversations (test-retest reliability with the same pair of conversational partners). These included the amount of speech contributed by each partner (speech units produced), the number of content words produced by the person with aphasia, the nature of the contributions (type of turn: substantive vs minimal) and the incidence of repair. However, the type of repair, types of error, number of topics covered and topics initiated by the person with aphasia were all not reliable across samples.

While the Herbert *et al.* analysis shows promise, particularly in its attempt to identify those aspects of conversation that might relate to/be affected by word-finding ability. It is of note that some of the measures that were found to be reliable are similar to those investigated in impairment level investigations, e.g. content word production (cf. Saffran, Berndt and Schwartz 1989). Similarly, Ferguson (2002) demonstrated that proportions of correct information units (Brookshire and Nicholas 1993) were stable across short conversational samples. Once again, despite being obtained in a conversational setting, this measure could be classed as an index of language function (impairment). Indeed while the assessment from which it was drawn is entitled the 'Discourse Comprehension Test' (Brookshire and Nicholas 1993), the test uses a story recall task and the measures (e.g. grammatical well-formedness; type:token ratio) are predominantly those associated with impairment-focused assessment. Hence it seems that while the strength of conversational and discourse analyses is that they can investigate the detail of communicative behaviour, methodologically, it is predominantly the more general measures that have been shown to have stability across samples (i.e., across samples taken in identical contexts; it is of course a strength of these approaches that they should show sensitivity to changes across samples, for example, with different conversational partners, or different discourse genres). Unfortunately however, more subtle pragmatic aspects of communication (e.g. clause complexity analysis; cohesion, conversational repair) appear less easy to quantify reliably (being more variable within and across individuals and conversational dyads).

In sum, Frattali's (1992) conclusion still holds – further research is needed to determine if and how assessments of language use can possess:

> Sensitivity to change over time; reliability within and across raters, and over time; sufficient range of performance measured to prevent threshold effects; usefulness across different methods of administration; usefulness during different phases of rehabilitation and relevance to function outside the clinical setting.

(1992, p. 79.)

Communication activities and participation II: quality of life/psychosocial issues

The previous section examined functional language use (including pragmatics), and while there is acknowledgement of the effects of context in this domain, the emphasis remains on the person with aphasia's role. This section will have a greater focus on the 'social approach' to aphasia. This approach is encapsulated in the philosophy of Life Participation Approaches to Aphasia (LPAA) (Chapey, Duchan, Elman *et al.* 2001), which focuses on enhancing the living of life with aphasia. Communication is not merely concerned with the exchange of information, but also fulfils social needs. Simmons-Mackie (2001) argues that because of the social significance of communication, disrupted communication entails social meanings and consequences. When social systems do not support communicative access for the individual with aphasia, psychosocial well-being and quality of life are reduced. For the social approach, these psychosocial dimensions are not viewed as separable but rather are seen as an integral part of aphasia and aphasia rehabilitation. Hence assessment is designed to provide insight into well-being, personal consequences and lifestyle effects of aphasia. While assessment within a social model also includes those functional and pragmatic tools described earlier, there can be a greater emphasis on the communicative skills of other people in the communicative environment of the person, and remediation may focus on the communicative partners to as great an extent as the person with aphasia (e.g. Kagan and Gailey 1993; Lyon *et al.* 1997).

While most clinicians would attempt to assess the impact of the aphasia on social and psychological well-being, and quality of life, this is often informal and part of the interview process (and continues with ongoing interactions with the person with aphasia). There are relatively few measures used routinely in the clinical setting to measure these factors. Moreover, the majority of the scales for rating quality of life and psychological well-being are not designed specifically for aphasia – e.g. Short-form-36 Health Survey (SF-36) (Ware and Sherbourne 1992); Ryff Psychological Well-being Scale (Ryff 1989); Stroke-Specific quality of life scale (SS-QOL) (Williams *et al.* 1999), although there have been attempts to make these scales aphasia-friendly (e.g. Hilari and Byng 2001). They are often broad-ranging; for example, the Dartmouth COOP charts (Nelson, Wasson, Kirk *et al.* 1987) measure health-related quality of life through the medium of nine charts of functional status assessing biological, physical, emotional and social well-being and quality of life. Hence, once again, with only nine ratings the issue of sensitivity of measurement is raised. The Code-Müller Protocols (CMP) (Code and Müller 1992) are one tool designed specifically for acquired communication disorders. The protocols use a ten item questionnaire to gain information on the perception of psychosocial adjustment from the point of view of the individuals with aphasia, their significant others and speech and language therapist. Its main product is a measure of optimism about psychosocial adjustment. However, Code, Müller, Hogan and Herrmann (1999) note that their function was not to diagnose and quantify psychosocial changes or adjustment or the emotional responses to aphasia. Another measure designed specifically for aphasia is the Visual Analogue Self-Esteem Scale (VASES) (Brumfitt and Sheeran 1999). The VASES is intended to overcome aphasic people's language impairments by using pictorial material (10 pairs of pictures) to represent thoughts and feelings relevant to self-esteem.

However, despite the clear utility of the VASES in assessing the self esteem of people with aphasia, self-esteem is only one potentially contributing factor to overall quality of life.

Cruice, Worrall, Hickson and Murison (2003; Worrall and Holland 2003) note that while it is generally assumed that communication is an important factor and/or determinant of quality of life, there is little research examining this assumption. importantly, there is also little research regarding the impact of impaired communication on a person's quality of life. In a review of previous studies, Cruice *et al.* (2003) suggest that physical functioning, emotional health or depression, social functioning, psychological functioning, well-being, communication, autonomy and relationships were all crucial to quality of life following a stroke with aphasia. Their own research also supported the idea that in addition to communication impairment, factors other than aphasia determined individual's participation and quality of life (see also Hilari *et al.* 2003a; Ross and Wertz 2002, 2003). Cruice *et al.* also sound a note of caution regarding assessment of quality of life. They note that existing quality of life assessments require modification for people with aphasia, and the reliability of these modified assessments is unknown (but see Hilari *et al.* 2003b). Moreover, they point out that communication and social relationships are generally underrepresented in such assessments. Hence, the sensitivity of these assessments to quality of life issues in aphasia, and the changes in these over time, must be questioned. In addition, the ability to measure change in quality of life and attribute this change to the effects of therapy, is likely to be difficult. By its very nature, quality of life is dynamic and changing dependent on multiple factors in the social/psychological/physical environment. Hence, while it is possible multiple baselines may show stability of quality of life prior to therapy, and improvement in some aspects after therapy, it will be harder to attribute these changes specifically to therapy and exclude the effects of other life influences. However, once again, these difficulties are more likely to be overcome if a treatment is aimed at specific aspects of psychosocial functioning, and the treatment is preceded by a detailed and sensitive assessment that discriminates between the target of treatment and other aspects of psychosocial functioning. Then efficacy of treatment can be demonstrated by changes in the targeted psychosocial areas but not others. That is, that a pattern of change is observed that can be specifically related to the intervention and is unlikely to occur by chance from the effects of other life events. While one school of thought might embrace any (positive) change in quality of life as a benefit regardless of its source, the fact remains that like all rehabilitation approaches, therapies aimed at improving quality of life must demonstrate their efficacy.

Outcome measures

It is common practice that rehabilitation outcome within an institution must be documented. However, there are grave concerns regarding the suitability of such assessments for adequately capturing change. For example, the Functional Independence Measure (FIM) (State University of New York, 1990) was designed as a minimum data set for a wide range of patient populations. However, Frattali (1992) notes that it is insensitive to capturing functionally important change in aphasia over time, and incapable of measuring aspects of communication other than those on a simple receptive/expressive dichotomy (e.g. pragmatics, gesture).[1]

The Therapy Outcome Measure (TOM) (Enderby and John 1997) aims to provide speech and language therapists with a tool specifically designed to measure outcomes of care. It comprises four dimensions (impairment, disability/activity; handicap/participation and well-being) each of which is rated on an 11-point scale (0–5 with half marks; well-being can also be rated from two perspectives: client and carer).

[1]To increase the sensitivity of the FIM two instruments have been subsequently developed, including the Functional Assessment Measures (FAM; Forer, 1990) and the Rehabilitation Institute of Chicago Functional Assessment Scale (RICFAS; Heinemann 1989).

John and Enderby (2000) investigated the reliability of this measure. While intra-rater reliability was relatively high for known cases, it was only with a relatively large degree of training (5 hours over 2 sessions and 12 cases rated) that adequate inter-rater reliability was obtained. In all cases there was less reliability (more variability) for handicap/participation and well-being in particular, and relatively greater concensus for impairment.

However, while outcome measures may reliably document gross changes associated with spontaneous recovery or long-term treatment effects, they remain lacking in sensitivity and are unlikely to be able to capture reliably the specific effects of a particular treatment.

Relationships between language function and limitations in communication activities and participation

The ultimate goal for everyone involved in the rehabilitation of aphasia is to produce meaningful (positive) changes for the person with aphasia in their daily life. Given this goal, one of the critical questions is whether we need to assess and treat at the level of impairment of language function? Is there any consistent relationship between the degree (and/or type) of impairment of language function and the limitations in language activities, restriction in participation and reduction in quality of life? Can we expect change at the level of language function to be reflected by change in activities, participation and quality of life?

There seems to be a general perception that there is no clear relationship between impaired language function and activity limitations and participation restrictions, although most would agree that impairment does generally impact on these levels. A number of papers have addressed these issues, predominantly using correlational techniques to examine the relationship between assessments of different types. In contrast to the generally negative perceptions, most studies have found a significant correlation between measures of language impairment (e.g. WAB aphasia quotient; Boston Naming Test) and measures of communication activities and participation (e.g. CETI; CADL) (e.g. Aftonomos, Steele, Appelbaum and Harris 2001; Cruice *et al.* 2003; Irwin, Wertz and Avent 2002; Ross and Wertz 1999; but see Ulatowska, Olness, Wertz *et al.* 2001). There is less consistency (and less research) in studies examining relationships between language impairment and quality of life (compare, for example, Cruice *et al.* 2003, and Ross and Wertz 2002). This seems unsurprising; as we discussed above, so much more impacts on quality of life than the language impairment – it would be naive to expect a simple relationship.

Whilst it is gratifying for an impairment-focused researcher to see correlations with more functional measures, I must quarrel with both the methodology and the meaningfulness of the results. It is now generally accepted that there is no single entity that is aphasia – individuals with aphasia have impairments that vary both quantitatively (in severity) and qualitatively in the pattern of impairments across and within modalities. Hence, to ask the question 'Does language impairment correlate with communication activities and participation?' is simplistic in the extreme. A more sensible question might be 'Which particular aspect of language impairment relates to which aspect of activity limitation/participation restriction?' Doesborgh, van de Sandt-Koenderman, Dippel *et al.* (2002) take just this approach, asking whether a lexical-semantic or a phonological impairment has the greatest impact on verbal communication. They used measures of semantic processing impairment (e.g. Semantic Association Test, Synonym Judgements) and phonological processing impairment (e.g. Repetition of words, Repetition of non-words), and a measure of functional language (ANELT scale A) for 29 individuals with aphasia. In a multivariate regression analysis, only the semantic measures appeared to contribute independently to the prediction of the ANELT-A. Hence, lexical-semantic impairment would appear to have a greater impact on functional language use, as measured by the ANELT, than phonological measures (yet both would contribute to overall aphasia severity).

Furthermore, no one would deny that, of course, there are multiple factors (over and above communicative competence) which affect activity and participation for an individual – some of these factors will have been evident before the aphasia (within the non-aphasic population there is huge variability in these domains), others may be affected by co-occurring symptoms of the brain damage. Hence these factors also complicate the relationship between measures of impairment and those of activity and participation.

These concerns remain valid when we turn to research examining the relationship between change in language impairment and change in more functional measures (see Marshall, Chapter 17 this volume). In addition, we have already raised concerns regarding the suitability and reliability of both aphasia impairment 'batteries' and many measures of functional language use, for documenting change over time. Hence, it is unsurprising that the majority of studies fail to find significant relationships between change in an impairment measure (e.g. WAB Aphasia Quotient) and a functional measure (e.g. CETI) (e.g. Aftonomos *et al.* 2001; Irwin *et al.* 2002; Ross and Wertz 1999). Once again, we need to use specific and reliable assessments that can allow us to determine whether a specific change in language impairment has a knock-on effect for relevant aspects of language activities, participation and quality of life (see for example Hickin *et al.* 2004 for an attempt to address this issue). Hence, improved written naming skills (impairment of function) may be observed to improve functional letter writing (activity) and consequently result in increased participation in social networks with significant others with whom communication has been predominantly via letter. However, the same reduced impairment would not be expected to impact on ordering a drink at a pub, nor on increased face-to-face social participation. Until we ask the right questions, we cannot hope to obtain the correct answers, and those answers we do get will be at best uninformative and at worst, misleading.

Summary

Assessment of acquired language disorders is and will remain a complex task. Indeed, as our knowledge and understanding of language and communication become increasingly sophisticated, so the opportunities for increasingly sophisticated assessment increase. It is argued here that because of its large scope

Table 15.6 Summary of recommendations for rehabilitation-focused assessment of aphasia

General principles for rehabilitation-focused assessment:
Assessment should be hypothesis-driven and goal-focused*   Broad-ranging, comprehensive assessments are inappropriate   ALL assessments must be critically evaluated for their adequacy for each specific situation prior to use.   Assessments need to be reliable (show consistent test-retest) and sensitive.
For documenting change over time and the establishing effectiveness of therapy:

Sensitive, reliable assessment requires the use of relatively large samples of behaviour
 Assessment should include measures predicted to change as a result of therapy and those
   NOT predicted to change.
 Identical assessments must be performed pre- and post-therapy.
 Ideally assessments should be repeated on more than one occasion pre-therapy (to establish
   baseline variability).

*Goal setting should be a collaborative process with the person with aphasia and their primary communicative partner
Note: These recommendations apply to rehabilitation focusing on any and every aspect of an individual and their social context that is, or might be, impacted by their aphasia. Specifically, they do not just refer to impairment level treatments but also to those focusing directly on functional language use, psychosocial issues and quality of life.

and complexity it is inappropriate to attempt a comprehensive assessment with every (or possibly any) individual with aphasia. Instead, assessment should be hypothesis driven, on the basis of observation and joint discussion/decision-making with that individual and their primary communication partners. Hence, the clinician's hypothesis might be one of impaired semantics. However, whether the further investigation of this hypothesised impairment and its functional consequences initially focuses on, for example, spoken production, written production or written comprehension, will depend on the relative priority of the skill as perceived by the individual with aphasia. Hence, for an individual for whom reading and understanding the newspaper each day is a high priority, investigation may focus more on written comprehension. In contrast, with the individual who feels the ability to exchange social greetings with neighbours is critical to their quality of life, initial assessment may focus on spoken language.

It is emphasised that the hypothesis-testing approach to assessment applies not just to language functions (identification of impairment) but to every aspect of an individual and their social context that is, or might be, impacted by the aphasia. The hypothesis drives the nature of the assessment. In particular it is stressed that to be of benefit for documenting change over time assessments need to be reliable (show consistent test-retest) and sensitive. Both of these criteria require a relatively large sample of behaviour (e.g. many items to name aloud; many observations of attempted conversational repair; multiple ratings of similar communicative behaviours e.g. ordering a pizza, ordering a taxi, ordering a curry).

Finally, it is suggested that the relationship between impairment of language function and restrictions in language activities, participation and quality of life is not straightforward. Moreover, current attempts to correlate change at one level with change at the other are fundamentally flawed (and not only because they use two or more imperfect measures). However, while there is no guaranteed relationship between degree of impairment to language function and the degree of restriction to communication activities and participation and quality of life, it is argued that it remains appropriate to assess (and focus rehabilitation) at the level of impairment. The lack of a relationship simply reflects that activity, participation and quality of life are impacted by many factors over and above the language impairment – illustrated by the fact that there is huge variability in these areas for the non-aphasic population.

To conclude, in order to effectively assess the individual with aphasia and use those assessments to track change over time, we must be acutely aware of the strengths and limitations of our assessment tools. We have a duty to all those involved in the rehabilitation process to strive to overcome these limitations and critically evaluate the efficacy of our therapies as part of routine clinical practice. As Kearns (1993) argues:

> Failure to apply scientific thinking and measurement during the clinical process is surely as misguided as leaving our empathy, clinical intuition, and caring attitudes behind as we enter the clinical arena.

(1993, p. 71).

Acknowledgements

Thanks to Beth Armstrong, Wendy Best, Madeline Cruice, Alison Ferguson, Peter Halligan, Jane Marshall, Derrick Wade and Linda Worrall for helpful comments and discussion during the preparation of this paper, and to Peter Halligan and Derrick Wade for inviting me to participate in the conference. The author was supported by an Australian Research Council Queen Elizabeth II fellowship during preparation of this paper.

16 Language deficits

The efficacy of the impairment-based treatment

Anna Basso

Abstract

This chapter reviews studies on efficacy of aphasia therapy regrouped according to how the problem was dealt with: studies on spontaneous recovery from aphasia, on recovery in treated chronic aphasic patients, studies comparing treated and untreated groups of patients, and studies comparing patients treated by speech therapists and volunteers. Results of these studies are conflicting and do not allow any firm conclusion about aphasia therapy efficacy, but they strongly suggest that long-lasting treatments are efficacious. Results of studies on the effect of duration and intensity of treatment are reported; they clearly indicate that length significantly affects recovery. In the last 10 years meta-analyses have repeatedly been applied to aphasia therapy studies. They confirm the efficacy of aphasia therapy. In the last part of the paper, studies on long-term outcome of aphasia are reviewed.

Introduction

Thirty years ago, in 1972, Darley asked an important question about aphasia therapy:

> Does language rehabilitation accomplish measurable gains in language function beyond what can be expected to occur as a result of spontaneous recovery? Or, stated differently, does therapy have a decisive influence on the course of recovery and the ultimate outcome?
>
> Darley (1972, p. 4)

I am persuaded that the answer to the question is 'yes', and I hope to show that there is by now sufficient experimental evidence for such an assertion.

Studies on the efficacy of aphasia therapy date back to the 1950s. At that time aphasiologists were interested in studying and treating the language disorder itself. Interest in the communicative aspect of language use came later and a clear distinction between the language impairment and its effect on daily living was drawn even later. According to the World Health Organization's (1980) *International Classification of Impairment, Disability and Handicap*, impairment refers to the damage at the level of the organ and disability is defined as the difficulty in carrying out everyday activities (see Chapter 4). No attempt will be made here to tease apart studies on recovery of the language disorder from studies on recovery of communication, but studies on efficacy of aphasia therapy are for the most part concerned with recovery from the language impairment and only rarely has communication been taken into consideration.

I shall review studies on spontaneous recovery, on recovery in treated chronic aphasic patients; studies comparing treated and untreated patients and therapists and volunteers, on the effect of intensity and duration of therapy, and on meta-analyses. Finally, I shall consider the question of long-term outcome.

Spontaneous recovery and clinical studies without a control group

Functional cognitive disorders consequent to brain damage undergo a variable degree of 'spontaneous' recovery in the first months post onset. Many factors – such as age, sex, handedness, aetiology, lesion size and site, and type and severity of aphasia – have been considered and studied in relation to recovery from aphasia but none of these, except severity of the aphasic disorder, has been proven to have an important effect on recovery and they will not be discussed here (for review see Basso 1992; Cappa 1998).

Important for the evaluation of aphasia therapy efficacy is the time course of spontaneous recovery. Although it has not been studied longitudinally in a group of patients, comparing the results of studies on spontaneous recovery in patients seen at different times post-onset (Sarno and Levita 1971; Hagen 1973; Pickersgill and Lincoln 1983; Lendrem and Lincoln 1985; Wade *et al.* 1986) some conclusions can be drawn with confidence.

Spontaneous recovery is steepest in the first 2–3 months after onset and flattens out in the following 3–4 months. No spontaneous recovery occurs after 6–8 months post-onset, although a few patients have been described who showed significant spontaneous improvement for longer periods of time (e.g., Hanson *et al.* 1989). The results of these studies are summarized in Table 16.1.

The first group of studies about the efficacy of aphasia therapy, however, were based on treated patients only and did not take into consideration the effect of spontaneous recovery. A summary of their results is reported in Table 16.2. All authors state that aphasia therapy is efficacious, but the lack of a control group renders these conclusions useless for the study of efficacy of aphasia therapy.

Chronic patients

The efficacy question can be addressed by considering recovery in chronic patients beyond the period of spontaneous recovery. Table 16.3 reports the main results of these studies.

Table 16.1 Studies on spontaneous recovery

Authors	No. of patients	TPO at testing	Recovery
Sarno and Levita (1971)	14	2 w, 3 m, 6 m	Higher in the first 3 m
Hagen (1973)	10	3 m, 6 m, 12 m, 18 m	In the first 6 m
Pickersgill and Lincoln (1983)	20	mean 3 – 4 m	Trend in comprehension
Lendrem and Lincoln (1985)	52	4 w, 10 w, 22 w, 34 w	Max within 10 w, slight between 10 and 22 w, none between 22 and 34 w
Wade *et al.* (1986)	545 stroke patients: 24 per cent aphasics, 28 per cent unass	7 d, 3 w, 6 m	At 3 w 9 per cent were unass and 20 per cent aphasics. At 6 m 3 per cent of survivors were unass and 12 per cent aphasic

D = day; w = week; m = month; TPO = time post onset; unass = unassessable (adapted from Basso 2003).

Table 16.2 Studies on therapy efficacy in treated patients without control group

Authors	No. of patients	Duration of therapy	No. of sessions	Results
Butfield and Zangwill (1946)	70	n.r.	5 to 290	70–80 per cent recovered
Marks et al. (1957)	159	1 to 12 m	1 to 110	50 per cent poor recovery, 21 per cent fair, 29 per cent good
Leischner and Link (1967)	116	n.r.	n.r.	5 per cent no recovery, 40 per cent slight-to-moderate, 55 per cent good
Sands et al. (1969)	30	2 w to 32 m (mean 7.5 m)	n.r.	mean: 10 points percentile on FCP
Sarno and Levita (1979)	34	3 to 12 m	3 to 5/w	improved in all modalities

W = week; m = month; n.r. = not reported; FCP = Functional Communication Profile (Sarno 1969) (adapted from Basso 2003).

Wepman's (1951) study is rather heterogeneous with respect to all other studies cited so far because of the homogeneity of the population studied and the regimen of the treatment, and because of its intensity and duration. The patients, young traumatic males first evaluated at least 6 months post-onset, were rehabilitated for 18 months, 6 hours per day. The reported results are striking, with 86 per cent of the patients showing improvement, demonstrating that aphasia therapy can also be efficacious after the period of spontaneous recovery. Although less striking, some improvement is reported in all the studies cited in Table 16.3.

A characteristic common to most of the previous studies is that recovery was evaluated subjectively, frequently by the same person who treated the patients. This fact obviously diminishes or even cancels the impact of these studies. Standardized evaluations were used in the following group of studies, which compared treated and untreated patients.

Table 16.3 Studies on therapy efficacy in chronic aphasics without control group

Authors	No. of patients	TPO	Duration of therapy	Treatment regimen	Results
Wepman (1951)	68	minimum 6 m	18 m	6 h/d5 d/w	51 per cent much improved; 35 per cent improved; 14 per cent unchanged
Broida (1977)	14	12 to 72 m	2–21 m (mean 9 m)	3–5 h/w	mean recovery: 11 points percentile
Aten et al. (1982)	7	mean 98 m	12 w	2 h/wgroup-therapy	sign improvement in CADL
Mackenzie (1991)	5	Minimum 9 m	4 w	5 h/d group-therapy	Good recovery in 3 patients; 2 unchanged

TPO = time post onset; h = hour; d = day; w = week; sign = significant; CADL = communicative. Abilities in Daily Living (Holland 1980) (adapted from Basso 2003).

Treated and untreated patients

Vignolo (1964) examined 42 rehabilitated and 27 non-rehabilitated patients. At second examination there was a trend towards a greater frequency of improved patients in the rehabilitated group (71 per cent vs 52 per cent). Hagen (1973) compared 10 vascular male patients rehabilitated for a year to 10 patients who were untreated due to shortage of speech therapists. After three months of observation only the rehabilitated patients continued to improve.

In a study by Basso et al. (1975), recovery of oral expression was studied in 91 rehabilitated and 94 non-rehabilitated patients subdivided according to time post-onset. The percentage of improved treated patients was significantly higher in the three time-groups.

Gloning et al. (1976) computed prognosis for individual patient in a group of 107 aphasics. The patients were tested three times: on entering the study, after one week, and approximately 18 months later. Speech therapy lasted at least six months and was found to influence prognosis positively. The authors, however, do not specify how many patients were treated nor the treatment regimen.

Levita (1978) compared 17 treated and 18 untreated aphasics, first evaluated three months post-onset and treated daily for eight weeks. No significant difference was found, but initial severity of aphasia in the two groups is unknown.

Basso et al. (1979) studied the effect of therapy, separately for oral and written production and oral and written comprehension in 162 treated and 119 untreated patients, most of whom lived far from Milan where the only existing aphasia rehabilitation unit was located. Rehabilitation proved to be significant in all four verbal behaviours; time post-onset had a significant negative effect on recovery but not on efficacy of aphasia therapy.

In Pickersgill and Lincoln's study (1983), 36 treated patients underwent an eight-week therapy course of unknown intensity, and 20 patients made up the control group. No significant difference between treated and untreated patients was found.

Lincoln et al.'s (1984) study is the only example of a randomized controlled trial in this group of studies. They assessed patients at 10 weeks post stroke and randomly allocated them to the treatment (n = 104) or no treatment (n = 87) group. The treatment group was given two sessions weekly for 24 weeks, but due to drop out only 27 patients were given more than 37 therapy sessions. Comparison was done by t tests and no significant difference was found.

Shewan and Kertesz (1984) compared recovery in two groups of aphasic patients treated by speech pathologists, a group treated by non-professionals and a self-selected no-treatment group. The first two groups improved significantly more than the no-treatment group. The group treated by non-professionals did not reach significantly greater recovery than the no-treatment group.

Poeck et al. (1989) compared amount of improvement of a group of 68 patients receiving therapy 9 hours per week over 6–8 weeks to the expected rate of spontaneous recovery as determined by a previous study (Willmes and Poeck 1984). About two-thirds of the patients showed greater improvement than expected by spontaneous recovery.

Finally, Mazzoni et al. (1995) compared recovery in 13 treated aphasic patients and 13 untreated matched controls. The number of recovered patients was significantly higher in the treated group seven months post-onset. Table 16.4 summarizes results from these studies. The results of these studies are conflicting, and do not allow any firm conclusion about aphasia therapy efficacy. Moreover, only in David et al.'s (1983) study were subjects randomly allocated to the treatment or no treatment group.

Random allocation of subjects prevents any bias in the assignment of patients and guarantees that the groups are comparable, but in behavioural sciences random allocation is not always possible. In aphasia therapy efficacy studies, ethical reasons prevent the formation of a no-treatment group; at best, a delayed-therapy group can be used but this implies a relatively short treatment.

Table 16.4 Studies on therapy efficacy in treated and untreated patients

Authors	N of patients		Duration of therapy	N of sessions	Results
	Rehab+	Rehab−			
Vignolo (1964)	42	27	Min 40 d	min 20	no sign difference
Hagen (1973)	10	10	12 m	12 h/w	after 3 m only treated patients improve
Basso et al. (1975)	91	94	Min 6 m	3 h/w	(oral production) higher percent of treated patients improve
Gloning et al. (1976)	107		Min 6 m	n.r.	sign effect
Levita (1978)	17	18	8 w	5 h/w	no sign difference (unknown severity at entrance)
Basso et al. (1979)	162	119	Min 5 m	3 h/w	higher per cent of treated patients improve
Pickersgill and Lincoln (1983)	36	20	8 w	n.r.	no sign difference
Lincoln et al. (1984)	104	87	max 24 w	2 h/w	no sign difference
	(randomized)				
Shewan and Kertesz (1984)	52	23	up to 12 m	3 h/w	sign difference
Poeck et al. (1989)	68	69	6–8 w	9 h/w	sign difference
Mazzoni et al. (1995)	13	13	6 m	4–5 h/w	no difference at 4 mpo; sign difference at 7 mpo
	(matched in pairs)				

H = hour; w = week; n.r. = not reported; sign = significant; mpo = months post onset (adapted from Basso 2003).

According to Robey *et al.* (1999), however, lack of random allocation of patients does not imply a lack of scientific rigor but 'rather it speaks to the complexity of the behavioural and social sciences' (p. 446).

Different therapeutic methods and different 'therapists'

The treated and untreated groups in the studies just reviewed did not differ for presence/absence of therapy only; they also differed in the amount of attention and conversational opportunities they were given. Studies comparing patients treated by speech therapists and patients treated by volunteers or family members, and studies comparing different treatments compare groups of patients receiving the same amount of attention. Table 16.5 reports an overview of these studies.

No significant difference was ever found when comparing results obtained by speech therapists to results obtained by volunteers, family members or counselling. The only significant difference found was between two therapy regimens: individual therapy being more effective than group therapy (Wertz *et al.* 1981).

The question about the efficacy of aphasia therapy remains unresolved. Studies without a control group always claimed that aphasia rehabilitation was efficacious but the conclusion was subjective and cannot be taken into serious consideration. In chronic patients beyond the period of spontaneous recovery, amelioration has been reported and in the studies comparing treated and untreated patients a difference has sometimes but not always been reported. Better recovery in treated than

Table 16.5 Efficacy of different therapists and methods

Authors	No. of patients	Treatments/ therapists	Duration of therapy	No. of sessions	Results
Sarno et al. (1970)	10–10–11	Programmed inst, classical, no treatment	3 m	80 ½ h	No sign diff
Meikle et al. (1979)	17 – 14 (randomized)	th vs vol	max 80 w (th: mean 36 w, vol: mean 21)	4 h/w	No sign diff
Wertz et al. (1981)	32 – 35 (randomized)	Group vs individual therapy	44 w.	8 h/w	Individual >group
David et al. (1982)	48 – 48 (randomized)	th vs vol	max 20 w	30 h	No sign diff
Wertz et al. (1986)	38 – 43 (randomized)	th vs trained vol	12 w	8–10 h/w	No sign diff
Hartman and Landau (1987)	30 – 30 (randomized)	th vs counselling	6 m	2 h/w	No sign diff
Marshall et al. (1989)	31 – 37 (randomized)	th vs trained family member	12 w	8–10 h/w	No sign diff

Inst = instruction; th = therapist; vol = volunteer; w = week; m = month; h = hour (adapted from Basso 2003).

untreated patients, as indicated by results of studies comparing speech therapists and volunteers, could be the result of the attention given to the patients and not a specific effect of rehabilitation.

However, careful reading of the literature suggests that whenever treatment lasted for long periods of time aphasia therapy was found to be efficacious (Hagen 1973; Basso et al. 1975, 1979; Gloning et al. 1976; Shewan and Kertesz 1984; Poeck et al. 1989; Mazzoni et al. 1995). It seems important, therefore, to study the effect of duration and intensity of therapy.

Duration of therapy

The five studies summarized in Table 16.6 were specifically concerned with duration or intensity of aphasia rehabilitation; they all show that number of sessions and intensity or duration of therapy significantly affect recovery. At this point a plausible conclusion is that therapy is efficacious if it is prolonged and/or intensive. The negative results found in some of the studies comparing treated and untreated patients, as well as lack of difference in recovery in patients treated by speech therapists and volunteers, may be explained by the short duration of treatment.

The Office of Technology Assessment Efficacy (OTA) drew a clear distinction between efficacy and effectiveness studies. Efficacy has been defined as 'The probability of benefit to individuals in a defined population from a medical technology applied to a given medical problem under ideal conditions of use' (Office of Technology Assessment, 1978, p. 16). Effectiveness, according to OTA, is the probability of benefit under average conditions. Thus, efficacy indicates that a treatment *can* work in clinical practice and effectiveness indicates that a treatment *does* work in clinical practice. Effectiveness studies should be carried out only after efficacy studies have proven the efficacy of a treatment in ideal conditions: if the treatment is not efficacious in ideal conditions it will not be effective in average conditions.

Table 16.6 Studies on duration and frequency/intensity of therapy

Authors	Patients	Treatment/method	Results
Marshall et al. (1982)	110	Studied effect of 11 factors, including number of sessions (range: 10–345)	Number of sessions is the most powerful predictor of improvement
Basso (1987)	95 non-rehab; 21 rehab 3 m; 58 more than 6 m	Studied effect of therapy and duration of therapy for oral production and comprehension	Rehab is sign more effective in patients treated more than 6 months
Brindley et al. (1989)	10 chronic Broca aphasics	12 weeks/2 sessions per week 12 weeks/25 hours per week	No improvement in the first period, sign improvement in the second
Denes et al. (1996)	17 acute global aphasics	Regular therapy: average 60 sessions Intensive therapy: average 130 sessions	Better results (sign only for writing) for the intensive therapy group
Basso and Caporali (2001)	3 pairs of matched patients	Control subjects: one hour daily for 14,23, 20 months (all reached a plateau) Experimental subjects: 2–3 h daily for 14, 36, 12 months (all still recovering)	Better test results and better use of language in daily life for the experimental subject

Treatment conditions were not ideal but were better than average in the studies that demonstrated a significant effect of therapy; they were average in those indicating that aphasia rehabilitation was not effective. In agreement with this interpretation is a statement by David et al. (1983, p. 74)):

> Both our own study and that of Meikle et al., as well as many others of similar nature, arose from the practical and organizational difficulties of the overpressed speech therapy service ... our main concern was to evaluate the existing standard speech therapy provision in Britain.

If this interpretation were correct, the obvious consequence would be to increase the number of therapy sessions delivered to all patients and not to negate therapy to aphasic patients because of its inefficacy.

Meta-analyses

In the last 10 years, meta-analyses have been applied repeatedly to aphasia therapy efficacy studies and they confirm the efficacy of aphasia therapy. Whurr et al. (1992) reviewed 45 studies carried out from 1947 to 1988 and concluded that the meta-analysis demonstrated a significant effect of treatment but that studies on efficacy of aphasia therapy suffer from lack of internal and external validity.

Robey (1994) reviewed 48 reports, 21 of which he included in his meta-analysis. He analysed results for patients seen before and after four months post-onset separately and concluded that treated patients improve more than untreated patients, and that the difference is larger in acute than chronic patients. In a second study, Robey (1998) examined a larger series of clinical trials and considered 55 studies eligible. He studied the effect of amount and types of treatment, severity and type of aphasia, and time post-onset. Results of the meta-analysis indicated that recovery in treated patients was superior to recovery in untreated patients and that the difference was higher in acute patients. Moreover, intensive treatment was found to be more effective than less intensive treatment.

Table 16.7 Meta-analyses

Authors	Studies reviewed	Results
Whurr et al. (1992)	45 (1947–1988)	Significant effect of treatment (but lack of internal and external validity in studies)
Robey (1994)	48; 21 eligible	Treatment is effective, more in acute than in chronic patients. The difference between treated and untreated patients exceeds medium size effect in acute patients and nearly reaches it in chronic patients
Robey (1998)	55	Treated patients recover more than untreated patients, the difference is higher in acute patients. Intensive treatment is more effective than less intensive treatment
Greener et al. (1999)	45 (1968–1998); 12 eligible (only randomized trials)	Too few studies to perform a meta-analysis: only 2 compare treated and untreated patients, and 4 compare professionals and volunteers

Greener *et al.* (1999) compared randomly allocated treated and untreated vascular patients, and patients treated by speech therapists and by volunteers. Only 12 of the studies published from 1968 to 1998 were considered eligible and only two compared treated and untreated patients (Lincoln *et al.* 1984; Wertz *et al.* 1986). A meta-analysis was obviously not performed and the authors' concluded that aphasia therapy has not been demonstrated as either clearly effective or ineffective.

Finally, the Brain Injury-Interdisciplinary Special Interest Group (BI-ISIG) of the American Congress of Rehabilitation Medicine has developed recommendations for the practice of cognitive rehabilitation (Cicerone *et al.* 2000). The studies reviewed were classified by the committee according to the soundness of their experimental methodology in Class I (prospective, randomized controlled studies), Class II (prospective cohort studies and clinical series with well-defined controls), and Class III (clinical studies without controls and single case studies with appropriate methodology). Recommendations for clinical practice were organized into practice standards (based on the highest level of evidence), practice guidelines, and practice options.

The committee concluded that there is enough evidence to recommend language and communication disorder rehabilitation as practice standards.

Long-term outcome

Recovery from aphasia has been intensively studied from different points of view but long-term outcome from aphasia has received little attention. I found only two studies concerned with long-term outcome.

Hanson *et al.* (1989) regularly examined 35 male aphasics from 3 to 55 months post-onset. All patients were initially rehabilitated, but rehabilitation never continued beyond two years post-onset. All patients improved in the first year and remained stable or continued to improve in the second year. In the third year, however, 10 patients started to regress and the decline continued for the following two years. The authors were unable to identify a specific cause for the patients' worsening.

Wahrborg *et al.* (1997) present results from a 10-year follow-up of eight relatively young aphasic patients. All patients participated in a 34-week educational program for aphasics and at the end of the treatment they all showed improvement. At follow-up ten years later, they were more severely aphasic than at the end of the course and in many cases aphasia was even more severe than at entering the course.

Caporali and Basso (2003) investigated the long-term course of aphasia in 52 patients, with at least three aphasia examinations and who were at least three years post onset at follow-up (mean length of illness was five years).

A methodological problem when studying the evolution of a cognitive damage is intrinsic to the upper-limited extent of the scale. A possible solution is to select only patients matched on their scores at the first of the two examinations that are to be compared. We chose this strategy and selected from the whole sample two groups of patients with comparable scores at the first of the two to-be-compared evaluations, thus comparing two groups of patients who shared the same starting point and the same range for recovery.

We compared results on the token test, oral and written confrontation naming, reading aloud and writing to dictation of words by *t* tests for differences between non-independent measures. All patients were rehabilitated between the first and the second evaluation, carried out when rehabilitation ceased (range: 4–20 months, mean = 8.7, SD = 4.2). No patient underwent rehabilitation between the second and the third evaluation, carried out long after the second (range 24–84 months; mean distance = 50.6, SD = 15.9). The differences in the first time interval were significant for all tasks, with higher scores at the second evaluation, but none of the differences reached significance in the second time interval. Our data confirm that, as a group, after an initial partial recovery aphasic patients reach a plateau.

We also considered the pattern of recovery in each patient. Ignoring slight variations of one or two points that can be due to levels of attention or fatigue, the direction of change in the first time interval is the same for all but one patient who slightly worsened in one task. In the second time interval the trend is less uniform. A few patients continued to improve, many patients were more or less stable and some showed some worsening. Worsening, however, was clinically evident in three patients only; in one patient it was evident in writing, and in another in reading. Only one patient with initial global aphasia showed a general decline of his language disorders.

To sum up, out of 52 patients with a mean length of illness of five years only a global aphasic clinically worsened (but his scores were still higher at final examination than at entrance in the study), the majority remained stable and some patients continued to improve, showing that the passing of time has no negative effect on chronic aphasic subjects.

Conclusion

This chapter briefly reviewed studies on efficacy of aphasia therapy regrouped according to how the problem was dealt with: clinical studies without a control group, treated chronic patients, treated and untreated patients, comparison of different methods, meta-analyses, and long-term outcome. I believe that the evidence is strongly in favour of efficacy of aphasia therapy, provided treatment is sufficiently prolonged.

The fact that no difference in recovery was ever found comparing patients treated by speech therapists and volunteers can be explained either by the relatively low number of therapy sessions (David *et al.* 1982; Hartman and Landau 1987) or by the fact that volunteers were supervised and trained by speech pathologists (Wertz *et al.* 1981; Marshall *et al.* 1989).

Interestingly, however, papers that published results suggesting that aphasia therapy is efficacious have not aroused widespread interest. For the most part they have been criticized for their limitations and rapidly dismissed. Prins *et al.* (1989), for instance, argue that the statement that two groups of treated patients made a significant improvement 'seems unwarranted, because the observed improvement can also be explained by test-retest effects' (p. 89). Schoonen (1991) argues that efficacy studies lack internal and external validity and wonders 'How can we explain the "significant" improvement in so many studies? One of the "explanations" is that these researchers were just lucky' (p. 460).

Pedersen *et al.* (1996) state 'It is only when no difference is found, that it is possible to draw a valid conclusion from a comparison with no treatment' (p. 130). On the other hand, the message that therapy provided by speech therapists is no better than simple counselling or therapy delivered by volunteers has been immediately accepted by the scientific community. I have no explanations for such a widespread scepticism, but I do hope to have shown that there is sufficient experimental evidence to demonstrate that aphasia therapy can significantly reduce the language impairment.

17 Can speech and language therapy with aphasic people affect activity and participation levels?

A review of the literature

Jane Marshall

Abstract

This chapter will briefly discuss how the International Classification of Functioning Disability and Health (ICF) (WHO 2001) applies to aphasia, and will consider the relationships between the different components of the system. It is argued that despite evidence of correlations, e.g. between impairment and activity measures, these relationships are complex. In particular, we cannot assume that change in one dimension will be accompanied by change in another. The chapter will argue that change at the level of activity and participation is the primary goal of rehabilitation, regardless of the approach taken. Therapy studies will then be reviewed for evidence that this change can be achieved. The first section will examine evidence from general group studies. Outcomes from specific approaches will then be reviewed, focusing on impairment therapies, compensatory therapies, conversational therapies, and group therapy. Therapy aiming to improve social participation is given its own section. In conclusion, it is argued that speech and language therapy should be multidimensional and driven by the life goals of the individuals involved. Diverse methods of evaluation are also required, which can explore changes in the dimensions of impairment, activity, and participation. The evaluation strategy should be driven by a hypothesis about the changes that are predicted from the therapy being administered. This approach will enable us to look for theoretically explicable change and will develop our understanding of how change in one dimension relates to change in another.

The ICF and aphasia

The ICF belongs to the family of health-related classifications developed by the World Health Organisation (see chapter 4). Key components in relation to disability are impairments, activity limitations and participation restrictions (see Figure 17.1 for definitions). Within the classification disability is conceived as an interaction between health condition(s) and contextual factors. So a person may be disadvantaged by a severe impairment, but equally by barriers in their physical or social environment.

A number of commentators have applied the WHO classifications to aphasia (e.g. see Rogers, Alarcon and Olswang 1999; Ross and Wertz 2002; Irwin, Wertz and Avent 2002; Worrall *et al.* 2002).

Impairments	Problems in body function of structure as a significant deviation or loss (were body functions include psychological functions)
Activity limitations	Difficulties an individual may have in executing activities
Participation restrictions	Problems an individual may experience in involvement in life situations

Figure 17.1   Definitions of terms used in the ICF.

Most use the term 'impairment' to mean the specific language deficit, as measured by tests like the Boston Diagnostic Aphasia Examination (BDAE) (Goodglass and Kaplan 1983) the Porch Index of Communicative Ability (PICA) (Porch 1967), Western Aphasia Battery (WAB) (Kertesz 1982), or Psycholinguistic Assessment of Language Processing in Aphasia (PALPA) (Kay Lesser and Coltheart 1992). Impairments can be defined in behavioural terms, such as 'a naming impairment' or 'a sentence comprehension impairment'. Alternatively, we can view the impairment as a point of breakdown within an abstract language processing system. For example, a person may have an impairment in the processes which access word phonologies, or which formulate the syntactic structure of sentences.

The activity limitations experienced by aphasic people may include difficulties in holding conversations, reading for pleasure, using email and following TV and radio. These limitations are typically measured by functional communication assessments like the Communicative Activities of Daily Living (CADL) (Holland 1980, CADL-2 Holland *et al.* 1998), American Speech and Hearing Association Functional Assessment of Communication Skills for Adults (ASHA-FACS) (Frattali *et al.* 1995) and Functional Communication Profile (FCP) (Sarno 1969; see Chapter 16 this volume for information about these tests). Other methods include structured interviews, such as the Pragmatics Profile (Dewart and Summers 1996) and conversational measures.

Participation restriction refers to the social exclusion experienced by aphasic people. Loss of social roles, such as the loss of a job and reduced involvement in parenting, falls within this dimension. Ross and Wertz (2002) claim that there is currently no assessment of participation restriction in aphasia. Others have argued for techniques like qualitative interviews, frequency counts of social contacts, and analyses of social networks (Simmons-Mackie 2001; Simmons-Mackie and Damico 2001). Quality of Life Questionnaires (e.g. Hilari *et al.* 2003a, b) are also of value here.

The different dimensions of aphasia call for different therapy approaches. Therapy can aim to reduce the impairment, e.g. by using naming or sentence processing tasks. Alternatively, therapy can be pitched directly at the activity and participation level, e.g. by working on conversation. Regardless of the therapy approach, most people would agree that achieving change at the level of activity and participation is a primary goal of rehabilitation. Certainly, when aphasic people and their relatives are asked about what constitutes change for them they tend to focus on everyday activities, rather than isolated language skills (Hoen *et al.* 1997).

The relationship between language impairment and activity limitations

There is evidence that scores on measures of language impairment and communication activity correlate (e.g. Holland 1980; Ross and Wertz 1999; Joseph *et al.* 2000; Irwin *et al.* 2002), suggesting that there is a relationship between these dimensions. In some ways, this concurs with our intuitions. So, for example, a severe naming impairment is likely to have profound consequences for the person's ability to undertake daily communication activities, such as using the phone or holding a conversation. This, in turn, has implications for rehabilitation. It suggests that if we can change a person's impairment, there may also be positive effects on activity levels.

However, there are a number of reasons for being cautious about this conclusion. First, although impairment and activity levels are clearly related, as measured by these tests, the nature of that relationship is much less clear. It is possible, for example, that the correlation reflects the general severity of the stroke, rather than any more precise relationship between the language impairment and function.

A second problem is that merely looking for correlations between measures ignores important individual differences. For example, two people with similar naming impairments may experience very different activity limitations, because of differences in their problem-solving abilities or differences in their environment. So, the person who sustains communication activities may use alternative communication strategies, or be surrounded by friends and relatives who cope well with communication despite the aphasia.

A third problem is that changes in test scores fail to uphold the correlation. Ross and Wertz (1999) tested 22 aphasic people on 3 aphasia tests. Two were impairment measures (PICA and WAB), and one was an activity measure (CADL). The tests were administered on entry to the study and at its conclusion, which was on average 4.8 months later. In line with previous studies, there was a strong initial correlation between impairment and activity measures. However, there was no correlation between the change scores. In other words, change in one impairment test failed to correlate with change on the other, or with changes on the activity measure (see Aftonomos *et al.* 2001 for similar findings from therapy outcome data).

The above studies suggest that even if therapy brings about changes in one dimension we cannot assume that benefits will generalise to another. Furthermore, although there is now quite extensive evidence that therapy can improve performance on impairment level assessments (see reviews in Hillis 2002 and Chapter 16 this volume), few studies have focussed on other dimensions of change.

This paper will review some of the available evidence in relation to communication disability. First, I will present evidence from general group studies. I will then focus on small group and individual studies, in order to explore the effects of particular types of therapy, and, crucially, whether these affect activity levels. The issue of whether social participation can be affected by therapy will be given its own section. Finally, I will suggest how future studies might explore these issues further.

General group studies

There have been numerous group studies exploring the efficacy or effectiveness of aphasia therapy, a selection of which are summarised in Table 17.1.

As can be seen from the table, the majority of studies do not employ activity measures. Furthermore, whether or not an activity measure is used is often difficult to predict from the content of therapy. So, for example, Denes *et al.* (1996) evaluated therapy that aimed to restore the use of language in conversation, and used conversation tasks in treatment. Despite this, only an impairment measure (the Aachen Aphasia Test) was used. In contrast, Sarno *et al.* (1970) administered impairment level language drills, yet included the FCP in their evaluations.

Six of the reviewed studies employed activity measures. Of these, only two show evidence of change that can be attributed to therapy (Wertz *et al.* 1981; Brindley *et al.* 1989). For example, Brindley *et al.* show that changes in the FCP and in analyses of conversational speech occur only after intensive speech and language therapy is provided, with performance during the baseline and maintenance period being stable.

Table 17.1 Group studies of aphasia therapy

Study	Design	Sample size	Random assignment to groups?	Type of therapy	Activity measures used?	Main findings
Basso et al. (1979)	Explored influence of 4 variables on recovery	281	No	Individual impairment based	No	Rehabilitation has positive effect on improvement in language skills.
Denes et al. (1996)	Compared intensive and non intensive therapy for global aphasia	17	Yes	Aims to restore use of language in a conversational setting; uses conversational tasks	No	Both groups improve more than predicted by spontaneous recovery. Improvements greater in the intensive group.
Hagen (1973)	Compared treated with un-treated patients	20	Yes	Intensive; group and individual; combines impairment based work and work on social-verbal interaction	No	Treated group better than controls on reading, language formulation, speech production, spelling and arithmetic
Hartman and Landau (1987)	Compared language therapy with supportive counselling	60	Yes	Language therapy comprises language drills. Supportive counselling discusses life events & communication problems at home, encourages independent problem solving	No	Groups achieve equal gains on PICA
Mazzoni et al. (1995)	Compared matched groups of treated and un-treated patients	26	No	Individual and impairment based	No	Treated group better than controls on expressive language measures.
Meikle et al. (1979)	Compared therapist administered with volunteer administered treatment	28	Yes	Intensive individual and group; unspecified content	No	No difference between groups on language measure (PICA)
Poeck et al. (1989)	Treated patients compared to untreated controls	160	No	9 sessions per week for 6 – 8 weeks; impairment based individual work plus group work working on 'transfer and consolidation'	No	Treated patients improve more than predicted by spontaneous recovery.

Study	Comparison	N	Randomized	Treatment		Results
Shewan and Kertesz (1984)	Compared 4 groups: Language oriented therapy, stimulation therapy, therapy administered by nurses, no treatment	100	No	1 hour per week for 1 year; stimulation or language orientation therapy	No	All treated groups are better than controls on WAB scores; no differences between the treated groups.
Wertz et al. (1986)	Compares 3 groups: therapy delivered by SLT, Volunteer administered therapy; deferred treatment	121	Yes	8 – 10 hours per week for 12 weeks; individual impairment based	No	Group treated by SLT improve more than deferred treatment group on PICA; No significant differences between volunteer treated group and the other two groups.
Brindley et al. (1989)	Compared intensive with non intensive therapy	10	N/A	Intensive therapy 25 hours per week for 3 months; impairment work and group therapy working on effective communication	Yes	Gains on FCP and in samples of conversational language, only when intensive therapy administered
David et al. (1982)	Compared therapist administered treatment with volunteer administered treatment	96	Yes	30 hours over 15 – 20 weeks; content not described	Yes	Both groups improve on FCP; no difference between volunteer and therapist treated
Lincoln et al. (1984)	Compared treated and untreated groups	191	Yes	48 sessions over 24 weeks; content not described	Yes	No difference between treated and untreated patients on FCP and PICA
Marshall et al. (1989)	Compares 3 groups: therapy delivered by SLT, Volunteer administered therapy; deferred treatment	121	Yes	8 – 10 hours per week for 12 weeks; individual impairment based	Yes	See Wertz et al. (1986); Volunteer treated patients and deferred treatment group no different on CADL
Sarno et al. (1970)	3 groups compared: programmed instruction, non-programmed instruction and untreated	31	No	80 half hour sessions; individual impairment based	Yes	No difference between treated and untreated patients
Wertz et al. (1981)	Compares individual with group therapy	67	Yes	8 hours per week for up to 48 weeks; individual therapy involved impairment work; group therapy targeted social language use	Yes	Both groups improve on all measures and beyond the period of spontaneous recovery; individual > group on PICA, but not on disability measures

Drawing firm conclusions from these studies is difficult, often because of quite profound methodological problems (e.g. see Pring 1986; Howard 1986). One tentative finding is that change seems contingent on the length or intensity of therapy. In essence, evaluations of large amounts of therapy often demonstrate change, including change on activity measures (e.g. Brindley *et al.* 1989; Wertz *et al.* 1981), while evaluations of small amounts do not (e.g. Lincoln *et al.* 1984).

These studies have little or nothing to say about the effects of different types of therapy. Usually only a very brief description of treatment is provided. Also, within the groups, participants often receive different therapies, according to their individual needs. So even if group effects are found, the source of those effects may be obscure.

Small group, or individual studies are a much better medium for exploring outcomes from particular treatments. The following sections will selectively review such studies of impairment therapy, compensatory therapy, conversational therapy and group therapy.

Impairment therapy

Impairment therapies aim to improve particular language skills, such as naming, sentence production, reading and writing. They typically involve abstract language tasks, which enable the person to develop and practice the target skill. There is now ample evidence that such approaches can improve performance on impairment measures (e.g. see reviews in Hillis 2002). Less clear is whether they have an impact on the person's ability to undertake communication activities, mainly because researchers rarely assess this dimension. Despite this, a few studies provide some positive hints. For example, Beeson *et al.* (2002) found that clients made novel uses of writing in their daily communication after a period of writing therapy, and Thompson (1998) found gains on the ASHA FACS (Frattali *et al.* 1995) after working on sentence production. A number of studies document improved narrative production after sentence therapy (e.g. Byng 1988; Marshall 1999).

Hickin *et al.* (in press) explored whether naming therapy can change two important communication activities: narrative and conversation. The aphasic participants in the study both had moderate/severe word finding difficulties. There were two phases of therapy. The first aimed to improve word retrieval using naming practice with phonological and orthographic cues. The second focussed more on communicative tasks, such as making functional lists, reminiscing and telling anecdotes. Therapy was evaluated with picture naming tests, a narrative task and videos of pre and post therapy conversations. The latter were analysed for aspects of word production, such as the number of words used by the aphasic person and the rate of lexical errors. Of interest was whether picture naming improved after therapy, whether this generalised to untreated words and, crucially, whether any effects were detectable in narrative and conversation.

The two individuals responded rather differently to therapy. Both showed significant gains in picture naming. With one of the participants, H.P., benefits were confined to items that had appeared in therapy. The other person, M.H., showed more generalised improvements, i.e. even with untreated words.

The narrative and conversational results also varied. H.P., whose naming improvements were confined to treated items, showed no changes on these tasks. M.H., however, did improve. For example, in conversation, he produced more nouns per turn after therapy and made fewer lexical errors (and after showing a stable baseline on this measure). Interestingly, these changes could be detected even after the first period of therapy or before the more functional communication tasks were introduced.

This study offers a preliminary attempt to explore the effects of therapy on two aspects of everyday language. The activity measures were clearly related to the content of therapy and the results are broadly explicable. In particular, they suggest that gains in narrative and conversational speech cannot follow item-specific gains in naming. Rather, they depend on the person recovering some generalised access to word forms.

Hickin *et al.* suggest that reducing the language impairment may, in some cases, have an automatic effect on communication activities. In other cases, specific work may be needed to help the aphasic person transfer skills learnt in the clinic to every day life. Robson *et al.* (1998) describe a therapy programme conducted with R.M.M., a woman with severe jargon aphasia. R.M.M. produced virtually no comprehensible speech and showed little awareness of her speech difficulties. In some respects her writing was equally impaired, since she could produce no written words spontaneously. However, R.M.M. could copy some words, even after a delay, and could sort anagrams using letter tiles. She also seemed able to monitor her writing, since she was dissatisfied by her errors and attempted to correct them. This suggested that writing was a promising target for therapy.

Therapy aimed to establish a written vocabulary, which would enable R.M.M. to communicate basic concepts to those in her environment (a nursing home) and which might help her to resolve communication breakdowns. The vocabulary was picked for its personal relevance in consultation with two of her close friends. The first phase of therapy aimed to develop written naming skills. Tasks included: sorting letter tiles to label pictures, delayed copying of picture names and picture naming with first letter cues. This brought about significant improvements in picture naming for treated items, which were maintained six weeks later. However, untreated items showed no change, and, crucially, R.M.M. made no use of writing in her daily communication (as observed by nursing home staff and her friends).

Subsequent therapy phases aimed to expand the number of words that R.M.M. could write, through further naming tasks, and promote the communicative use of writing. The latter involved tasks such as writing words in response to conversational questions, conveying information about recent events in her life to a third person, and writing a list of things to take on holiday. In the third phase 'Message Therapy' was used, which aimed to connect the single words that R.M.M. could now write to messages that she might want to convey. For example, a written message was read aloud to R.M.M. (such as 'the laundry is late'). She was then shown three pictures, one of which was related to the message: shirt, shoes, walking stick. R.M.M. had to pick the associated picture and write its name. Feedback emphasised that this word might act as a clue to the message.

Communicative writing was evaluated with novel assessments, which required R.M.M. to write words in response to questions ('Where did you go on holiday?'), or to convey messages ('What could you write if you wanted to say that the curate had called?'). R.M.M. improved significantly on both tasks after therapy, but only when she was able to use treated words. Most optimistically, her friends and staff were able to report uses of writing in daily communication, such as when she wrote 'hair' to indicate that the hairdresser had not called.

Robson *et al.*'s study again shows that we can improve the picture naming abilities of an aphasic person through therapy, this time in writing. It also demonstrates that therapy can enable the person to use the acquired vocabulary in more open tasks, like answering conversational questions. There is a hint that this may have an impact, albeit a small one, on the person's daily communication. Furthermore, a subsequent study replicated this finding with other people with jargon aphasia (Robson *et al.* 2001).

In summary, it is now well established that 'impairment level' therapy can improve performance on specific language tests such as picture naming (Raymer and Gonzales Rothi 2002) and sentence production (Marshall 2002). A few studies suggest that such skills may generalise to more open conditions (e.g. Robson *et al.* 1998; Beeson *et al.* 2002) and conversation (Hickin *et al.* in press). However, this generalisation is by no means guaranteed. The work of Robson and her colleagues highlights the processing differences between the constrained tasks used in therapy and open communication. They show that being able to write a word like 'park' in order to name a picture is very different from being able to use the same word to describe what one did on Saturday afternoon. Here an entire event is being processed, even if not expressed. The person has to condense this complex idea into single concept, which can be mapped onto the one word available. We cannot assume that aphasic people will make this leap automatically. Rather, therapy should help them to apply their skills to the messy business of daily life.

Clearly more evaluations of impairment therapy are needed, which explore generalisation to the level of activity. Researchers need to form a hypothesis about which language skills will be changed through therapy and how this might affect daily communication. This, in turn, will almost certainly require the creation of novel tests exploring transfer to conversation and other daily uses of language.

Compensatory therapies

Impairment therapies aim to rebuild specific language skills, in the hope that this will have an effect on communication activities. Another approach is to develop strategies that enable the person to communicate despite their impairment. Typical strategies include gesture, drawing, using communication books and pointing to symbols. Several commentators have advocated this approach to therapy, often with creative ideas for its execution (e.g. Lyon 1995; Hunt 1999; Lawson and Fawcus 1999; Pound *et al.* 2000), but evaluations are rarer. One exception is the paper by Sacchett *et al.* (1999). This study involved seven people with severe aphasia, most of whom had minimal written or spoken output. Therapy consisted of one group and one individual session per week for 12 weeks. It aimed to establish communicative drawing, or the use of drawing to convey novel information during interactions. Some of the tasks aimed to develop specific drawing skills, like adding distinguishing features to drawings in order to improve their clarity, but most focused on the use of drawing in conversation. In line with the aims of therapy, relatives were involved, with a view to their developing strategies for interpreting drawings. For example, they were shown how to ask 'homing in' questions about a drawing, and how to elicit clarifying details.

Therapy was evaluated mainly through a novel drawing assessment, which asked clients to draw a solution to a problem. This was either presented in the form of a photograph (e.g. a photo of a woman with a cut finger, for the target plaster) or a conversational cue ('I have cut my finger and it is bleeding, what do I need?'). The task was administered twice prior to therapy (with an intervening gap of six weeks), once after therapy and again six weeks later.

Participants' drawings were scored for recognisability (judged by students who were otherwise not involved in the project) and rated for quality (by different external assessors). After therapy, both measures improved, and the gain was maintained after therapy ceased. There were no changes in the baseline period and there were no changes in language measures unrelated to the content of therapy.

Clearly therapy improved participants' ability to generate drawings in response to a problem-solving task. On the face of it, it seems that the skills needed to complete this assessment are similar to the skills needed for everyday communicative drawing. So, in the task, the person has to interpret a problem, conjure up a possible solution to that problem and draw that solution. If they can do this, they might also be able to use drawings in daily communication, if only at a rather basic level. To explore whether this was the case, the researchers also attempted to evaluate uses of drawing outside the clinic. One procedure asked relatives to keep communication diaries, recording conversations with the aphasic person that occurred between therapy sessions. However, most relatives found these diaries impossible to keep. The other involved administering the Pragmatics Profile (Dewart and Summers 1996), which is a structured interview exploring the communication behaviours of the aphasic person in different situations. Although informal, several interviews suggested that drawing was making a novel impact on communication difficulties at home.

Conversational therapies

Many of the therapies described so far attempted to improve the skills of the aphasic person, e.g. in performing specific language tasks or in using a compensatory strategy. The therapists either assume that these skills will carry over into conversation, or incorporate activities to promote such carry over. This section will review studies in which conversation is not only the goal of therapy, but also its medium (e.g. see Lyon *et al.* 1997; Holland 1991; Boles 1998; Booth and Perkins 1999; Lock *et al.* 2001a; Kagan *et al.* 2001; Garrett and Huth 2002; Lustig and Tompkins 2002; Hopper *et al.* 2002; Rayner and Marshall 2003).

One challenge in conversational therapy is to develop a means of evaluation. Most studies use before and after therapy recordings of conversations between an aphasic person and a partner. These may be rated by observers (e.g. Kagan *et al.* 2001; Lustig and Tompkins 2002), or scored for features like the number of main concepts conveyed (Hopper *et al.* 2002) or the number of successful exchanges (Garrett and Huth 2002). Several studies use Conversational Analysis (CA) to provide a qualitative evaluation, particularly in terms of the conduct of repair (e.g. Booth and Perkins 1999; Lock *et al.* 2001a, b). CA can also yield quantitative evidence of change. For example, the percentage of turns spent in repair may decline after therapy, and there may be a reduction in the length of repair sequences (Booth and Perkins 1999).

All conversational measures need to control for extraneous sources of variation. One means of doing this is to use multiple baselines, and aim to show that measures only change after therapy, or training, is introduced (e.g. Hopper *et al.* 2002; Lustig and Tompkins 2002; Rayner and Marshall 2003). Another is to use a control group of subjects to show that only those receiving intervention change (Kagan *et al.* 2001). However, it is a criticism of this area of work that some studies have no experimental control (e.g. Lesser and Algar 1995; Wilkinson *et al.* 1998; Booth and Perkins 1999).

There are different approaches to conversational therapy. Some promote strategies on the part of the aphasic person, which can be used to facilitate conversation. Lustig and Tompkins (2002) worked with an aphasic and apraxic person (L.G.), who was more able to write than speak. L.G. made occasional use of writing to resolve difficulties in conversation. The therapy aimed to promote this strategy, first in private conversations with the clinician, then in conversations held with the clinician in a public place, and finally in conversations with strangers. In therapy, L.G. practiced holding conversations using topic cards as stimuli. Whenever she struggled to produce a word, she was cued to attempt writing (mainly by the clinician making a 'stop' gesture). Therapy progressed from conversations with the clinician to conversations with strangers. The study used a multiple baseline design, in which videos of L.G. in conversation were rated by speech and language therapy students. The conversations were also scored for how often L.G. used the target strategy and for how often communication targets were abandoned. Ratings of conversations improved with therapy, although only when short clips were used. Strategy use also improved, and there were fewer abandoned targets after therapy.

A different approach includes the main conversational partner in therapy, and aims to change their behaviours as much as the aphasic person's (e.g. Lesser and Algar 1995; Boles 1997; 1998; Lyon 1998; Booth and Swabey 1999; Lock *et al.* 2001a, b; Maneta *et al.* 2001). Hopper *et al.* (2002) worked with two couples, where one member had moderate or severe aphasia. Therapy was based on the principles of Conversational Coaching (Holland 1991). The aphasic person watched a clip of TV, which s/he had to re-tell to the conversational partner. The therapist advised on strategies to aid re-telling, such as communicate the main idea first, draw, gesture, write, and provide feedback. These strategies could be for the aphasic person, but equally for the partner. The couples were observed during re-telling, with the therapist offering further feedback and advice. Evaluation involved pre- and post-therapy clips of the couples carrying out the task (with multiple baselines), and pre- and post-therapy administration of the CADL. The video clips were scored by students for the number of main concepts conveyed. Both couples improved on this measure, with one also improving on the CADL.

Booth and Perkins (1999) only included the conversational partner in therapy. They worked with the brother of a severely aphasic man (J.B.), and based therapy on the results of Conversational Analysis. The pre-therapy analysis, carried out on a recorded conversation between the brothers, found that conversation was dominated by repair. Many of these repairs were directed at errors that had not, in themselves, obstructed communication. Furthermore, rather than being collaborative, which is the normal pattern in repair, the non-aphasic brother often withheld collaboration. So, for example, he might insist on his brother saying a word correctly, even when he had already understood the target. Therapy consisted of a 12 hour carers' training course (attended by the brother and three other carers). This covered general features of aphasia, psychosocial aspects, and the specific difficulties of J.B. Conversational strategies were taught, and particularly strategies for collaborative repair. A post therapy recording of a conversation between the brothers showed dramatic changes. Conversation was much less dominated by repair, and there were no repairs when the non-aphasic brother already knew the target. Encouragingly, J.B. also played a more active role in the conversation, in that he was more likely to initiate topics.

One weakness of this study is the lack of any experimental control. It is possible, therefore, that the differences between the pre- and post-therapy conversations are part of normal variation. The authors argue against this, on grounds of the magnitude of the changes. There is the further difficulty that the abnormal patterns observed in the pre-therapy conversation may have been induced by the investigation procedure. For example, the brother may have changed his behaviours because of (mistaken) beliefs about what the therapists wanted him to do. However, similar patterns have been documented by other researchers and in other settings (e.g. Wilkinson *et al.* 1998; Lindsay and Wilkinson 1999; but see Laaksko 2000 for different findings). This suggests that some of the obstructions in aphasic conversation may be due to distorted reactions to the aphasia, as much as the aphasia itself. Therapy, therefore, can usefully eliminate these reactions.

The above studies involved friends or relatives as conversational partners. Others have given this role to volunteers (Kagan and Gailey 1993; Lyon 1989; Lyon *et al.* 1997). This has the merit of widening the social circle of aphasic people and can give individuals access to conversation even when they have no close friends or relatives. Kagan *et al.* (2001) carried out a systematic evaluation of volunteer training. Their study involved 40 volunteers who were randomly assigned to experimental and control groups. The experimental group received a one day workshop in supported conversation together with supervised conversational practice with aphasic people. The control group watched an information video about aphasia and had the opportunity for unsupervised interaction with aphasic people. Each volunteer was videoed at the outset and at the end of the study while holding a conversation with an aphasic individual. Videos were rated by experienced speech and language therapists, in order to capture the skills of the volunteers and the level of participation of their aphasic partners. Results showed that, unlike the controls, the trained volunteers achieved significant improvements in ratings, and this was matched by improvements in participation of the aphasic people. The volunteers in Kagan's study were new recruits to aphasia work. A subsequent, smaller study has shown that similar techniques can significantly improve the conversational skills of long standing volunteers (Rayner and Marshall 2003).

For most people, conversation is one of the most important communication activities undertaken. This brief review showed that therapy can give aphasic people useful conversational strategies, and/or can change the behaviours of their communication partners. The latter seems to improve aphasic peoples' participation in conversation.

Several of the above studies involved widening the focus of therapy, in that the conversational partner was an equal or sole participant in the treatment (see also Togher, McDonald, Code and Grant 2004). In line with the ICF, this approach assumes that the problems of aphasia do not reside solely with the aphasic person. They are also a product of an environment that is poorly adapted to his or her needs. An obvious implication is that therapy aiming to make a difference to activity levels is unlikely to work if it only involves the aphasic person. We must also tackle the communication barriers faced by aphasic people in their daily lives. Working with friends, relatives and volunteers is, at least, a move in that direction.

Group therapy

Many clinicians argue that group therapy is a particularly strong medium for promoting daily communication skills, and reducing the psychosocial consequences of aphasia (e.g. Johannsen-Horbach *et al.* 1993; Penman 1999; Kearns and Elman 2001 and see Elman 1999). Groups provide opportunities for increased socialisation, they offer a forum for sharing emotions and a supportive environment in which to practice communication strategies.

What evidence is there that group therapy can reduce activity limitations? Wertz *et al.* (1981) compared the efficacy of individual and group therapy. The former is described as traditional stimulus-response type treatment, including auditory comprehension, reading, speaking and writing tasks. The latter aimed to facilitate language use in a social setting and involved group discussions and recreational activities, but not specific language tasks. After therapy, both groups improved on language impairment and activity measures. This is argued to be a therapy effect, since the participants were beyond the period of spontaneous recovery.

Subsequent evaluations of group therapy have provided further evidence that this form of treatment can improve communication activities, as assessed by the CADL (e.g. Aten *et al.* 1982; Bollinger *et al.* 1993; Elman and Bernstein Ellis 1999). Two of these also brought about changes in measures of language impairment (Bollinger *et al.* 1993; Elman and Bernstein Ellis 1999). As in Wertz *et al.*, the therapies used in these studies attempted to mimic natural communication, with tasks like discussing current affairs, sharing personal experiences, discussing TV programmes, and role playing real life situations.

Therapy aiming to improve social participation

So far, this review has made minimal reference to the dimension of participation. This is mainly because few evaluation studies address this area. Yet there is considerable evidence that aphasic people experience profound social exclusion, even if rehabilitation has been provided (e.g. Parr *et al.* 1997; Le Dorze and Brassard 1995).

Many commentators use such evidence to argue that increased social participation should be one of the main goals of therapy (e.g. Byng, Pound and Parr 2000; Pound *et al.* 2000; Simmons-Mackie 2001). These commentators subscribe to the social model of disability. They argue that the disadvantages experienced by aphasic people are not solely attributable to the language disorder, but equally arise from disabling attitudes and barriers within society. Dismantling such barriers becomes a prime target for intervention.

As yet, evaluations of this approach are rare. Lyon *et al.* (1997) investigated a programme aiming to re-integrate aphasic people into community activities. The therapy involved 10 triads, each of which consisted of an aphasic person, his or her main carer and a volunteer communication partner. In the first stage of therapy (six weeks) the aphasic person and volunteer developed communication strategies, which were practiced with feedback from the clinician. In the second stage (14 weeks), the aphasic person identified home based or community activities that they would like to resume. These activities were discussed in clinic then attempted, with a follow-up review.

Evaluation measures included a language impairment test, a language activity measure and three questionnaires exploring psychosocial well being and communication use. The results showed no changes in the impairment or activity measures. There were changes on two of the questionnaires, although a small 'deferred treatment' control group also improved on these. The one positive outcome was in the range of new activities undertaken by the aphasic participants. Furthermore, these were often sustained beyond the duration of the study.

Simmons-Mackie and Damico (2001) present a single case evaluation of therapy aiming to improve social participation. The study involved Karen, an aphasic woman who was two years post onset and had been discharged from previous therapy because she had 'functional communication'. Despite this, an interview assessment showed that Karen was now extremely socially isolated. She had minimal participation in former or new activities and her social network was almost entirely restricted to family members. Karen expressed profound dissatisfaction with this state of affairs, contrasting it unfavourably with her pre-stroke life:

Clinician: Can you give me an example of something you did before the stroke?
Karen: Teaching…teaching…always. I love it…it's me.

Clinician: What is a typical day like for you now?
Karen: (shrugs) nothing…here (points to television)

Therapy aimed to expand Karen's social activities. It focussed on reducing external barriers, e.g. by training communication partners, and on reducing personal barriers, e.g. by increasing Karen's confidence and maximising her use of compensatory strategies. One aspect of the intervention involved introducing Karen to voluntary work at a local day centre. Therapy helped Karen use her communication strategies in this setting and provided training for staff members, so that they could communicate successfully with her.

Therapy was evaluated with interviews, conducted with Karen and other key family members before and after therapy. These demonstrated some dramatic changes in the range of activities undertaken by Karen after therapy, and in the constitution of her social networks. She, and her family members, also expressed much more positive feelings about her situation after therapy.

Karen: Busy…maybe too busy now (laughs)
Husband: She's a different person now. She laughs a lot and I don't feel so put upon – oh that sounds selfish but I mean, she has a life! She's not so afraid to do things.

Less positively, the authors do not assess the maintenance of change in this study, or whether or not Karen sustained her new activities after therapy was withdrawn. This seems a crucial issue for therapy aiming to promote participation.

Discussion and Recommendations

Few people would argue that effective speech and language therapy should demonstrate change at the level of activity and participation. Less clear is how to achieve this change. Many evaluations of impairment therapy, aiming to develop specific language skills, fail to probe for change at the activity level. However, this review identified some evidence that such approaches may improve everyday communication, particularly if therapy encourages the person to use the skills beyond the clinical setting. Alternatively, therapy may be pitched at the activity level from the outset, as is the case in many conversational and group therapies. Some studies demonstrate improvement in participation. Here therapy takes a very different approach, e.g. by using volunteers to re-connect aphasic people with their local community.

An ideal therapy package may involve a series of different types of input to tackle these different levels. So impairment therapy might aim to improve the production skills of the individual, followed by conversational therapy, which would engage the main conversational partner, with further participation therapy aiming to widen the person's social networks and activities.

A more integrated approach is advocated by Duchan and Black (2001). They argue that therapy should be based around life goals, identified by the aphasic person. Therapy is therefore pitched at an activity/participation level from the outset. This does not preclude impairment assessment or therapy. Rather, these components act as servants to the therapy goals. Duchan and Black give the example of a client who wishes to resume her human rights activities in Central America, activities that previously involved extensive reading. There are different means of attaining this goal. Some might involve volunteer support, and so bypass the need for reading on the part of the client. Alternatively, the client may wish to access written information more independently, in which case impairment level work, in the form of assessment and treatment of reading, may become a component of the intervention.

A final question relates to evaluation. Investigating change at the level of impairment is relatively straightforward. It typically entails pre- and post-treatment administrations of specific language tests, with controls provided by repeated baselines or the measurement of untreated tasks and items. Measuring change at the level of activity is more difficult. For example, it is difficult to sample daily communication without distorting that communication, and conversational measures are fraught with problems of scoring and variability. Some well-designed activity tests are available, although these have been criticised for not reflecting the realities of daily communication or the personal priorities of clients (Worrall et al. 2002). Measuring participation is even more difficult. Some aspects can be quantified, such as the number of social contacts experienced by an aphasic person. However, this dimension is probably more sensitively evaluated by qualitative procedures, like interviewing. These, for example, enable us to explore the quality of social interactions and the aphasic person's feelings about them.

No single procedure can overcome the difficulties. Rather, a comprehensive evaluation should employ a number of different measures, which explore change within the different dimensions. We should also formulate hypotheses at the outset about what changes we would expect as a result of the particular therapy being administered. This should enable us to look for theoretically explicable change, and begin to address the question of how change in one area relates to change in another. Studies of this kind should develop our knowledge not only about which therapies are effective for which impairments, but also about how to make a real difference in the lives of aphasic people.

Acknowledgements

I am grateful to Deborah Cairns, Katerina Hilari and Tim Pring for their comments on an early draft of this paper.

Section 5

Executive disorders

18 Theories of frontal lobe executive function: clinical applications

Paul W. Burgess and Jon S. Simons

Abstract

Many of the symptoms that are particularly difficult to treat are associated with damage to the frontal lobes. There are a very large number of symptoms which are collectively referred to as 'dysexecutive symptoms'. These are not only problematic in themselves, but can also affect a patient's ability to benefit from therapy aimed at ameliorating other forms of deficit (e.g. physical therapy), and are often associated with a generally poor response to treatment (Alderman 1991). Considerable treatment advances have been made in this area in the last few years. However, in order to develop new methods we need to understand the causes of the particular symptoms. This chapter has four aims: (1) To describe some of the latest findings about the functional anatomy of the frontal lobes; (2) to describe the main clusters of frontal lobe symptoms, how they relate together, and their relative importance; (3) to explain the main theories of how the frontal lobe executive system works and how they relate to the symptoms you can expect to see day to day, and (4) to give some 'blue-sky' predictions about which therapeutic methods might be worth pursuing based on these theories.

Aim of this chapter

The frontal lobes of the human brain are involved in a myriad of functions, including language, motor and high-level perceptual skills. Critically however, they also play an important role in what are known as 'executive functions'. These are the abilities that allow a person to adapt to new situations and develop and follow their life goals. In this regard, 'executive functions' is an umbrella term for a host of functions such as those that allow people to plan and organise themselves over long periods of time; make complex high-level and abstract judgements; and organise and control their memory processes. The way these functions interact with the environment and are supported by the brain are not straightforward. As such this is a theoretically complex area, and going from pure theory to practical clinical application is therefore not always easy. However this does not mean clinical practice cannot on occasion be informed by basic science in the area. Accordingly, this chapter presents an outline of the practical rehabilitation implications of current theories and models of executive function, outlining some 'provisional principles' for the rehabilitation of the dysexecutive patient. These are not as yet empirically supported findings, but are hypotheses developed from theorising which we hope may one day be testable. As the reader will see, these principles are not especially surprising, and in fact generally correspond to the sorts of approaches that are good practice in everyday rehabilitation settings. But this is how it should be. After all, the gifted intuitions of many rehabilitation professionals have honed the approach to the treatment of the dysexecutive patient. And if current theorising has any validity, then its implications should correspond to what has been found to work in practice.

The aim of this chapter is to try and describe why it is that these procedures have been found to work. For further information about the rehabilitation methods mentioned in this chapter the reader is directed to Burgess and Alderman (2004); Alderman and Burgess (2002); Mateer 1999; Robertson 1999; Sohlberg *et al.* 1993; and chapters in this book by Jon Evans and Andrew Worthington: Chapters 20 and 21 respectively.

Introduction

There is little doubt that deficits in the executive functions of the frontal lobe are of major concern for the rehabilitation professional. Many of the symptoms that are particularly difficult to treat are associated with frontal lobe abnormalities (e.g. apathy; Okada *et al.* 1997). Moreover, it has been argued on many occasions that frontal executive dysfunction can affect a patient's ability to benefit from therapy aimed at ameliorating other forms of deficit (e.g. physical therapy), and is often associated with a generally poor response to treatment (e.g. Alderman 1996; Tamamoto *et al.* 2000). However, the theory of how rehabilitation of executive functions might work is not as developed as for other areas of therapy (e.g. speech and language therapy; physiotherapy) or indeed other areas of cognitive rehabilitation (e.g. amelioration of memory deficits). This is largely a consequence of two interlinked factors: the myriad of symptoms of executive dysfunction, and the theoretical complexities involved in investigating (and therefore understanding) them.

For the range of symptoms of executive dysfunction, consider Table 18.1. This lists the twenty most commonly reported symptoms of frontal lobe dysfunction that were described by Stuss and Benson (1984, 1986). There are also many other symptoms that may be less common but which could also have been included (e.g. utilisation behaviour, Shallice *et al.* 1989; bizarre behaviour, Burgess and Shallice 1996a; multitasking problems, Shallice and Burgess 1991a, Burgess *et al.* 2000), attentional difficulties (Stuss *et al.* 1999; Robertson *et al.* 1997). In addition, one might also include the difficulties with spoken language, visual perception and motor control that can occur following frontal lobe damage (see Fuster 1997; Passingham 1993 for reviews) but which are traditionally considered under other topic headings in cognitive neuroscience, and so are not outlined here. A pragmatic solution is to include all of these symptoms under one topic heading (e.g. 'executive (dys)function'), but there is a danger that this implies the possibility of finding a single unifying explanation for them, and therefore a single rehabilitative method. The present evidence suggests that this will not be possible, and that the practicing clinician will need a range of techniques which can be applied to different symptoms.

What can we learn from theories of frontal lobe function?

For the reasons just described, there is often a sizeable gap between empirical evidence and theorising in this area, and its implications for rehabilitation. This chapter will try to bridge this gap as far as is currently possible. After all, every good therapy needs a theory of what is being treated, and how the intervention will work. For this reason, our theories about frontal lobe function should crucially influence the manner of our intervention. What, therefore, do current theories tell us about how we should treat our dysexecutive patients?

Table 18.1 Frequencies of reporting dysexecutive symptoms[3]

Symptom	Patients reporting problem (per cent)	Carers reporting problem (per cent)	Rank of disagreement[1]	Scaled disagreement in ranks[2]
Poor abstract thinking	17	21	16.5	−9
Impulsivity	22	22	19.5	−10
Confabulation	5	5	19.5	+3
Planning	16	48	1	+8
Euphoria	14	28	5	+7
Poor temporal sequencing	18	25	15	−8
Lack of insight	17	39	3	+5
Apathy	20	27	13	−5
Disinhibition (Social)	15	23	13	−3
Variable motivation	13	15	18	−7
Shallow affect	14	23	10.5	+1
Aggression	12	25	6	+6
Lack of concern	9	26	4	+9
Perseveration	17	26	10.5	−1
Restlessness	25	28	16.5	−6
Can't inhibit responses	11	21	9	+4
Know-Do dissociation	13	21	13	−2
Distractibility	32	42	8	+1
Poor decision-making	26	38	7	−3
Unconcern for social rules	13	38	2	+10

[1]This number represents the rank size of the disagreements (in proportions reporting the symptom) between patients and controls, where 1 = largest disagreement. In other words, 1 means that carers reported this symptom much more often than patients.

[2]This number reflects the relative disagreement in rank frequency of reporting between patients and controls, scaled from −10 to +10, with 0 being absolute agreement in rank position of that symptom. On this scale, −10 means that this was a commonly reported symptom by patients, but not by carers; and +10 means that carers reported this symptom frequently, but it was relatively uncommon for patients to report it.

[3]Only ratings of 3 or 4 (out of a maximum of 4) for each item on the DEX questionnaire (Burgess et al. 1996a) were considered as indicating a problem. These correspond to classification of the symptom as 'often' or 'very often' observed. These results are based on data gathered as part of the study by Wilson et al. (1996).

Most current 'theories' of frontal lobe function may be (in the terms of Morton and Bekerian 1986) more accurately characterised as frameworks than falsifiable theories. For this reason, they are often of rather distant help when faced with a specific symptom. However, some general principles emerge. The greatest level of distinction as regards implications for rehabilitation method concerns the way in which the theory was developed. The main differences are between single account theories, 'construct-led' theories, multiple-account theories and single symptom theories. We cannot cover all of the theories in this chapter, so we have chosen a few illustrative ideas.

Single system theories

Cohen's contextual information theory

Single system theories are those that hold that damage to a single process or system is responsible for a number of different dysexecutive symptoms. A good example is the theory of Cohen and his colleagues (Cohen *et al.* 1990; Cohen and Servan-Schreiber 1992; Cohen, Braver and O'Reilly 1998), which is derived from connectionist modelling of simple tasks such as the Stroop paradigm. Cohen *et al.*'s theory is that prefrontal cortex (PFC) serves an adaptive, task-dependent function, representing 'context information', which they define as the 'information necessary to mediate an appropriate behavioural response' (Cohen *et al.* 1998, p. 196). This information may be a 'set of task instructions, a specific prior stimulus or the result of processing a sequence of prior stimuli (i.e. the interpretation resulting from processing a sequence of words in a sentence)' (ibid.). Different functions of PFC, such as behavioural inhibition and active memory, may therefore reflect the operation of the context layer under different task conditions. Under conditions of response competition, when a strong response tendency must be overcome for appropriate behaviour, the context module plays an inhibitory role by supporting the processing of task-relevant information. On the other hand, when there is a delay between information relevant to a response and the execution of that response, then the context module plays a role in memory by maintaining that information over time.

Cohen and colleagues acknowledge that their theory is incomplete (Cohen *et al.* 1998). They maintain that for a more general account of cognitive control (as opposed to one that is constrained chiefly to explaining patterns of Stroop performance), mechanisms are required that deal with the management of interference, the identification of task-relevant information and the representation of many different information types. A strength of this theory, however, is that various aspects of it can be tested empirically. For instance, Cohen *et al.* make the prediction from the model that memory deficits should emerge earlier than inhibitory deficits in schizophrenia.

Grafman's structured event complex theory

Jordan Grafman's theory (e.g. Grafman 2002) is different from many others which seek to understand how the executive system works because it focuses not on adaptive processes supported by the frontal lobes but on the nature of representations stored within this region of the brain. Grafman terms these representations 'structured event complexes'. A structured event complex (SEC) is 'a set of events, structured in a particular sequence, that as a complex composes a particular kind of activity that is usually goal-oriented' (Grafman 2002, p. 298). A SEC is a knowledge representation of all the typical actions and sequences of events that go to make up a common event. For instance the structured event complex for going to a restaurant with a friend might include the sequence of events such as getting in your car and driving to the restaurant, ordering the meal, food being served and so forth. Grafman believes that there are many SECs within the frontal lobes, categorised according to the posterior cortical or subcortical regions to which particular frontal lobe areas are connected. This theory predicts that damage to the frontal lobes of the brain can cause deficits in a wide range of situations, depending on which set of SECs has been affected. Thus a rehabilitation suggestion from this theory is that one needs to study carefully the situations in which the patient experiences problems and then work with them one by one, without expecting much generalisation of gains to other situations.

Implications for rehabilitation

These accounts both have the advantage of parsimony. They make different predictions, however, about patterns of impairment, and therefore approaches to rehabilitation. Cohen's theory holds the promise that apparently quite different symptoms might share a common cause, and thus treatment might lead to improvement in a range of situations. In contrast, Grafman's theory suggests that behavioural impairments in particular situations may have different underlying causes (depending on the locus of the damage), and thus predicts a more restricted outcome for rehabilitation, with each problematic situation needing to be tackled separately. However they both encourage careful consideration of the precise demands of the situations in which patients demonstrate their impairment, and both theories suggest that it might be difficult to predict the exact form of improvement in any one case. In practical terms, Grafman makes the useful point that his theory has the advantage of being easily understood by family members. He suggests that therapists might want to target for rehabilitation an (impaired) activity that has a 'mid-range frequency of experience by the patient. This gives the patient some familiarity with the activity, but the activity is not so simple…'. He suggests training using behaviour modification methods, working on situations that are targeted at specific activities relevant to the patient's daily life (for examples of these methods see Alderman and Burgess 2002).

By contrast, Cohen's theory suggests that dysexecutive patients might be helped by a system for reminding patients what they are supposed to be doing, and how far they have so far progressed in achieving their goal. A moment by moment feedback system, in other words. A system of this kind has been used by Nick Alderman and his colleagues at St Andrew's Hospital in Northampton, in the UK. Alderman *et al.* (1995) described a programme of Self-monitoring Training (SMT) which had two specific aims: first, to improve the ability of the individual to attend to multiple events; and second, once this has been established, to reduce the behaviour of concern using an appropriate operant strategy. They argued that the latter will only be effective when the ability to attend to multiple events, and in particular, to monitor one's own behaviour and modify it in response to change in the environment, is possible. The training involved the following five stages:

- *Stage One – Baseline:* The therapist first obtains a baseline of the target behaviour.
- *Stage Two – Spontaneous self-monitoring:* In the second stage, the participant was instructed to monitor the target behaviour whilst conducting some background task over a discrete time period. The participant was given an external counting device to enable them to achieve this (a mechanical 'clicker', whereby each time a button is pressed, a number display is advanced by one digit). At the same time, the therapist discretely monitored the behaviour using a similar device. At the end of the trial, the therapist compared their recording with that of the participant.
- *Stage Three – Prompted self-monitoring:* Stage two was repeated with one modification: each time the participant engaged in the target behaviour but did not record it, the therapist gave a verbal prompt that they should do so. The purpose of this stage of the training was to encourage the participant to monitor their own behaviour more accurately and get into the habit of routinely making a recording whenever it occurred.
- *Stage Four – Independent self-monitoring and accuracy reward:* The purpose of this stage was to withdraw external structure and facilitate self-monitoring by reinforcing accuracy within gross limits. This involved explaining to the participant that they would receive a reward at the end of the trial providing the recording they made was accurate to within 50 per cent of that made by the therapist. During the trial itself, prompts to record would not be given to the participant.
- *Stage Five – Independent self-monitoring and reduction of the target behaviour:* The aim of the final stage of training was to encourage inhibition of the target behaviour using an appropriate operant strategy. To this aim, the patient receives reward at the end of a trial providing they had met a specified criterion (e.g. a certain number of occasions of the target behaviour). During the training period, they continue to use the external counter to monitor behaviour in an effort to keep within the limit that has been set. With success, this target is gradually reduced until the target behaviour is eliminated, or occurs infrequently. Of course, the point is that successful participation in the operant stage of the training is only possible because it has been preceded by improvement in the accuracy of multiple-monitoring skills.

In the original case described by Alderman *et al.* (1995), considerable reduction in a very frequent, disruptive target behaviour was achieved using SMT. It had not been possible to develop inhibitory control over this behaviour previously using other operant approaches due to a gross impairment in monitoring skills. Furthermore, this improvement was still evident when reassessed some months after the training had been completed. (See also an example of SMT to treat confabulation: Dayus and Van Den Broek 2000.)

Construct-led theories

Construct-led theories are those that propose a cognitive construct[1] such as 'working memory' or 'fluid intelligence' as a key function of the frontal lobes. Usually they are predicated on various patterns of performance on experimental tasks, or a characterisation of the demands of those tasks. Investigators typically go in search of the critical brain structures that they think support this construct (e.g. Duncan *et al.* 2000).

The most prevalent ideas of this type are the working memory theories of frontal lobe function. Two of the most commonly encountered are those by Petrides and colleagues (e.g. Petrides 1994) and by Goldman-Rakic and colleagues (e.g. Goldman-Rakic 1995) (see also Baddeley and Della Sala 1998).

Working memory theories

Petrides's position concerns the roles of the mid-dorsolateral and mid-ventrolateral aspects of the frontal lobes. He argues that the mid-dorsolateral region (areas 9 and 46) supports a brain system 'in which information can be held on-line for monitoring and manipulation of stimuli' (Petrides 1998, p. 106). By 'monitoring' he refers to the process of considering a number of possible alternative choices. This system enables the evaluation and monitoring of self-generated choices and the occurrence of events. The mid-ventrolateral region, on the other hand, 'subserves the expression within memory of various first-order executive processes, such as (the) active selection, comparison and judgement of stimuli' (p. 107). It plays a role in the maintenance of information in working memory, as well as the explicit encoding and retrieval of information from long-term memory. The distinction between frontal lobe areas involved in monitoring and manipulation on the one hand, and maintenance on the other, is supported by evidence from patients with frontal lobe damage (Petrides and Milner 1982; Owen *et al.* 1990).

In contrast, Goldman-Rakic argues that the various different frontal lobe regions all perform a similar role in working memory, but that each processes a different type of information (Goldman-Rakic 1995). Working memory is defined as the ability to 'hold an item of information "in mind" for a short period of time and to update information from moment to moment' (Goldman-Rakic 1998, p. 90). It is argued that dysfunction of this system can cause a variety of deficits. Problems on the verbal fluency and Stroop tasks are explained as a failure to suppress a prepotent response due to an inability to use working memory to initiate the correct response. Perseveration and disinhibition may result from the 'loss of the neural substrate necessary to generate the correct response' (p. 93). This theory is based largely on electrophysiological recording in animals (e.g., Wilson *et al.* 1993) and functional neuroimaging studies in humans (Courtney *et al.* 1996).

An interesting aspect of these theories is that they are the ones that most strongly make a connection between function and neurochemistry. Links are consistently made between working memory, dorsolateral PFC and dopaminergic systems (See Diamond 1998, for a review). Indeed, there is a link

---

[1]'Construct' here just refers to an idea. A theoretical characterisation of, or explanation for a set of empirical results. It is unusual for such ideas in this area of science to be expressed in a form where there could ever be a single disproof. Often they are post-hoc explanations of patterns of data, and only rarely does one construct compete directly with another. On occasion, many different constructs may be evoked as explanations of the same data set.

here with Cohen's theory, where dopaminergic neuro-modulation is also a critical aspect of the account (e.g. Cohen *et al.* 1998, pp. 207–8).

Implications for rehabilitation

Two possible avenues for rehabilitation emerge from the working memory accounts of dysexecutive symptoms. The first is drug therapy, as suggested by the link between working memory deficits and dopaminergic system dysfunction. The uses of drugs that alter the action of dopamine in the brain are of course well developed for schizophrenia. They are less well developed for the treatment of brain injury, although evidence is now beginning to emerge (e.g. Karli *et al.* 1999; Powell *et al.* 1996; Kolb 2002). However, these theories suggest that a role might be found for patients whose pattern of deficits is consistent with working memory problems. The second possibility arising from these theories is the use of simple and varied instructions, and quite basic methods of reinforcement. The argument goes as follows:

Let us assume that Petrides is correct, and the root of many dysexecutive patients' problems is that they cannot either (i) hold in mind a number of things at one time, and/or (ii) select, compare and make judgements upon incoming stimuli. Let us also assume that Goldman-Rakic might be correct, and that working memory systems might be information- or modality-specific (e.g. verbal, visual, tactile etc.). These characterisations have quite straightforward implications for the way that rehabilitation should be conducted: keep instructions simple and unambiguous. Reasoning with someone about their behaviour requires the person to track the various arguments as they are being said, and to compare the various aspects of the argument. This may well be beyond the capabilities of the patient with working memory problems, and suggests that one should consider using simple reinforcement and reward techniques if possible.

Petrides maintains that the ventrolateral WM system is implicated in encoding and recall of complex material. If this system is damaged, the patients may have difficulty encoding for themselves the salient aspects of the learning situation. So it may be better if verbal reinforcement alone is not relied upon; actual acts of reward may be more effective. Moreover, it may be unwise to rely for treatment effect on the patient's ability to encode and actively later remember the content of previous sessions. Gradual behavioural shaping may be a better solution. Above all, one might expect just saying to a patient 'it would be better to do X because. ... ' or general talking therapies to be relatively ineffective for dysexecutive symptoms that may be secondary to WM impairment. According to Goldman-Rakic, this might include disinhibition, which as Table 18.1 shows, is a quite common dysexecutive symptom.

Duncan's Theory of 'g'

Another construct-led theory of frontal lobe function is Duncan's frontal lobe theory of 'general intelligence' or 'g'. (e.g. Duncan 1995; Duncan *et al.* 2000). This is quite different from the working memory theories. It suggests instead that the principal purpose of the frontal executive system is to support a single function that is used in many situations, called 'fluid intelligence' or Spearman's g.[2] As its implications for rehabilitation are considerable, it is worth outlining in a little detail.

Duncan's concept takes as its starting point the almost universal finding that if a very large number of (healthy) people are given a very large range of psychometric tests, the resulting correlation matrix will tend to show more positive correlations than one would expect by chance. This effect is known as

---

[2]Current working memory theories of frontal lobe function might also be included under this category, given that it has been used to explain such a wide range of dysexecutive symptoms (especially in non-human primates), and performance in such a wide range of situations.

'positive manifold'. Duncan follows Spearman (1927) in interpreting this positive manifold as evidence for a single cognitive process or function that is used in many (if not all) apparently different situations. This process, ability or function was called 'g' by Spearman (short for 'general intelligence'; see Duncan and Miller 2002 for further details).

It has been known for many years, however, that a single underlying function is not the only possible explanation of positive manifold. It is perfectly possible to get the same effect if there are many (but a limited number of) different cognitive processes involved in different tasks, and any one task samples from a different subgroup of them. In short, positive manifold is not proof of a single core cognitive process, yet the notion of 'g' (or fluid intelligence) persists to this day as one possible explanation of a very prevalent finding.

So what is the evidence that Duncan uses to demonstrate that the frontal lobes play a critical part in 'g'? The first is his demonstration using three frontal lobe patients. These people showed planning and organisational problems in everyday life despite normal performance on executive (e.g. verbal fluency, WCST), memory, language or perception tests, and also performed normally on the WAIS (Duncan, Burgess and Emslie 1995). However they performed poorly on Cattell's Culture Fair intelligence test, which was designed as a measure of 'fluid intelligence'. They also performed poorly on multitasking tests such as the Six Element Test (Burgess *et al.* 1996b) and the Multiple Errands Test (Shallice and Burgess 1991a).

In a second study, Duncan *et al.* (1996) found that a small group of frontal patients showed increased 'goal neglect' on a difficult speeded task involving searching arrays whilst also maintaining attendance to switching signals. Goal neglect was defined as 'disregard of a task requirement even though it has been appreciated verbally' (Duncan *et al.* 1997, p. 716). The patients also showed decrements in Cattell's intelligence test. Duncan *et al.* argued that this association of deficits, together with the finding that in the normal population performance on their goal neglect task is closely related to *g*, suggests a link between fluid intelligence or *g*, goal neglect, and the frontal lobes. Or perhaps more correctly, between fluid intelligence, the frontal lobes, and whatever *prevents* goal neglect. This process (i.e. which when damaged leads to goal neglect) is described as a 'frontal process of … constructing an effective plan by activation of appropriate goals' (Duncan *et al.* 1997, p 716).

In a study a year later, Duncan *et al.* (1997) showed generally stronger correlations in a group of 24 head-injured patients between Cattell's Culture Fair test performance and three executive tasks (Six Element Test, Verbal Fluency, and Self-Ordered Pointing) than between the executive tests themselves.[3] Finally, and most recently, Duncan *et al.* (2000) report rCBF changes in lateral frontal cortex when people are performing so-called 'high-*g*' tasks relative to 'low-*g*' ones. This result is used to argue that 'general intelligence results derives from a specific frontal system important in the control of diverse forms of behavior' (p. 399).

Implications for rehabilitation

A prediction from Duncan's view is that if one could somehow improve, circumvent, or provide compensatory aid for the damaged function (i.e. *g*), then one would expect to see benefit across a whole range of situations. Another way of putting this is that you would expect to see good generalisation of gains. If a task could be found that tapped the crucial processing aspect eeffectively, regardless of whether it bore any resemblance to real-world situations, then any improvements on the training task

---

[3]However this result was largely due to the very low correlation between Verbal Fluency and the Six Element Test (see also Burgess 2000). In fact the correlation between the Six Element Test and the Self-Ordered Pointing Task was actually larger than for two of the three correlations that involved Cattell's test.

would be reflected in changes in many activities of daily living. Indeed a logical conclusion would be that if one could improve a subject's performance on the measure of fluid intelligence he uses (Cattell's Culture Fair Test), then they should also show improvement in everyday life.[4]

Is there any evidence then that such generalisation occurs? Stablum *et al.* (2000) trained 10 closed head injury (CHI) and 9 anterior communicating artery aneurysm (ACoAA) patients on a dual task paradigm. Training consisted only of performing the task, and was given once a week for five weeks. Stablum *et al.* report gains in dual-task performance for both patient and control groups. This is not especially surprising since one would expect some practice effect. More surprising however was the improvement of both groups on neuropsychological tasks (e.g. Paced Auditory Serial Addition Task (PASAT), Continuous Performance Test (CPT)) that were not trained. However, there are caveats that could be applied to the results of this study (e.g. there was not a no-treatment patient group, or multiple baseline-type design; improvement on real-world tasks was not measured). Nevertheless it does provide an interesting suggestion worthy of larger-scale investigation.

Alderman (1996) gives a complimentary finding. He administered a series of dual-task paradigms to a group of head-injured patients on admission to a rehabilitation unit that specialises in the treatment of severe behavioural problems. He found that the patients who subsequently failed to benefit from rehabilitation showed significantly greater dual-task decrement (i.e. the amount that performance on one task is affected by having to do another at the same time) at admission than those who did benefit. There was no significant difference between the groups in performance in the single task conditions (which were digits forwards and backwards, the temporal judgement subtest of the BADS, and conversation). There were also small differences between the groups on other executive measures (cognitive estimates, verbal fluency, WCST and Trail-Making). The link between dual-task decrements, dysexecutive behavioural symptoms and frontal lobe lesions is supported by Baddeley and Della Sala (1998), who report that a group of frontal lobe patients with behavioural disturbance showed significant dual-task decrements relative to a frontal lobe group without dysexecutive behavioural disturbance. Performance on verbal fluency or WCST was not significantly different between the groups, although there was a non-significant trend for the patients with dysexecutive behavioural disturbance to be poorer. So perhaps one marker of a resource that is important for many situations in everyday life with executive requirements is dual-task decrement.

If these kinds of accounts are true, there is a potential consequence that clinicians might wish to consider. If no more than merely performing an executive task (as in the Stablum *et al.* 2000 study) can cause training effects that generalise to other executive tasks, then this has implications for assessment as well as treatment. Theoretically, if in one's standard assessment, five executive tasks (for instance) were administered (and in our laboratory we routinely give more than twice this number), one would expect to see order effects in performance on the tasks. Moreover assessment of change over time and the determination of its cause would be problematic. The upside is that one could bask in the knowledge that by giving a patient a standard assessment, one was also rehabilitating them at the same time!

Clearly it is important for rehabilitation that we should know whether this account of the frontal lobe executive system is a good one, since if it is true it should inform our whole treatment approach. However, Burgess and Robertson (2002) outline a series of problems for any single account theory:

1. In group studies of either neurological patients or healthy subjects, correlations between performance on different executive tasks are typically very low (see e.g. Burgess and Shallice, 1994; Robbins 1998; Miyake *et al.* 2000).
2. Group studies also show that different behavioural symptoms of the dysexecutive syndrome tend to cluster together rather than all loading on one factor (Burgess *et al.* 1998).

---

[4]Of course the suggestion is not that 'training' someone in the performance of a specific version of this test would be helpful. The improvement would need to be such that it could be demonstrated on versions of the test that had not previously been encountered.

3. At the single case level, symptoms such as confabulation or multitasking deficits may be seen independently of virtually any other signs (e.g. Shallice and Burgess 1991a; Burgess and McNeil 1999; Burgess *et al.* 2000).

4. Also at the single case level, deficits such as response suppression and initiation problems can doubly dissociate (Shallice 1988) on executive tests (e.g. Burgess and Shallice 1996c).

5. Different behavioural symptoms are associated with performance decrements on different clinical executive tasks (Burgess *et al.* 1998).

6. As a group, frontal lobe patients can show a range of different forms of error on the same executive test (e.g. Burgess and Shallice 1996a, c; Stuss *et al.* 2000).

7. Brain lesions in different parts of the frontal lobes can be associated with decrements on different executive tasks, and with different types of failure (e.g. Burgess *et al.* 2000; Stuss, Eskes and Foster 1994; Stuss *et al.* 1999; Stuss and Alexander 2000; Troyer *et al.* 1998).

8. Functional imaging and electrophysiological studies of the frontal lobes suggest potential fractionation of the executive system (see Picton, McIntosh and Alain 2002; D'Esposito and Postle 2002).

Together, these results suggest that although there may well be cognitive control/executive processes that are used in many different situations as the single process and construct-led accounts claim, it is doubtful that they can be complete accounts of the entire frontal cognitive system (as the authors themselves generally admit). As a consequence, some theorists have presented more complex models that attempt to take these potential fractionations into account: the multiple process theories.

Multiple process theories

These are theories that propose that the frontal lobe executive system consists of a number of components that typically work together in everyday actions, but can be examined relatively independently in experimental studies. There are large aspects of common ground amongst the various models. They take (often implicitly) as a starting point an automatic/routine vs. controlled/novel distinction in the organisation of thought and behaviour. Frontal lobe cognitive processes are aligned with the operation of controlled processing, and the purpose of these processes is to deal with novelty.

Fuster's temporal integration framework

Fuster (1997; 2002) provides one of the most concisely articulated examples of this type of theory. This states that

> The prefrontal cortex is essential for the formulation and execution of novel plans or structures of behaviour. These gestalts of action, with their goals, are represented in neuronal networks of this cortex in the form of abstract *schemas*. The simpler components of those structures of action are represented in frontal or subcortical networks at lower levels of the motor hierarchies.
>
> Fuster (1997, p. 251)

The frontal cortex exerts its influence through connective and reciprocal links with posterior cortical regions, and the overall frontal system performs three functions:

1. Working memory: the provisional retention of information for prospective action. This function is mainly supported by dorsolateral prefrontal cortical areas (DLPFC).

2. Set: The selection and preparation of particular (established) motor acts. This is also supported by DLPFC, and also the anterior medial cortex.

3. Inhibitory control: This function serves to suppress interference, either from external distractors, or from internal inappropriate sensory and motor memories, and is supported primarily by the orbitomedial PFC.

Stuss's anterior attentional functions

The idea in Fuster's model that the frontal lobes serve control functions over more basic schemas[5] is one of the enduring ideas in modern frontal lobe theorising (e.g. Luria and Homskaya 1964; Norman and Shallice 1986). Recently, Stuss *et al.* (1995) expanded upon how they see the relationship between the schema and the executive system might operate (see also Stuss *et al.* 2002).

Stuss *et al.* (1995) describe a schema as a network of connected neurons that can be activated by sensory input, by other schemata,[6] or by the executive control (i.e. frontal lobe) system. In turn, it can recruit other schemata to cognitive control processing so as to produce its required response(s). In addition they suggest that schemata provide feedback to the executive system concerning its level of activity. Different schemata compete for the control of thought and behaviour by means of a process called 'contention scheduling' (a concept described originally by Norman and Shallice 1986) and is mediated by lateral inhibition. They suggest that each schema contains multiple internal connections, some of which provide internal feedback. Once activated, a schema remains active for a period of time depending upon its goals and processing characteristics. This might be only a few seconds in situations such as reaction-time tasks. But over longer periods that require activity without triggering input, activation has to be maintained by repeated input for the executive control system.

The focus of Stuss *et al.*'s theorising is attention. They propose seven different attentional functions, each of which have their own neuronal correlates:

1. sustaining (right frontal),
2. concentrating (cingulate),
3. sharing (cingulate and orbitofrontal),
4. suppressing (DLPFC),
5. switching (DLPFC and medial frontal),
6. preparing (DLPFC), and
7. setting (left DLPFC).

Shallice's supervisory attentional system

The notion that the frontal lobes are crucially involved in attention is also reflected in one of the most influential modern theories of frontal lobe function. This theory was developed by Shallice and his colleagues over the last 20 years (e.g. Norman and Shallice 1986 [initially published as a technical report in 1980]; Shallice 1988; Shallice *et al.* 1989; Shallice and Burgess 1991a, b, 1993, 1996; Burgess and Shallice 1997; Burgess *et al.* 2000). The use of the term attention in this theory is broad, and refers in a general sense to the allocation of processing resources (Shallice 1988).

The first version of this theory (Norman and Shallice 1986) was principally concerned with outlining in broad terms the organisation of the executive control system over well-rehearsed behavioural (and thought) routines. There were four levels of increasing organisation. The first level consisted

---

[5]The term 'schema' as used in these theories is generally equivalent to Piaget's (1952) notion of 'schema'. Other practically equivalent terms used in this area are 'scripts' or 'memory organisation packets' (see Schank 1982; Grafman *et al.* 1995).

[6]'Schemata' is the plural of 'schema'.

merely of 'cognitive or action units', which were the basic abilities one has (e.g. reaching for an object, reading a word). Schemata existed at the second level. These were nests of these units that had come to be closely associated through repetition, as described above. The third level was a process called 'contention scheduling'. This was the basic triggering interface between incoming stimuli (including thoughts) and the schemata. Its purpose was to effect the quick selection of routine behaviours in well-known situations. However, of course, many situations (or aspects of them) that we encounter are not well-rehearsed. In this situation one has to consciously decide what one has to do. The cognitive system that effects this conscious deliberation was called the 'supervisory attentional system' (SAS).

In the early versions of the theory, the SAS was merely represented as a single entity. This was not because it was thought that the system comprised only one process or construct, but merely that there was little empirical evidence at that time concerning potential fractionation (see points 1–7 above). Most recently, the putative organisation of the SAS has been articulated in more detail (Shallice and Burgess 1996). In this model, the SAS plays a part in at least eight different processes: working memory; monitoring; rejection of schema; spontaneous schema generation; adoption of processing mode; goal setting; delayed intention marker realisation; and episodic memory retrieval (see Figure 18.1).

Implications for rehabilitation

The strength of the multiple process theories is that they encapsulate the results from many different types of studies, and they attempt to explain behaviour in many different kinds of situations. As such they stand a better chance of explaining a variety of dysexecutive symptoms (see Table 18.1). Their disadvantage is that they are difficult to disprove. If a new dissociation between tasks or symptoms is found, it is easy to either bolt on another process to the theory, or explain it as a refinement of one of the existing concepts. It is difficult to see at what stage such a theory would ever be completely rejected.

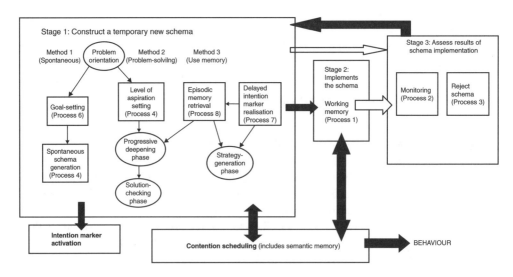

Figure 18.1 The Shallice and Burgess (1996) update of the Norman and Shallice (1980) "Supervisory Attentional System" model. Temporally distinct phases of supervisory system processing are depicted by circles. An operation (i.e. a change of state of one or more control variables) is depicted on a solid rectangle/square. Solid lines depict flow of control, unfilled lines represent information transfer.

For rehabilitation the suggestions of these models is more complex than for the single-process or construct-led theories. These theories suggest that one first needs to isolate the locus of the impairment(s). In practical terms, this would require administration of the sets of procedures upon which the model was based (or as close as is practically possible). This is likely to be a much more time-consuming procedure than for the other types of theory: however it is less likely that an important impairment would be missed. Moreover, a number of the hypothesised processes are only tapped in certain situations, and one needs to assess a patient in a wide range of them.

Rehabilitation efforts can then be targeted to the specific situations in which the patient has problems. In this way, the implications for rehabilitation of the multiple process models are quite different from the previous theories, the suggestion of which is that rehabilitation could be performed out of the everyday situations in which the patient has problems. So are there any grounds for establishing a basic minimum set of investigations that should be performed as a first stage assessment of the dysexecutive patient?

The results of a study by Burgess *et al.* (1998) may give some hints. In this study, the carers or relatives of 92 mixed aetiology neurological patients were given a questionnaire (the DEX) (Burgess *et al.* 1996a) which asked them to rate the frequency of occurrence of the 20 most common dysexecutive symptoms in the patients they knew well. These symptoms are listed in Table 18.1. When the results were subjected to factor analysis (orthogonal rotation), five factors were selected: Inhibition (principally problems with response suppression and disinhibition); intentionality (everyday deficits in planning and decision-making); executive memory (e.g. confabulation, perseveration); and two purely affective factors – positive (e.g. euphoria) and negative (e.g. apathy) affective changes. A range of neuropsychological tests was also administered to the patients, which allowed examination of the relationships between the scores for these behavioural symptom factors and individual psychometric test performances. Burgess *et al.* found a distinct pattern of relationships between test performances and the behavioural symptoms. Performance on none of the psychometric tests was associated with either of the affective symptom factor scores. However performance on many executive tests (Cognitive Estimates, Verbal Fluency, Trail-Making and the Six Element Test of the BADS) was significantly associated with Inhibition factor scores, as were WAIS Full-Scale IQ scores. Modified Wisconsin Card Sorting Test (MWCST) performance and verbal fluency was associated with the Executive Memory factor scores. And only one test (out of a total of 22) was significantly associated with the Intentionality factor scores: the Six Element Test (Shallice and Burgess 1991a; Burgess *et al.* 1996b). From these results, Burgess *et al.* (1998) recommended that at the very least an assessment of a dysexecutive patient should include tests that measure each of these symptom clusters (the affective aspects will be dealt with below). Broadly, these would include:

1. A general measure of inhibitory abilities (impairments of which are detected by a wide range of tasks including those of intellectual function).
2. Measures of executive memory abilities both short-term (i.e. working memory) and long-term (i.e. accuracy of episodic recollection).
3. A measure of multitasking ability (the subcomponents of which will be described in detail below, but include planning, and prospective memory – including task switching).

The degree of concordance of these empirical results with the multiple-process theories outlined above is striking. Two of Fuster's three temporal integration functions are closely replicated, and if one takes a broad view of the preparatory set, then there is further agreement. Stuss's inhibition, switching, preparation and attention maintenance aspects are also all reflected in these empirical findings. Shallice's model copes particularly well. It explicitly mentions, as separate processes, inhibition (in the form of both schema rejection and adoption of processing mode); both working memory and episodic retrieval; and both components of multitasking (prospective memory as 'delayed intention marker realisation', and planning as the set of processes in method 2 of new schema formation). Thus the multiple-process theories cope generally well with explaining the multitude of symptoms that can follow frontal lobe damage.

They also suggest a general approach to investigating the root causes of everyday dysexecutive impairments. Following formal assessment of function as outlined above, one would examine how the particular impairments contribute to disability in everyday life. This requires componential analysis of the situations that present the greatest problem (as identified, for instance by ABC analysis). It is at this point that it is most unfortunate that experimental paradigms are so often unlike real-world situations (as addressed above), since if this were not the case, much of the work would already have been done for the rehabilitation specialist and this stage would be largely redundant. The final stage would of course be intervention, the exact method of which would depend on the nature of the impairment, the situation in which it manifests itself, the *intact* abilities the patient shows, and other relevant clinical variables. In the next section we will consider examples of the treatment of each of the main variables isolated here (inhibition problems, executive memory problems, and multitasking problems).

However, the foregoing argument raises two important and interconnected matters for the rehabilitation of executive function. The first concerns the relative importance of the various symptoms, and the second concerns the patients' awareness of them. If one considers Table 18.1, it is apparent that some symptoms are reported more frequently than others by carers of dysexecutive patients. Indeed, some (e.g. planning problems) are reported as a problem by relatives in almost half of the cases that formed the sample in the study from which this data was taken (Burgess *et al.* 1998). This is even more remarkable when one considers that this group of patients was not specifically selected because they showed dysexecutive symptoms, but merely because they represented a cross-section of the sort of neurological patients that might typically be encountered in clinical practice (consisting of 59 per cent head injury; 13 per cent dementia; 8.5 per cent CVA; 6.5 per cent encephalitis; 13 per cent other conditions). Clearly one would ideally first develop treatment methods for, and target efforts towards, those symptoms that are most often observed, since these are *ipso facto* most likely to be problems in everyday life.

A frequently encountered problem, as Table 18.1 shows, is that patients are often unaware of the extent of their problems. This is not a problem that is confined to executive dysfunction: many amnesics or people with neglect etc. may be unaware of their problems, at least in the early stages of their disability. However, it is a difficulty that is both prevalent and persistent in this area, as Table 18.1 shows (see also Prigatano 1991). This should at least in part guide the agenda for dysexecutive patients' rehabilitation. All other matters being equal, treatment of a problem that the patient does not notice or acknowledge will always be more problematic than for one about which the patient complains. Table 18.1 shows that two of the symptoms where there is typically greatest disagreement between patients and carers both involve a lack of concern. This presents an interesting conundrum: how does one make a patient concerned that they are unconcerned? Perhaps considering the item of greatest absolute disagreement between patients and carers provides an answer: planning problems. One might in a simple-minded fashion suggest that a consequence of not considering the future, or the future consequences of one's actions, is likely to be a lack of concern. So if one can first facilitate this planning function, the problem with concern is likely to show concomitant improvement. So in this example, it would make most sense to target one's rehabilitation efforts first towards the deficits in planning. This argument suggests a further dysexecutive rehabilitation principle should be that when choosing which dysexecutive behaviour to treat first, do not just consider which is the most troublesome. Also consider the order in which the symptoms should be treated (see the example of Alderman and colleagues' SMT training above).

Single-symptom theories

It is probably significant for this area of science to note that there are a greater number of general theories that seek to explain many dysexecutive symptoms at once, than there are theories more modest in their ambitions. Nevertheless there are a few areas where theorising about specific symptoms has developed to the point where it could be used to suggest rehabilitation methods. A full review of the rehabilitation implications of all possible theories of all possible dysexecutive symptoms would be beyond the scope of this article. However, as an example we will take two symptoms that are both quite common, and also for which theorising is reasonably well developed: confabulation and multitasking deficits.

Confabulation

One of the more detailed theories of confabulation is given by Burgess and Shallice (1996b). They reasoned that if confabulation is a consequence of damage to the memory control processes involved in autobiographical recollection, one should be able to demonstrate their influence in people who do not confabulate. So a group of subjects were asked to reflect aloud upon their thought processes as they tried to answer a series of simple autobiographical questions such as 'What were you doing for the two hours before lunchtime last Sunday?' The participants' reflections were then transcribed and each statement was classified as belonging to one of 25 different utterance types. By examining the probability of the frequency of any two statements following in sequence, it was possible to establish a prototypical recollection structure. It was found that there were three broad classes of control processing statements that were relevant to the recollection process. They could be defined in terms of their decreasing proximity to memories in the recollection structure, respectively: 'descriptor elements' (i.e. specifications of what it is that is being asked of the memory store); 'editing elements' (i.e. verification, checking and comparison operations) and 'mediator' elements (i.e. problem-solving routines). On the basis of these findings, Burgess and Shallice (1996b) proposed the model shown in Figure 18.2, and argued that the consequence of failure of these memory control processes would be confabulation. Indeed, it was argued that some of the errors that normals quite commonly make are similar to some of those that can be seen, with greater frequency, in confabulation. In this way, the Burgess and Shallice model is a synthesis of aspects of many other leading theories of confabulation (e.g. Papagno and Baddeley 1997; Dalla Barba *et al.* 1997; Moscovitch and Melo 1997). It predicts that a variety of forms of confabulation may be seen, either singly or in combination: those who show problems with self-initiated retrieval; those whose retrieval processing is insufficiently constrained; and those who cannot distinguish between real memories and fantasies and other thoughts. The Burgess/Shallice theory has since been used to explain the pattern of confabulation in a number of cases (e.g. Burgess and McNeil 1999; Dab *et al.* 1999; Worthington 1999).

Implications for rehabilitation

Most confabulators tend to stop confabulating of their own accord (Schnider *et al.* 2000). However some do not, and clinical experience suggests that the speed of recovery in those who will in any case improve may well be increased by cognitive intervention. Different treatment approaches are suggested by the Burgess/Shallice theory. Those whose problems are principally at the descriptor level are characterised by the ability to remember information if given sufficient cues. They are probably best helped therefore by methods to ameliorate the need for self-initiated retrieval, e.g. training in the strict use of a diary, and with reminders such as the Neuropage system (Evans, Emslie and Wilson 1998). Fortunately these methods are also likely to be of benefit for those with 'editor' impairments,

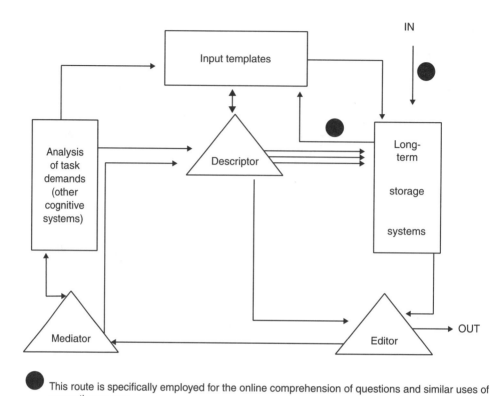

This route is specifically employed for the online comprehension of questions and similar uses of semantic memory.

Figure 18.2 The Burgess and Shallice (1996b) model of the control processes involved in autobiographical recollection.

whose memory system tends to run unfettered. But experience suggests that the key element for these patients is feedback: knowing one has a tendency to produce erroneous memories soon leads to a more cautious approach to recall, which is sometimes all that is needed. The most difficult group of confabulators is likely to be those with mediator-type impairments. These patients suffer from more generalised dysexecutive impairment, one aspect of which is manifested in their memory recall. It is likely that these patients would be helped by a more general approach rather than one which just aimed to deal with their disability in this one situation.

These predictions are largely speculative at present, and are presented in the spirit of trying to suggest links between theory and practice. However there is some early evidence for the effectiveness of these simple methods. For instance, Burgess and McNeil (1999) report the successful treatment of a patient (B.E.) who confabulated following an operation to clip an anterior communicating artery aneurysm. His particular form of confabulation was unusual in that it was stable and restricted to just one part of his life, as the following description shows:

> On one of the first days after returning home, B.E.'s wife found him getting out of bed in the morning and dressing in formal clothes. This was rare for him since he was a shopkeeper. However in addition to his shopkeeping, he used to earn extra money by performing stock-takes for other shops with his business partner. On these occasions he used to dress more formally. B.E.'s wife was alarmed, and asked him what he was doing. He replied that he had a stock-take to perform for a local shop. His wife pointed out that he had only just returned from hospital after recovering from major surgery, and told him that no arrangements had been made for his

involvement in stock-taking for the foreseeable future. However B.E. said that he remembered having a conversation with his business partner the day before when he had arranged to do some stock-taking. His wife knew that this was false, but B.E. was only stopped when he finally was at the door ready to leave (despite his wife's protestations), but couldn't remember exactly where it was that he thought he should be going.

The remarkable thing about this case was that these events occurred every day (and sometimes twice a day) for three weeks until intervention was instituted. This was causing great difficulty between him and his wife.

For treatment, B.E. was trained to keep a diary in which he wrote a detailed account of his daily activities including meals he had eaten, television programmes he had watched, and particularly any telephone calls he had made or received, however trivial they seemed at the time. This helped in two ways. First it provided a record he could check to see if had actually had the telephone conversations he was erroneously remembering. But it also helped because the additional details in his diary served as a cue for him to be able to remember things about the day before that he could not remember without prompting (i.e. a 'descriptor impairment', above). This enabled him to piece together the events of the day and usually remember a real memory that conflicted with the erroneous one. He could then reject the confabulatory memory with more confidence. This simple technique had dramatic effects in a relatively short period of time (five weeks). Although at the end he reported that he sometimes still 'felt' like he might have performed a stock-take recently, he did manage to stop himself acting on the confabulations, and the conflicts with his wife no longer occurred.

This theory-motivated intervention was just a first step. Moreover, it is clear that some paramnesic phenomena are less amenable to current treatment methods than others (see Burgess et al. 1996c). However it does at least suggest that our theoretical understanding of this fascinating disorder is beginning to reach the level of sophistication where rehabilitative methods might soon be developed that will be effective for at least some confabulators.

Multitasking deficits

Mesulam (1986) articulated an observation that had been discussed clinically for many years, but never formally investigated. This was that some frontal lobe patients may show marked problems with higher-level cognitive functions such as planning and organisation in everyday life, but appear normal or near-normal on formal laboratory testing. The years since Mesulam's observation have seen considerable interest in these cases, partly because they have presented a problem for rehabilitation and medico-legal assessment of disability, and partly because they are good evidence of the potential fractionation of the executive system.

As a consequence, we now know a fair amount about the neuropsychological profile of these cases (see Burgess 2000a, for review). The problems that are noticed in everyday life by carers and relatives are typically reported as: tardiness and general disorganisation, unreliability, absent-mindedness (by which is usually meant prospective memory failures) and failures to complete even quite basic tasks such as shopping or preparing a meal. Typically, tasks are started but never completed, with patients often breaking off in the middle of one task to start another, but never returning to the first. Despite these obvious difficulties in everyday life, they may fail none of the traditional tests of executive function (e.g. WCST, fluency, cognitive estimates, Tower of London; Stroop; Trail-Making), nor show any problems on formal testing with WAIS Full-Scale IQ, language, memory, motor or visuospatial perception.

Shallice and Burgess (1991a) explained this pattern as being due to the fact that traditional neuropsychological tasks are typically very well-structured (see Goel et al. 1997; Burgess et al. 2005, for discussion on this point). More specifically, they do not typically require the following: the creation, maintenance and execution of delayed intentions; the ability to recognise the need for, self-initiate and carry out complex meta-strategies; dovetailing of tasks to be time-effective; prioritisation of tasks; and deciding for oneself in the absence of feedback whether a result is satisfactory. In other words, traditional executive tests do not measure many of the abilities that make a person effective in the real world.

The cardinal situation that does tap these characteristics, however, can be called 'multitasking'.[7] Burgess (2000b) describes eight features of the situation, the first five of which are axiomatic, plus a further three (6–8) that are usually true of everyday life multitasking:

1. Many tasks: A number of discrete and different tasks have to be completed.
2. Interleaving required: Performance on these tasks needs to be dovetailed in order to be time-effective.
3. One task at a time: Due to either cognitive or physical constraints, only one task can be performed at any one time.
4. Delayed intentions: The times for returns to task are not signalled directly by the situation.
5. No immediate feedback: there is no moment by moment performance feedback of the sort that participants in many laboratory experiments will receive. Typically, failures are not signalled at the time they occur.
6. Interruptions and unexpected outcomes: Unforeseen interruptions, sometimes of high priority will occasionally occur, and things will not always go as planned.
7. Differing task characteristics: tasks usually differ in terms of priority, difficulty and the length of time they will occupy.
8. Self-determined targets: People decide for themselves what constitutes adequate performance.

The most typical multitasking test used in the clinic is the Six Element Test (see above). In this test, participants are given three simple sets of tasks (e.g. dictation, writing down the names of some common objects), each of which has two sub-components, A and B. (For instance A and B of dictation task are describing a holiday and describing any memorable event). Subjects are given 10 minutes for the task overall, and are told three things: First, it is not possible to do everything in the allotted 10 mins; second, but you must try to do at least some of each subtask. Third, you are not allowed to do an A section of a task followed immediately by the B section of the same task.

Clearly, dealing with situations like these may require a number of different behavioural stages. However, since a given process may be used at many different stages, it may be that the processing demands may be characterised more simply than might at first be imagined. In fact there is some evidence that this is the case. Burgess *et al.* (2000) administered a procedure similar to the Six Element Test (called the Greenwich procedure) to 60 people with circumscribed cerebral lesions and 60 age- and IQ-matched controls. In addition to the basic test measures, the task was given in a way that allowed consideration of the relative contributions of task learning and remembering, planning, plan-following and remembering one's actions to multitasking performance. A basic finding was that this sort of procedure is sensitive to a range of cognitive problems – despite no differences between the controls and patients on measures of premorbid (NART) or current fluid intelligence (Raven's Advanced Progressive Matrices), the patients showed significant impairment on most of the variables (a similar finding is reported by Levine *et al.* 2000). At a more specific level, lesions in different brain regions were associated with impairment at different stages in the multitasking procedure. Lesions to a large region of superior posterior medial cortex including the left posterior cingulate and forceps major

[7]Multitasking can be distinguished from 'multiple-task' performance principally by the 'ill-structuredness' of the situation, and by the requirement of the activation of delayed intentions (see Goel and Grafman 1995 and Burgess 2000b for discussion).

gave deficits on all measures except planning. Remembering task contingencies after a delay was also affected by lesions in the region of the anterior cingulate, and rule-breaking and failures of task switching were additionally found in people with lesions affecting medial and more polar aspects of Brodmann's areas 8, 9 and especially 10. A theory of the relationships between the cognitive constructs underpinning multitasking was tested using structural equation modelling. The results suggest that there are three primary constructs that support multitasking: retrospective memory, prospective memory and planning. Burgess *et al.* (2000) tentatively suggested that left anterior and posterior cingulates together play some part in the retrospective memory demands, while the prospective memory and planning components make demands upon processes supported by rostral PFC and RDLPFC respectively.

It seems likely that the principal contribution of the PFC to multitasking lies with supporting the planning and especially the prospective memory that is required. Impairment of this prospective memory component typically manifests itself in two ways on tasks such as the Six Element Test (SET). First, subjects may fail to switch tasks when they intended.[8] Second, they may break the task rules (in the case of the SET, this means doing two subsections of the same type consecutively). Interestingly, a recent study by Alderman *et al.* (2003) suggests that these two types of failure might be unrelated. Fifty mixed aetiology neurological patients were given a simplified version of Shallice and Burgess's (1991a) Multiple Errands Test (MET). The MET is a real-world shopping test, carried out in a shopping precinct. Participants have to buy several items and carry out errands whilst following a set of quite arbitrary rules. Alderman *et al.* found that the patient group could be divided into those who tended to forget to carry out tasks, but did not break rules, or those who broke the rules but completed tasks. This suggests that different rehabilitative methods should be used for the two groups.

Mechanisms of recovery

We have discussed some of the leading theories of how the frontal lobes exert their control over behaviour. And we have outlined in broad terms some of the implications for the rehabilitation of patients with executive control deficits. In some cases the form of rehabilitation might be termed 'cognitive prosthetics': in other words the aim is to improve function rather than ameliorate the cognitive impairment by the use of external aids (e.g. the Neuropage system (Wilson *et al.* 1997)). In other cases, rehabilitation may reduce the need for the impaired ability by changing the environment. A third type aims to establish behaviour patterns that rely on intact systems: in other words to alter the construct demands of the old function (for illustration, a rather simple example might be where a patient with severe speech production problems is encouraged to write messages to communicate). A fourth type, however, aims to improve the actual cognitive impairment itself. But how might such an improvement occur in the damaged brain?

The current primary evidence comes from studies of motor skill deficits. In a recent study by Liepert *et al.* (2000), the cortical motor output area of a hand muscle was mapped in thirteen stroke patients using transcranial magnetic stimulation before and after treatment. The rehabilitation consisted of twelve days of constraint-induced movement therapy. They found that before treatment the cortical representation area of the affected hand muscle was significantly smaller than the contralateral side. However, following treatment the muscle output area in the affected area was significantly enlarged, and the motor performance of the paretic limb was improved. Liepert *et al.* (2000)

---

[8]Switching an abnormally large number of times also occurs in patients. However the relation of this rare pattern to switch failures is not known.

claim that the shift in the centre of the output in the affected hemisphere was suggestive of the recruitment of adjacent brain areas (see also Traversa *et al.* 1997).

However, the positive effect afforded by functional reorganisation has an enemy. Nudo *et al.* (1996) discuss how a subtotal lesion confined to a small portion of the representation of one hand can result in a further loss of hand territory in the adjacent, undamaged cortex (in squirrel monkeys). Fortunately however, retraining of skilled hand use resulted in prevention of the loss of hand territory adjacent to the infarct, and in some instances the hand representations expanded into regions formerly occupied by representations of the elbow and shoulder. These results give a strong impetus for early rehabilitation intervention: it is possible that treatment is not only about recovery of function, but also about prevention of further loss of function (see Kolb 2002, for further discussion).

Interestingly, this may provide one explanation for a common sequence of events in patients who have sustained frontal lobe damage, but are otherwise quite intact. This is an early presentation of mildly euphoric and disinhibited behaviour that may continue for the early years. However as insight into their situation is gained, this can be replaced by a depression. Commonly there is some social withdrawal at this point, which is more usually the result of loss of goodwill amongst friends and relatives, who have often had enough of the tiresome behaviour, and the patient's failure to move on in their lives. This may settle into a longer-term mild to moderate social isolation, with the patient seeming more impaired many years on than they were initially, thus contradicting the truism of rehabilitation that some spontaneous recovery can always be expected. The most obvious explanation for this sequence of events is the interaction between the patient's behaviour and its social and financial consequences. However the recent experimental findings raise the possibility that following the initial insult, there is further detrimental neural change.

In any case from a theoretical standpoint there is good reason to be concerned about the onset of social isolation. Many theorists believe that a principle function of the frontal lobes is to deal with novel situations (see Burgess 1997 for a review). For this reason, finding tasks that can serve as foci for rehabilitation efforts is difficult: once someone has performed a given problem-solving task, it becomes less novel, and therefore stresses less the processes one intends to address. However, social interaction fulfils most of the criteria one would want as a 'rehabilitation exercise' since no two interactions are exactly the same (novelty). Moreover, successful interaction requires representing the states of mind, moods and emotions of others, self-generation of thoughts and words, fine judgement, and often some basic planning, inhibition and so forth. In other words very many of the functions of the frontal lobes. For this reason, there is good theoretical reason to recommend as important for rehabilitation that the dysexecutive patient receives much social interaction.

Discussion

The predictions from pure theory for rehabilitation that have been covered in this chapter are summarised in Table 18.2. These are extractions from pure theoretical work and as such should be treated with caution: they certainly do **not** have the status of being clinically tested guidelines. Our aim is, however, to try to bridge the gap between the basic scientific research in the area and clinical practice. This gap often appears very large, perhaps insurmountable. However it is our contention that this is a mirage created partly by the differences in terminology between the two areas and partly by the differing demands, concerns, and priorities of researchers and clinicians.

It is trite to state that it is difficult to understand how the executive system of the brain works, but true nevertheless. The executive system is the high-level interface between the person and the environment. It is the way that people decide what they want to achieve, decide how they will go on to achieve it, and then assess the level of their own success. In this way the behavioural outcome at any one stage

Table 18.2 Suggestions for rehabilitation emerging from pure theory of executive functions

1. Consider the use of feedback systems to modify dysexecutive behaviour, especially symptoms of disinhibition and distractibility (i.e. loss of goal).
2. Some dysexecutive patients fail to carry out intended tasks despite being able to recall (when prompted) what it is that they have to do. Consider the use of simple interrupts in their treatment.
3. Keep instructions and advice simple and unambiguous.
4. Use simple reinforcement and reward techniques if possible.
5. Pre- and post-treatment evaluation of dysexecutive problems requires assessment of competence in a wide range of situations.
6. Generalisation in improvement from one situation to another might be limited.
7. When deciding which dysexecutive problem to treat first, do not necessarily start with the most troublesome.
8. Consider also the best order, since in the long term treatment of certain problems may benefit greatly by initial groundwork elsewhere.

is influenced by the person's past experience and their current perception of their situation, as well as their pure executive function abilities, and abilities in other areas. It is little wonder therefore that there is such variety in the symptoms that patients will show, and variability in the effects of brain damage to any one region. However this should not mean that there are no underlying guiding principles, and the clinician is in a good position to discover them. As for the importance of developing behavioural and cognitive therapies for rehabilitation of executive dysfunction, it is clear that this should be a priority. Some theorists have argued that the greatest advance in rehabilitation for this area still awaits us: perhaps some practical application of stem cell research, for instance, that will enable the affected area of the brain to 'repair' itself physically. What is often missed in this speculation is that even if structural repair were perfectly achievable, this alone will never lead to *functional* repair. The processes and representations in the brain have evolved over a person's development since birth, and it is implausible that structural repair alone would replicate the effects of this complex process. Instead it seems likely that the analogy would be with physiotherapy, for instance, after successful surgery to repair a serious limb injury. Even though the limb may now have the potential to be functional, it still needs in most circumstances to be trained, and that training has to progress in a safe and progressive way, guided by the principles extracted from our understanding of how the limb, and other relevant structures, operate. This means that even if we do put faith in pure science research to achieve what we cannot at present (i.e. to produce perfect structural repair to the damaged brain), we will still need to understand the principles behind enabling the brain to once again be functional.

It is almost certain that there is no one rehabilitative method alone that is suitable for all impairments, and although for the critical (damaged) processes to be targeted, the training situations don't have to be real-world ones, we need first to know that they tap the processes that are actually used in the real world. In this regard it is vital that practical rehabilitative research continues, and that clinicians and theorists meet and share ideas with each other.

Acknowledgements

Preparation of this manuscript was supported by a grant from the Wellcome Trust number 061171. It is based in part on ideas first presented in Burgess and Robertson (2002). We are grateful to Barbara A. Wilson, Nick Alderman, Jon J. Evans and Hazel Emslie for letting us describe data collected as part of their study in Table 18.1.

19 Assessment of executive dysfunction

John R. Crawford and Julie D. Henry

Abstract

Executive deficits typically have a much more profound effect on recovery and adjustment than the more circumscribed deficits that arise from posterior lesions. However, the behavioural features of executive dysfunction have proven hard to capture formally. In keeping with the emphasis in this book on the use of quantitative evidence to guide practice, this review focuses on the measurement properties of putative tests of executive dysfunction and on validity information (e.g. data comparing anterior lesion cases with controls or posterior cases are used to calculate effect sizes for commonly used tests). The tests reviewed range from long-standing clinical tests (e.g. verbal fluency and the Wisconsin Card Sorting Test) to more recent tests that are more explicitly derived from theory, such as the Cognitive Estimation Task, the Brixton and Hayling Tests, dual task methods, and the Behavioural Assessment of the Dysexecutive Syndrome (BADS). The issue of the ecological validity of tests is discussed as is the need to consider a patient's premorbid ability when assessing executive functioning. Finally, the rating scales and questionnaire methods of assessing executive problems and disability (e.g., the DEX, PRMQ and FrSBe) are briefly reviewed.

Assessment of executive dysfunction

Executive deficits: serious problems and seriously problematic

Executive deficits arising from damage to the prefrontal cortex and related structures typically have a much more profound effect on a client's prospects for successful adjustment and independent living than the more circumscribed deficits arising from posterior lesions. However, these deficits have proven difficult to quantify and as such can be regarded as the most problematic area in neuropsychological assessment (Crawford *et al.* 1998).

In a rehabilitation setting the reasons for conducting a comprehensive assessment of executive functioning are largely self-evident. Given the impact of executive problems on a client's quality of life, rehabilitation efforts are often targeted directly at the executive problems themselves; this cannot be done successfully without identifying the nature and quantifying the severity of such problems. In addition, the presence or absence of significant executive problems are important determinants of the approach taken to rehabilitation of other functions. Moreover, when attempting to arrive at a formulation of what may appear to be other, more specific difficulties, it is crucial to consider the extent to which they may be a reflection of a broader executive dysfunction.

For example, as Bradley, Kapur and Evans note (Chapter 11, this volume), a patient's everyday memory problems may largely stem from difficulties in self-organisation and initiation rather than represent a core memory deficit. An empirical demonstration of the need to consider executive deficits in this context was provided by Crawford et al.'s (2000b) study of executive dysfunction in Huntington's disease (HD). They reported that the HD sample was severely impaired on the California Verbal Learning Test (CVLT) (Delis et al. 1987). However, controlling for executive dysfunction (using a composite measure of performance on executive tasks) completely abolished the group differences on the CVLT; group membership (i.e. HD versus controls) accounted for 90 per cent of the variance in CVLT performance, this fell to 0.001 per cent when executive dysfunction was controlled for. Furthermore, this effect was specific to the executive composite as large group differences in memory remained when general intellectual ability was controlled for using WAIS-R IQ. Similar effects, although less dramatic, were reported by Crawford et al. (2000a) in their study of memory, executive functioning and general ability in normal ageing.

Clinical skills and experience are of greater importance in the assessment of executive problems than in any other area of neuropsychological assessment. However, in keeping with the overall emphasis of this book on the quantitative evidence-base for clinical practice, and in view of space constraints, this chapter will focus primarily on evaluating formal ability tests and rating scales of executive functioning in terms of their measurement properties and their validity.

One common means of assessing the validity of putative executive measures is to compare the performance of patients with frontal lesion against healthy controls and posterior cases; the presence of a frontal lesion is taken as a proxy for the presence of executive problems (although all would recognise that it is a very imperfect proxy, as is the use of posterior cases as a proxy for the absence of executive problems). In the present work particular emphasis will be placed on quantifying the effect sizes for such studies and those from other types of validity studies. It is increasingly recognised that there has been an overemphasis on significance tests and a consequent neglect of the magnitude of effects (American Psychological Association, 2001). However, despite strongly worded recommendations to report effect sizes, this is still rarely done in research papers and test manuals.

A simple and commonly used index of effect size is r, the (point-biserial) correlation between group membership and test performance. This effect size can readily be calculated from routinely reported summary statistics (the means and SDs of the groups being compared). Although not commonly used for reporting purposes, the square of this effect size gives an even more meaningful measure; it tells us the proportion of variance on the measure of interest that can be attributed to group differences.

Effect sizes are particularly useful when evaluating and comparing neuropsychological tests. A highly significant difference between controls and a patient sample (or between two patient samples) may nevertheless be associated with a modest effect size (particularly if the Ns were large) and may still mean that the test will have limited utility when used in the individual case; i.e., the overlap in score distributions may still be very substantial. Similarly, when evaluating the sensitivity of two or more tests, the results of their individual significance tests is not very informative whereas expressing the group differences as effect sizes is immediately enlightening (for example, see the presentation of effect sizes for BADS subtests in Table 19.3; there were significant group differences on all these subtests but it can be seen that the magnitude of effects vary substantially).

The tests to be reviewed were selected on the basis that they are either currently used widely in clinical practice or have actual or at least potential advantages over their more common counterparts; Table 19.1 summarizes some of the strengths and weaknesses of these tests. The review will commence with two clinical tests and then move on to consider tests stemming from theories of the executive system (see Burgess and Simons, Chapter 18 this volume) and those aimed at providing measures that possess superior ecological validity (i.e. relate to everyday problems); happily some tests are grounded in theory and exhibit this latter quality.

Table 19.1 Summary of some strengths and weaknesses for selected tests of executive dysfunction

Test	Strengths	Weaknesses
Wisconsin Card Sorting	Extensive research base Good norms Moderate sensitivity Moderate ecological validity	Poor specificity Potentially confusing for clients
Verbal fluency	Extensive research base Good norms High reliability Quick and easy to administer and score Moderate sensitivity Normally distributed Moderate ecological validity	Low specificity Highly influenced by premorbid verbal IQ
Cognitive Estimation	Derived from theory	Poor sensitivity Poor specificity Poor ecological validity Poor psychometric properties Poor norms
Brixton Spatial Anticipation Test	Derived from theory Moderate sensitivity Moderate specificity Quick and easy to administer and score Normally distributed	Modest normative sample Coarse-grained scoring (Sten scores) Limited research base as yet
Hayling Sentence	Derived from theory Moderate sensitivity Moderate specificity	Modest normative sample Coarse-grained scoring (Sten scores) Limited research base as yet
Behavioral Assessment of the Dysexecutive Syndrome	Derived from theory Very high ecological validity Moderate sensitivity (six elements)	Limited research base as yet Low sensitivity (most subtests) Specificity unknown
Dual task methods	Derived from theory High ecological validity Good specificity	Not yet fully standardized and normed Potential problem with unreliability

An old warhorse: The Wisconsin Card Sorting Test (WCST)

The WCST (Grant and Berg 1948; Heaton 1981) has complex task demands but primarily measures concept formation, the ability to shift between these concepts, and the ability to utilise feedback to modify responses. Testees have to sort cards by the attributes (colour, shape and number of objects) they share with a set of stimulus cards. The rule to be applied is not specified and changes as the test progresses; testees are informed whether each card sort is wrong or right. A modified version of the Wisconsin was developed by Nelson (MCST) (Nelson 1976). The modifications were primarily aimed at reducing the confusion that testees can experience when performing the original version. Thus, in the MCST, cards sharing more than one attribute with a stimulus card are removed and testees are informed when the rule has changed.

Existing reviews (Mountain and Snow 1993; Reitan and Wolfson 1994; Parker and Crawford 1992) of the sensitivity and specificity of the WCST have concluded that the test has limited utility. For example, Mountain and Snow (1993) stated that

> The evidence that frontal patients perform more poorly than nonfrontal patients is weak. There is insubstantial evidence to conclude that the WCST is a measure of dorsolateral-frontal dysfunction. The clinical utility of the test as a measure of frontal-lobe dysfunction is not supported.
>
> (p. 108)

Studies published subsequent to these reviews have yielded results that reinforce their conclusions.

A particularly important study was conducted by Axelrod *et al.* (1996) using the WCST standardization data (356 healthy controls and 343 patients, including samples of patients with focal lesions). Axelrod *et al.* reported that the WCST achieved a modest degree of overall discrimination between patients and controls but did not discriminate between the different patient samples, i.e. the performance of frontal cases was not appreciably poorer than anterior cases; the effect size (r) for this latter comparison, calculated by the present authors, was 0.24. There has been much less evaluation of the MCST. In Nelson's (1976) original study a cut-off of 50 per cent perseverative errors had high specificity (but low sensitivity) for frontal lobe lesions. However, subsequent studies have reported patterns of results that mirror those found for the WCST. For example, van den Broek *et al.* (1993) found that although, overall, neurological patients could be differentiated fairly successfully from controls, the performance of anterior and posterior cases was indistinguishable.

Thus it would appear as if the WCST and its variants, although moderately impairment sensitive, have poor specificity for the presence of anterior lesions. Set against these disappointing results, there is some evidence that these tests have moderate ecological validity. Burgess *et al.* (1998) found that the MCST correlated significantly (0.37) with ratings made by the relatives of neurological patients ($N = 92$) on the Dysexecutive Questionnaire (DEX) (Wilson *et al.* 1996). There is also evidence that the WCST is a moderate predictor of the level of functional independence achieved following discharge from acute rehabilitation (Hanks *et al.* 1999); for example, the correlations between the WCST and measures of subsequent community integration and level of disability were −0.32 and −0.42 respectively.

Another old warhorse: phonemic fluency

Phonemic fluency requires the generation of words by initial letters under time constraints (normally 60 seconds per each of three letters). This test is also known as the Controlled Oral Word Association Test (COWAT) (Benton and Hamsher 1976), the FAS test (because these are the three letters commonly used), or is simply referred to as verbal fluency. Large scale normative data are available, including extensive data for the elderly (Ivnik *et al.* 1996), the internal consistency and parallel form reliability of these tests are very high, as is their inter-rater and test-retest reliability (e.g. see Spreen and Strauss 1998). Furthermore, the test is quick and easy to administer and score.

Perret (1974) suggested that phonemic fluency was sensitive to executive dysfunction (and more sensitive than semantic fluency) because normally we retrieve words based on their meaning; the requirement to retrieve by initial letter is non-routine and also requires suppression of words that are semantically related to previously produced words. Evidence from dual-task studies in healthy participants indicates that phonemic fluency imposes significant executive demands. Martin *et al.* (1994), reported a cross-over interaction when studying the effects of secondary tasks designed to activate either temporal structures (a semantic decision task) or frontal structures (a motor sequencing task) on phonemic and semantic fluency. Phonemic fluency was severely disrupted by the sequencing task but much less so by the semantic decision task; the converse pattern was observed for semantic fluency.

The evidence from focal lesion studies has provided further support for the position that phonemic fluency imposes significant executive demands, but the literature is full of contradictions (Reitan and Wolfson 1994). As sample sizes in these individual studies are often modest, many of these contradictions may simply reflect sampling error. In an attempt to clarify the literature, Henry and Crawford (2004) conducted a meta-analysis of focal lesion studies. When focal frontal lesion samples were compared to controls, a large mean effect size ($r = 0.52$) was obtained for phonemic fluency (the effect size for samples consisting exclusively of cases with *left* frontal lesions was even larger) but the effect size for semantic fluency was of an equivalent magnitude. In posterior lesion cases the effect size for phonemic fluency was smaller than that observed for frontal samples but the semantic fluency effect size was substantially larger (i.e. there was a cross-over interaction between fluency type and lesion location). Therefore, if one takes the presence of a focal frontal lesion as an (imperfect) proxy for the presence of executive dysfunction, these results suggests that phonemic and semantic fluency impose comparable executive demands. However, semantic fluency is more sensitive to a compromised semantic system.

Henry and Crawford (2004) also obtained effect sizes for other cognitive measures in order to provide context for the fluency results. For focal frontal lesions, the effect sizes for psychomotor speed (Trails A), and for IQ were modest indicating that (a) impaired fluency performance was not simply a reflection of a general slowing in psychomotor speed, and (b) was disproportionate to the general level of cognitive impairment in the frontal samples. The effect size for the WCST was also markedly smaller than that obtained for phonemic fluency, indicating that fluency is the more sensitive of the two measures. Importantly, the above evidence for a differential deficit on phonemic fluency was not apparent in posterior cases; i.e., the effect sizes for these other measures and phonemic fluency were broadly comparable. These results reinforce the view that, like all tests of executive dysfunction, phonemic fluency tests must be interpreted in the context of a client's overall pattern of current performance (and in the context of their premorbid level of ability; see the later section on p. 239).

A meta-analysis of verbal fluency following traumatic brain injury revealed that the pattern of performance across phonemic and semantic fluency and the other cognitive measures referred to above was remarkably similar to that found in focal frontal cases. Figure 19.1 presents the effect sizes

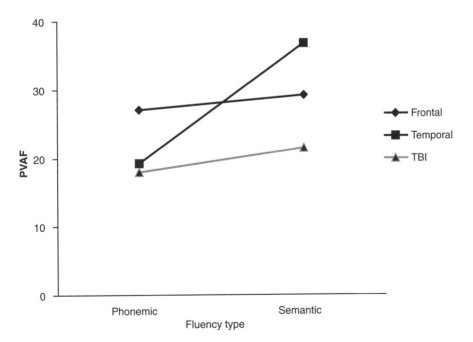

Figure 19.1 Effect sizes for phonemic and semantic fluency following focal frontal or temporal leisons or TBI; data are drawn from meta-analytic studies by Henry and Crawford (2004a) and Henry and Crawford (2004b) and are presented as the percentage of variance accounted for (PVAF) by group membership, i.e. clinical versus control.

on phonemic and semantic fluency for TBI and focal frontal and temporal lesions; the effect sizes are presented as the percentage of variance in the fluency measures accounted for by group membership (i.e., clinical group versus controls). The extensive primary literature on verbal fluency tasks in other neurological and psychiatric disorders has also recently been subjected to meta-analysis, with results that are both of theoretical and practical interest (Henry *et al.* 2004, in press, Henry and Crawford 2004a, b, 2005a, b).

There is some evidence that phonemic fluency has ecological validity as a measure of executive functioning. In the study by Burgess *et al.* (1998) referred to earlier, phonemic fluency was significantly correlated with ($r = 0.35$) with ratings of everyday executive problems as measured by the DEX. Similarly, in Hanks *et al.*'s (1999) study, phonemic fluency was a strong predictor of the level of functional independence achieved following discharge from acute rehabilitation; e.g. the correlation with the Disability Rating Scale was −0.52.

Alternatives to conventional fluency

There are a number of alternatives to conventional phonemic fluency tests. These alternatives hold promise because, in principle at least, they impose greater demands on the executive system. Alternating fluency requires switching between retrieval by phonemic and semantic probes. Downes *et al.* (1993) have shown that in Parkinson's disease, a disorder associated with executive deficits, alternating fluency was differentially impaired relative to conventional, non-alternating fluency.

Warrington (2000) developed a verbal fluency task she entitled the Homophone Meaning Generation Test (HMGT). The task involves providing multiple definitions for a series of homophones (e.g., bear/bare). The task was standardized on 170 normals (Warrington 2000), has good reliability (alpha = 0.82), and yields scores that are normally distributed (Crawford and Warrington 2002). Warrington has argued that the HMGT imposes greater executive demands than conventional fluency tasks and existing set-shifting tasks (such as the WCST) because it requires constant switching between concepts. Anterior cases were significantly impaired on this task (effect size r, calculated by the present authors, was 0.44 when compared to healthy controls); posterior cases did not differ significantly from controls and, encouragingly, the corresponding effect size was very small ($r = 0.07$). An unusual and useful feature of this fluency task is that it is untimed; as a result, and unlike conventional verbal fluency tasks, the clinician can be confident that impaired performance is not down to a general decline in speed of processing.

Crawford *et al.* (1995) developed an excluded letter fluency task (ELF) that requires generation of words that do not contain a specified vowel (e.g., testees have to generate words that do not contain the letter *e*). In keeping with Perret's (1974) argument reviewed above, the test was designed to involve non-routine retrieval (no matter how the lexicon is organised, it is not organised by the absence of letters) and, in addition, to impose greater demands on self-monitoring. Crawford *et al.* (1995) found that head-injured participants committed many more errors on this task than controls; in contrast the error rates on conventional fluency tasks were equivalent across the groups. In comparison to phonemic fluency, ELF is less dependent on crystallised knowledge and is more sensitive to ageing and slowed information processing. Normative data from 399 healthy participants have been provided by Shores *et al.* (submitted); these data include normative data on change on retesting.

To the present author's knowledge, Zangwill (1966) was the first to identify the potential of ideational fluency tasks as a means of capturing executive problems. The Uses for Common Objects task (UCO) (Getzels and Jackson 1961) or 'alternate uses' task requires the generation of unusual uses for everyday objects (e.g. a brick). This task therefore attempts to capture the problems in self-initiation and diminished creativity that characterise many patients with executive dysfunction; in clinical practice many patients are encountered who find it hard to move beyond the well-consolidated, conventional, uses for the stimulus objects.

Butler *et al.* (1993) compared frontal cases and controls on UCO and on phonemic fluency and reported that UCO was more sensitive; the UCO effect size (*r*), calculated by the present authors, was 0.53, versus 0.39 for phonemic fluency. Crawford *et al.* (1995) found that this task yielded the largest difference between head-injured patients and controls from among a battery that contained conventional fluency measures (i.e., phonemic and semantic fluency). Eslinger and Grattan (1993) reported that UCO performance was severely impaired in patients with frontal lesions (effect size *r*, computed by the present authors, was 0.76) whereas a posterior sample did not differ significantly from controls (effect size = 0.22).

Finally, drawing on evidence that naming verbs is disproportionately disrupted by frontal lesions, Piatt *et al.* (1999) suggest that action naming fluency is a potentially useful measure and have provided evidence consistent with the task imposing executive demands.

The importance of premorbid ability when assessing executive deficits

The vast majority of tests of executive function have moderate to high correlations with general intellectual ability in the healthy population (Obonsawin *et al.* 2002), where exceptions to this rule occur it usually reflects poor measurement properties of the tasks (such as ceiling effects). This has important theoretical implications, e.g. Duncan *et al.* (1995) have argued that executive functions and fluid intelligence are essentially synonymous, but it also has very practical implications for assessment. A client's performance on executive tasks must be interpreted in the context of their general level of *premorbid* ability; an average score on a particular executive task can represent a significant decline from a previously higher level in a patient of above average premorbid ability.

Verbal fluency tests provide a clear example of the need to consider this factor as they are highly correlated with verbal IQ in the general healthy population (Crawford *et al.* 1993). Furthermore, Borkowski *et al.* (1967) found that brain-damaged patients with high Verbal IQs outperformed healthy controls of below average IQ on verbal fluency tests.

A number of formal methods of estimating premorbid ability are available, of which the most common is the National Adult Reading Test (NART) (Nelson and Willison 1991). The NART is an oral reading test consisting of 50 words that violate grapheme-phoneme correspondence rules (e.g., *chord*). NART performance correlates highly with IQ (Crawford *et al.* 2001), and is robust in the face of many neurological and psychiatric disorders (Crawford 2004; O'Carroll 1995). The available evidence suggests that NART performance is relatively unaffected by focal frontal lesions (Bright *et al.* 2002; Crawford and Warrington 2002) or closed head injury (Watt and O'Carroll 1999).

The NART can be used to provide a general estimate of premorbid IQ. However, NART-based regression equations have also been developed specifically to provide comparison standard for a patient's performance on executive tasks. For example, Crawford *et al.* (1992) built a regression equation which can be used to estimate premorbid performance on phonemic fluency and a similar equation is available for the homophone fluency test (HMGT) referred to earlier (Crawford and Warrington 2002). In clinical practice the NART estimated premorbid fluency score is compared to the actual fluency score obtained on testing; a large (and statistically significant) discrepancy in favour of the former is taken as an indication of acquired impairment. Support for the utility of this approach is provided by results from a hierarchical discriminant function analysis in which inclusion of the NART as an index of premorbid ability significantly improved the ability of the HMGT to differentiate between frontal cases and healthy controls; the effect size (*r*) when the NART was included was 0.53 versus 0.44 for the HMGT alone.

The Cognitive Estimation Task

The Cognitive Estimation Task (CET) (Shallice and Evans 1978) requires selection of an appropriate plan for generating an approximation and monitoring of the result prior to production. In its original form it consists of 15 questions (e.g., 'How fast do race horses gallop?') that either do not have precise answers or, if they do, would go beyond the knowledge of most individuals. A revised 10-item version, for which norms are available, has also been employed (e.g. see O'Carroll *et al.*, 1994). Shallice and Evans (1978) reported that a sample of patients with anterior lesions performed significantly more poorly on the CET (an effect size for this difference was not reported and insufficient information is provided to permit its calculation from other statistics).

Subsequent evaluation of the measurement properties and validity of this test have been generally very disappointing. O'Caroll *et al.* (1994) reported that the reliability of the test was low (Cronbach's alpha = 0.40) in a sample of 150 healthy controls. Furthermore, although the CET yields a global score, O'Carroll *et al.* extracted five factors from 10 items; i.e., the scale is factorially impure. The available evidence suggests that the test's sensitivity to the presence of executive problems is also poor. Taylor and O'Carroll (1995) found that a sample of patients with anterior lesions did not differ significantly from a posterior sample. Moreover, these authors reported that the performance of a wide variety of neurological samples (including the anterior sample) did not differ significantly from controls; the one exception was a sample of patients with Korsakoff's syndrome. Crawford *et al.* (2000b) found that CET performance was significantly impaired in Huntington's disease (a condition associated with executive problems), but significantly less so than WAIS-R IQ (a measure relatively insensitive to executive problems). The CET was one of the few putative measures of executive function that failed to correlate significantly with rated everyday executive problems in the study by Burgess *et al.* (1998) referred to earlier. In conclusion, although the CET may occasionally yield clinically useful qualitative information, it cannot be recommended.

Brixton Spatial Anticipation Test

Conceptually the Brixton Spatial Anticipation Test (Burgess and Shallice 1997) has some similarities with the WCST. It requires testees to discover the rules underlying the placement (apparent movement) of a blue circle among a grid of unfilled circles; after a given pattern is established the rule changes.It has been argued (Burgess and Shallice 1997) that the Brixton has a number of practical advantages over other measures of set-shifting; namely that it is less time-consuming and less stressful for patients, and yields scores that are normally distributed in the general population. The normative sample is relatively modest ($N = 121$) and the reliability (internal consistency) of the test is only moderate (0.62). However, the validation data are impressive. Burgess and Shallice (1997) reported a highly significant difference between a sample of cases with frontal lesions and healthy controls; the effect size for this comparison, calculated by the present authors, was large ($r = 0.50$). Furthermore, frontal cases were significantly more impaired on the Brixton than cases with posterior lesions; the effect size for this comparison was moderate ($r = 0.34$). Finally, posterior cases did not differ significantly from healthy controls and the corresponding effect size was small ($r = 0.16$); i.e. posterior cases had relatively little difficulty with the task. This provisional evidence of the sensitivity and specificity of the Brixton for anterior lesions stands in contrast to the results obtained for other set-shifting tests; i.e., see Axelrod *et al.*'s (1996) study of the WCST referred to earlier.

One limitation of the Brixton is the use of Sten scores as a metric to express performance. Although Sten scores have the advantage of simplicity, they are coarse-grained (the difference between Sten scores correspond to 0.5 of an *SD*) and thus potentially meaningful differences between raw scores are obscured. However, normative data in the form of T scores, based on an enlarged normative sample ($N = 222$), have recently been developed (Crawford *et al.* in preparation); this study also includes a method of testing for changes in Brixton scores on retesting.

Hayling Sentence Completion Test

The Hayling Sentence Completion Test (Burgess and Shallice 1997) is primarily aimed at detecting difficulties in suppressing pre-potent responses and consists of two parts. In the first, the subject has to complete sentences with the pre-potent response e.g. providing the word 'ship' when presented with the sentence 'The Captain went down with the sinking ...'. In the second part the subject has to suppress the pre-potent response and complete the sentences with an unrelated word. The test yields four indices, all of which are expressed as Sten scores derived from the same healthy sample used to norm the Brixton ($N = 121$). The indices are: completion latency for the pre-potent responses (Hayling 1), latency of completion in the suppression condition (Hayling 2), number of errors in the suppression condition (Hayling 2 errors), and an overall score. The reliabilities of the test are generally very high in impaired groups (0.72 to 0.93) and the test has moderate to high temporal stability (0.62 to 0.76) in normals (Burgess and Shallice 1997).

The validity of the Hayling has been assessed by comparing the performance of frontal lesion cases with controls and cases with posterior lesions. Expressing these group differences as effect sizes (Table 19.2) is revealing: when comparing anterior cases against controls there is only a very modest difference between the effect size on Hayling 1 (0.39) and Hayling 2 (0.41). In other words latencies in providing the *pre-potent* responses were just as effective in differentiating healthy and anterior cases; this suggests that an overall slowing of response, rather than a problem with inhibition, may lie underlie the effect in the anterior cases. However, the suppression condition comes in to its own when the frontal and posterior cases are compared. The effect size for errors under suppression (0.37) is markedly larger than the effect size for basic initiation (0.23); therefore the anterior cases had disproportionately greater difficulties than posterior cases in inhibiting the pre-potent response. It can also be seen that, on all indices, the effect sizes for posterior cases versus controls are small, thereby providing encouraging evidence of the Hayling's specificity for anterior lesions.

Behavioural Assessment of the Dysexecutive Syndrome (BADS)

Many existing formal neuropsychological tests fail to detect important core components of executive dysfunction, such as problems in initiation and self-organisation, because they are highly structured. As Shallice and Burgess (1991) note:

> The patient typically has a single explicit problem to tackle at any one time ... the trials tend to be very short ... task initiation is strongly prompted by the examiner and what constitutes successful trial completion is clearly characterised.
>
> (pp. 727–728)

Table 19.2 Effect sizes[a] (anterior cases versus controls and versus posteriors) for the Hayling Test

Hayling Index	Anteriors vs. controls	Anteriors vs. posteriors	Posteriors vs. controls
Hayling 1 (Time 1)	0.39	0.23	0.17
Hayling 2 (Time 2)	0.41	0.32	0.04
Hayling 2 errors	0.42	0.37	0.03
Overall score	0.48	0.41	0.06

[a]Effect sizes calculated by present authors using data presented in Burgess and Shallice (1997).

The BADS test battery was developed in an attempt to address some of these limitations. It consists of six subtests: the Zoo Map test (a planning task); the Modified Six Elements Test, which is a simplified version of the Six Elements Test developed by Shallice and Burgess (1991) and taps planning/self-directed organisation; the Temporal Judgement Test, which is akin to the CET reviewed above, and requires the application of intelligent guesswork and error checking; the Rule Shift test, which measures set shifting and the ability to inhibit previously established responses; the Action Program test, a novel practical problem solving task; and the Key Search test, which taps self-directed organisation.

The norms for the BADS are derived from a sample of 216 healthy individuals aged between 16 and 87 years. Scores on the individual subtests are categorised on a four-point scale (0 to 4); these are summed and converted to yield an overall Profile score which is expressed on an IQ metric (mean 100, SD 15). With regard to the measurement properties of the test, the inter-rater reliability of the subtests are uniformly excellent, with coefficients ranging from 0.90 to 1.00 (the majority being 0.98 or above). The test-retest reliabilities of most subtests are moderate in magnitude (0.64, 0.67 and 0.71) but the remainder are low ranging from –0.08 to 0.39. Although these latter coefficients look alarming, two factors must be borne in mind. First, these coefficients were obtained from healthy participants, and given that they would exhibit ceiling effects (and hence limited variability), this would attenuate the coefficients; the coefficients would be substantially higher in an impaired sample. Second, difficulties in coping with novelty is a central feature of patients with executive dysfunction and the BADS seeks to capture this. Thus, the task demands on a second testing are very different from those on first exposure. As a result, and as is the case for many other putative tests of executive dysfunction, it is not realistic to expect the BADS to exhibit high test-retest reliability (Crawford 2004).

Internal consistency data for the BADS are not reported in the test manual but Cronbach's alpha for the Profile score can be calculated from other information that is provided (i.e., the means and SDs of the raw Profile score and the means and SDs of the subtest scores contributing to the Profile score). Alpha in the patient sample recruited for validation purposes was moderate (0.70).

The BADS manual reports the results of significance tests comparing controls to the patient sample but it is perhaps more informative to express the differences between these samples as effect sizes. These were calculated by the present authors and are presented in Table 19.3. It can be seen that, with one noteable exception, the effect sizes for the individual subtests are small to moderate in magnitude. However, it must be stressed that, unlike most of the other effect sizes reported in this chapter, these effect sizes are derived from comparing healthy controls to a *general* sample of neurological patients rather than a sample of patients with frontal lesions. Therefore, many of the patients in this sample would not be expected to exhibit significant executive problems and it follows that large effect sizes would also not be expected.

Table 19.3 Effect sizes (*r* for patients versus controls) for BADS subtests and Profile score and correlations with DEX ratings of everyday executive problems

BADS test	Effect size (*r*)[a]	*r* with DEX[b]
Action program	0.25	−0.37
Key search	0.12	−0.31
Six elements	0.53	−0.40
Rule shift cards	0.21	−0.45
Zoo map	0.15	−0.46
Temporal judgement	0.24	−0.40
Profile score	0.38	−0.62

[a]Effect sizes calculated by present authors using data presented in Wilson *et al.* (1996).
[b]Data from Wilson *et al.* (1996).

The effect size for the overall Profile score is larger than all but one subtest and is moderate- to large in magnitude (0.38). It is to be expected that a composite measure would have a larger effect size than its components. In this particular example, the results are consistent with a fractionation of the executive system (see Burgess and Simons, Chapter 18 this volume). In other words, the small effect sizes for individual subtests may arise because only a proportion of cases exhibited deficits on any one subtest and these were often not the same cases who exhibited deficits on the other subtests. Having said that, it is also clear that the source of much of the effect for the Profile score stems form the inclusion of the Modified Six Elements Test; this subtest has by far the largest effect size (0.53). The practical implications of these results are that the full BADS should be administered when feasible and that performance on the Six Elements test should be weighted highly when arriving at a formulation.

The major strength of the BADS lies with its demonstrated relationship to everyday executive problems. In the BADS patient validation sample all subtests correlated significantly with executive problems rated by relatives (these correlations are reproduced in the second column of Table 19.3). It can also be seen that the overall Profile score has a very strong (negative) correlation (-0.62) with everyday problems; this correlation is substantially larger than that obtained for a measure of general ability (WAIS-R IQ) in the same sample (-0.42) thereby providing evidence of specificity.

Dual tasks in the assessment of executive dysfunction

All major theoretical models of the executive system stress its role in the coordination of activity (see Burgess and Simon, Chapter 18, this volume). Baddeley and colleagues (e.g. Baddeley *et al.* 1997) have lain particularly strong emphasis on this aspect of the executive system and have explored the potential of using dual tasks to capture executive deficits. In Baddeley *et al.* (1997) patients with frontal lesions were assigned to one of two groups on the basis of whether they exhibited a dysexecutive syndrome (as assessed independently by two clinicians from a review of the medical notes). Dual task performance was assessed by combining digit span with a concurrent paper-and-pencil tracking task; the dependent variable was an index that compared single-task performance on these two tasks with performance on the tasks under the dual-task conditions.

On traditional clinical tests of frontal function (phonemic fluency and the WCST) the majority of both frontal groups were in the impaired range. However, the dysexecutive group was not significantly more impaired on these tasks than the non-executive group. In contrast, they did exhibit a significantly larger dual-task decrement than the non-executive group and the effect size (r) for this difference (calculated by the present authors from the reported t value for this comparison) was substantial (0.58). This effect size is particularly impressive as it is based on a comparison of groups both of which had frontal lesions as opposed to the other effect sizes reported (which are based on comparing frontal groups with either controls or posterior lesion samples). Further important evidence of the ecological validity of dual task decrements and their relevance to rehabilitation planning has been provided by Alderman's (1996) study of severely head-injured patients. A large dual-task decrement was associated with a poor response to behavioural intervention.

A potential problem with the use of dual tasks in individual assessment is that the key variable is a difference score (i.e. the dual task decrement). Difference scores have lower reliability than the components from which they are derived, particularly when, as is liable to be the case in the present context, the two components are highly correlated (Crawford 1996). However, the results reported above demonstrate that the effects are sufficiently large to overcome attenuation due to measurement error; furthermore, given the unreliability of differences, it can be concluded that the 'true' effect is considerably larger even than that obtained. In conclusion, dual tasks have great potential to capture what is a core executive process but their routine use in clinical practice awaits development of fully standardised tests and accompanying large-scale normative data.

Disability rating scales

Disability rating scales play a crucial role in quantifying the impact of cognitive deficits on everyday functioning and, particularly in the case of executive deficits, in identifying difficulties not captured by formal ability tests. As ratings can be carried out by patients and their relatives, they are also useful in identifying and quantifying diminished insight.

A promising rating instrument for assessing executive dysfunction is the Dysexecutive Questionnaire (DEX) (Wilson *et al.* 1996) which comes bundled with the BADS test reviewed earlier. The questionnaire consists of 20 items and comes in self-rating and proxy rating versions. The underlying structure of the instrument remains to be clarified; a principal components analysis reported in the test manual obtained a three factor solution consisting of factors labeled as *Behaviour, Cognition* and *Emotion*. Burgess *et al.* (1998) reported a five factor solution (*Inhibition, Intentionality, Executive Memory, Positive Affect,* and *Negative Affect*) in a neurological sample and provided some evidence that these factors related differently to formal tests of executive ability. Chan (2001) also obtained a five factor solution in a healthy sample: these factors had many similarities, but were by no means identical, to those obtained by Burgess *et al.*

The authors of the DEX view it primarily as a qualitative instrument, but it clearly has the potential to also yield quantitative information; currently the only healthy normative data consist of the mean and SD of members of the BADS standardisation sample, however, a patient's score can be compared against percentiles from the patient sample. The strength of the DEX stems from the previously reviewed evidence that it correlates with formal measures of executive functioning; i.e. the presence of these sizeable correlations simultaneously provides evidence of convergent validity for both the formal tests and the DEX. Further evidence of convergent validity can be found in Chan's (2001) study of the DEX and other executive tasks.

A recently developed rating instrument that has many impressive and useful features is the Frontal Systems Behavior Rating Scale (FrSBe) (Grace and Malloy 2001). It consists of 46 items that yield a total score and score on three subscales *Apathy, Disinhibition,* and *Executive Dysfunction.* There are self-rating and proxy (i.e. family member) rating versions and it is also available in Before (i.e. pre-injury) and After (post-injury) formats. The normative sample is impressive consisting of 436 persons with an age range of 18 to 95; ratings on the scales are converted to T scores and are stratified by gender, age and education.

The reliabilities of this instrument are generally high (Cronbach's alpha ranged from 0.72 to 0.95). The available validation data are also positive. A factor analysis of the FrSBe and found support for the allocation of items to the three subscales (Grace and Malloy 2001). Grace *et al.* (1999) compared scores on the proxy rated versions for samples of healthy controls and patients with either frontal or non-frontal lesions. There were highly significant differences between the Before and After ratings in the frontal sample. In addition, the frontal cases were scored significantly higher than both normal controls and non-frontal cases. In summary, this instrument has the capacity to yield much clinically useful information and has good normative data and sound measurement properties.

Finally, rating scales that assess other aspects of cognition and behaviour can also be useful in assessing patients with executive problems. For example, and as noted, executive dysfunction can produce memory difficulties, particularly when the everyday memory task imposes heavy strategic/organisational demands or involves prospective memory. A number of memory self and proxy rating scales are available including the Everyday Memory Questionnaire (Sunderland *et al.* 1988), and the Cognitive Failures Questionnaire (Broadbent *et al.* 1982); the coverage of the latter instrument falls midway between that of memory rating scales and dysexecutive rating scales.

A recently developed questionnaire for assessing memory problems that, because of its systematic coverage of retrospective and prospective memory, may have particular relevance to assessing patients with executive problems is the Prospective and Retrospective Memory Questionnaire (PRMQ) (Smith *et al.* 2000). This scale, which consists of 16 items, has high reliability (Cronbach's alpha = 0.89), comes in self- and proxy-rating versions, has normative data (expressed as *T* scores) from a sample of 555 healthy controls aged from 17 to 94, and has a latent structure that is consistent with the allocation of items to the Prospective and Retrospective subscales (Crawford *et al.* 2003).

Conclusion

A comprehensive assessment of executive dysfunction is fundamental in planning any neurorehabilitation attempt. This area of assessment is very challenging; only recently have formal tests become available that combine adequate psychometric properties, ecological validity and a sound theoretical basis. Although the emphasis in this chapter has been on formal ability tests and disability rating scales, clinical skills and experience are crucial in and in integrating these diverse sources of information to achieve a formulation of a client's difficulties and to draw out their implications.

20 Can executive impairments be effectively treated?

Jonathan J. Evans

Abstract

This chapter addresses the question of whether impairments of executive functioning can be effectively treated. The conclusion that is drawn from a review of the literature is cautiously positive, but there are many caveats. Executive functions are poorly defined and theoretical inconsistency makes evaluation of rehabilitation studies difficult and has probably limited the number of studies undertaken. There is some evidence that pharmacological approaches may have some value, but this is mostly anecdotal or from studies with very small numbers of participants. Attempts to train problem-solving or goal management skills have had some success, though it is not clear that such training can be considered to restore executive functioning to normal or act as a form of compensatory strategy for managing impulsivity. Some of the most convincing work addressing rehabilitation of executive functions has been undertaken with people with a diagnosis of schizophrenia. Studies of the use of external alerts, which may compensate for impaired attention and support goal maintenance, have shown promising results. Nevertheless, much work is still required to determine whether specific aspects of executive functioning can be improved through carefully targeted interventions.

Introduction

This chapter addresses the question of whether impairments of executive functioning can be effectively treated. Following the structure of this volume, the aim is to focus on examining the evidence that executive skills, rendered dysfunctional by brain injury, can be restored through the application of interventions that specifically target the impaired cognitive skills. Studies where the focus was on reducing the disability or level of handicap caused by executive impairments are examined separately by Worthington (Chapter 21 this volume).

There are several problems associated with addressing the question of whether executive impairments can be effectively treated. However, probably the most fundamental problem is the lack of agreement as to exactly what constitutes executive functions. It has been noted (Baddeley 1986) that one of the reasons for the lack of theoretical coherence in the concept of executive functions is that much of the theorising in this area has been focused on understanding what the frontal lobes do. This has led to the assumption that executive skills are the tasks or processes for which the frontal lobes are responsible. Given that the frontal lobes constitute a third of the brain cortex, that they have a role to play in a wide range of cognitive processes, and that lesions cause a huge range of potential deficits, it is not surprising that this approach to understanding executive functioning has been problematic. However, over the last two or three decades some common themes have emerged regarding the key elements of executive skills. These include concepts of planning, problem-solving and goal management (Shallice and Burgess 1996, Duncan 1986, Baddeley 1986, Baddeley and Wilson 1988, Burgess and Simon, Chapter 18 this volume). Subsumed under these broad concepts are also concepts of self-monitoring, task initiation, and task switching. Although the level of theoretical inconsistency remains problematic, nevertheless, these concepts are useful and to some extent can be mapped on to the problems faced by people with brain injury. This chapter will therefore focus on examining the evidence that deficits in planning, problem-solving, and goal management can be effectively treated.

Three different treatment approaches will be considered. The first is the use of pharmacological agents. The second is re-training approaches where the aim is to re-train problem-solving or goal management skills through practice and cognitive exercise. The third approach is where an internal or external strategy is used that is specifically targeted at reducing the impact of an executive impairment, although not specifically aimed at eliminating the impairment.

Pharmacological interventions

The evidence that pharmacological interventions can be used to improve executive functioning in adults with acquired brain injury is almost non-existent and certainly not conclusive. However, the major reason for this situation is the lack of studies. The two neurotransmitter systems most associated with modulation of frontal lobe functioning are the dopaminergic and the noradrenergic systems. There is evidence from studies of the use of methylphenidate, which increases levels of available dopamine and norepinephrine, that working memory and planning skills can be improved in children and adults with Attention Deficit Hyperactivity Disorder (see Mehta *et al.* 2001 for a review). There was evidence of improved executive performance with the administration of bromocriptine (McDowell *et al.* 1998; Powell *et al.* 1996) and amantadine (Kraus and Maki 1997; van Reekum *et al.* 1995), both of which increase dopamine levels. The McDowell *et al.* study was a double blind placebo controlled group study of 24 people who had suffered traumatic brain injury. The Kraus and Maki study was a single case study of a 50-year-old woman who had suffered a severe head injury, and who demonstrated impulsivity, irritability and was physically aggressive. Treatment with amantadine and then additionally with L-dopa brought about improvement in general behaviour, memory, attentiveness and concentration, and decreases in impulsivity and perseveration. This study, however, lack experimental control. There was also evidence for improvement in executive functioning (planning and problem-solving) in studies by Sahakian *et al.* (1994) and Coull *et al.* (1996) in which they used the alpha-2 antagonist idazoxan with a small number of patients with dementia of frontal type. Performance was shown to improve on a problem-solving task (the Stockings of Cambridge task, which has the same format as the Tower of Hanoi test), though generalisation was not studied. The studies of Powell *et al.* (1996) and van Reekum *et al.* (1995) both focused on the effects of increasing dopamine availability on initiation and activity, with the Powell *et al.* study also looking at a small number of cognitive and mood measures.

In summary, a small number of studies of pharmacological agents have provided some promise that this approach to treating executive deficits may have some merit. However, the evidence to date is limited, many studies lack sufficient control, and many also lack evidence of generalisation to day to day functional situations. For this reason the administration of such pharmacological agents is not yet justified.

Retraining approaches

Several studies have reported some success in improving aspects of executive functioning using a skill re-training approach. Such approaches work on the basis that practicing a particular cognitive function through tasks and exercises will enable that function to return to working in a more or less normal fashion. von Cramon *et al*. (1991) and von Cramon and Matthes-von Cramon (1992) described a group-based approach which they termed Problem Solving Therapy (PST). They note that the aim of the treatment is to enable patients to be more effective in breaking down problems, adopting a slowed down, controlled and step wise processing approach, in contrast to the more usual impulsive approach. The therapy explicitly draws on the problem-solving framework of d'Zurilla and Goldfried (1971) who used this approach in teaching adults with mental health problems to be more effective in mood management. The specific aim of the treatment group is to enhance patients' ability to perform each of the separate stages of problem-solving. Tasks were designed to exercise skills in:

- Identifying and analysing problems
- Separating information relevant to a problem solution from unimportant and irrelevant data
- Recognising the relationship between different relevant items of information and if appropriate combining them
- Producing ideas/solutions
- Using different mental representations to solve a problem
- Monitoring solution implementation and evaluation of solutions.

von Cramon *et al*. (1991) compared a group of patients who received problem-solving therapy (n = 20), with a group of patients who received a control 'Memory Therapy' (n = 17). The control group allowed for the possibility that clients might benefit from general advice and group activity, rather than specifically from the tasks aimed at exercising executive skills. They showed that patients who underwent problem-solving therapy showed some improvement in tests of general intelligence and problem-solving (Tower of Hanoi) compared with control participants, who were in the memory group. von Cramon and colleagues demonstrated some generalisation of problem-solving skills to untrained test tasks, but there was no evidence presented in relation to generalisation to everyday situations. von Cramon and colleagues also noted that a small number of patients actually deteriorated on tests. They hypothesised that this was due to an increased awareness of the complexity of problems on the part of the patient, leading to confusion about how to respond. By contrast, such patients had a pre-treatment propensity towards premature or ill-considered actions, some of which would have been correct by chance.

Executive impairments are considered to be one of the core deficits in schizophrenia and in recent years a number of studies have examined whether a form of retraining referred to as Cognitive Remediation Therapy (CRT), can improve cognitive and social functioning in this client group (Wykes 1998; Wykes *et al*. 1999, 2002; Penades *et al*. 2002; Bell *et al*. 2001). CRT (Delahunty and Morice 1993) includes exercises focused on cognitive flexibility (set shifting), working memory and planning. The programme involves 40, one-hour individual sessions, with three to five sessions per week. Wykes and colleagues have undertaken several evaluations comparing CRT with intensive occupational therapy, to control for non-specific therapist contact effects. The common finding has been that patients undergoing the CRT show greater improvement on some, though not all, executive tests (e.g. Wisconsin Card Sorting and Six Elements Tests) than those with the control therapy. The CRT group also showed greater improvements on a measure of self-esteem. However, there was no overall difference on measures of social functioning, though there were indications that the CRT group was more likely to reach a threshold of change in cognitive performance that appeared to be necessary for a change in social functioning to occur. In the most recent study, Wykes *et al*. (2002), also studied the impact of CRT on brain functioning using functional magnetic resonance imaging (fMRI). They found that CRT was associated with increased activation levels in right inferior frontal cortex and visual cortex bilaterally when doing a working memory task and that increased activation levels on this task were associated with improvements in performance on other working memory tasks.

It appears therefore that in a group of patients (people with a diagnosis of schizophrenia) for whom executive deficits are present along with a range of other symptoms, a cognitive exercise-based programme may bring some benefits. Once again the potential of such techniques to bring about generalised and sustained improvements in everyday functioning is much less clear. One of the possibilities that needs to be considered in relation to this approach is the question of how generalisation is fostered. If a treatment approach has brought about some fundamental improvement in executive skills, it might be argued that those skills should be available for use in any situation and therefore 'generalisation training' should not be necessary. However, another possibility is that skills are 'available', but their use is not triggered by situations that have come to be routinely undertaken in a more impulsive, less planful manner. It may be therefore that the development of skills is one matter, but the automatic application of those skills is another, requiring systematic training.

Levine *et al.* (2000) described the use of a Goal Management Training (GMT) technique, devised by Robertson (1996). The GMT technique was derived from Duncan's (1986) concept of 'goal neglect'. The principle is that patients with frontal lobe damage fail to generate goal (or sub-goal) lists of how to solve problems (and achieve goals), and/or may fail to monitor progress towards achieving sub- or main goals. The concept of working memory and goal management is illustrated using a metaphor of a 'mental blackboard' upon which tasks and subtasks are written, but which are also vulnerable to being rubbed off, leading to a failure to achieve intended goals. The training has five stages, which are first defined for the patient. These are illustrated in Figure 20.1.

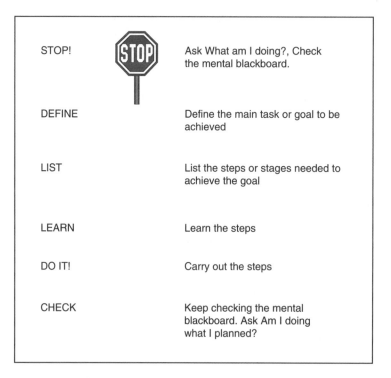

Figure 20.1 An illustration of the stages in Robertson's (1996) Goal Management Training.

After each stage is introduced, illustrative examples from the patient's own life are used as well as mock examples. Levine *et al.* evaluated the efficacy in two studies. Study 1 evaluated the technique with a group of head-injured patients on paper-and-pencil tasks. The second study described the use of this technique with one post-encephalitic patient seeking to improve her meal preparation abilities. In the first study, the GMT was applied in a single one-hour session, with testing on several target tasks undertaken afterwards. Levine *et al.* showed improved performance on three paper and pencil tasks, but generalisation to everyday life was not examined. Study 2 addressed the question of application of GMT in a more practical task. Patient K.F. suffered from a meningo-encephalitic illness, which resulted in some general intellectual decline, attentional, memory and executive functioning deficits. A particular problem for K.F. was meal preparation, with four specific areas of difficulty; failure to assemble the necessary ingredients, misinterpretation of written instructions, repeated checking of instructions and sequencing/omission errors. The measure used to evaluate the efficacy of GMT was the number of problem behaviours evident during meal preparation tasks (as well as performance on the paper and pencil tasks used in Study 1). GMT was applied over two sessions, and was adapted so that tasks relating to meal preparation and involving the various stages of GMT were created. The results of the study were that K.F. showed a significant reduction in errors in meal preparation stages over the course of the intervention. Although baseline data were collected that indicated the problem with meal preparation was clearly evident and this improved post-training, the lack of control variable information means that spontaneous recovery cannot be ruled out, especially given that she was only five months post-illness at the time of the study. Nevertheless, the study does raise the possibility that GMT may be a useful technique (especially considering the apparent efficacy based on a relatively small amount of training time).

Evans (2001) describes a group approach, adapted from von Cramon's PST and from the Goal Management Training. The Attention and Goal Management group is one component of a holistic rehabilitation programme. The first few sessions of the group (which runs twice a week for 8–10 weeks) primarily address attentional difficulties, and the later sessions are used to introduce a problem-solving framework to the clients. This framework is presented as a paper-based checklist of the stages of problem-solving. An accompanying template is also provided that can be used to proceed through the stages using a written format, but clients are encouraged, through practice at using the framework with the template, to internalise the framework so that in time the use of the framework becomes more automatic. No formal evaluation of this group has yet been undertaken, but the successful use of this framework by one client is described in Evans (2003).

One recent study of the impact of a problem-solving training group is that of Rath *et al.* (2003). They compared outcome for 27 patients who undertook the problem-solving training with a control group of 19 patients who underwent what they described as 'conventional' treatment. The conventional treatment combined general cognitive remediation training and psychosocial work and involved 24 sessions, with 2–3 hours per week contact. The problem-solving group also involved 24 sessions, with one two-hour group per week. The group programme was divided into two 12-session blocks. In the first 12 sessions, the focus was on what Rath *et al.* describe as 'problem orientation'. In this phase they addressed issues of affective reactions, attitude and motivation towards dealing with problems arising from the consequences of brain injury. The second 12-session block focused on the more specific problem-solving training, addressing the various stages of problem-solving as in the von Cramon group described earlier. The impact of the group was measured with a range of neuropsychological tests, questionnaires (e.g. Sickness Impact Profile, Community Integration Questionnaire, Rosenberg Self Esteem Scale), and also a role-play of a problem-solving scenario that was rated by independent raters. Rath *et al.* found that the problem-solving training group improved (and the conventional group did not) on Wisconsin Card Sorting Test performance, on self-assessed ratings of problem-solving skills, clear thinking and emotional regulation, and perhaps most importantly on the observer ratings on the role-played scenario. Improvement was also maintained at a six-month follow up. The major limitation of the study is of course the lack of evidence of generalisation to everyday life, but as noted already, this is a major difficulty for studies of this kind.

Self-monitoring is an important element of problem-solving and goal management, and although not easy to measure directly, frequently appears to be compromised following frontal lobe damage. The question arises as to whether self-monitoring skills can be re-trained. Alderman *et al.* (1995) reported use of a self-monitoring training (SMT) procedure with a man, H.C., who had suffered anoxic brain injury, and acquired a range of physical, cognitive and behavioural problems. He was described as having a complete disregard for social norms, and lack of inhibition. He produced very frequent verbalisations that were inappropriate for the situation. During meal times he made frequent requests for food and drink, even whilst eating. Behaviour modification programmes were unsuccessful. So, a SMT was commenced. This was a five stage process:

- **Stage 1:** A baseline measure of H.C.'s inappropriate behaviour was carried out.
- **Stage 2:** H.C. was given a counting device and asked to record whenever he made requests for food and drink. At the end of the trial his recordings were compared with those of a therapist, who had made simultaneous recordings. Inevitably initially his recordings were discrepant from those of the therapist.
- **Stage 3:** H.C. was prompted to record his behaviour each time it occurred. Accuracy increased, unsurprisingly.
- **Stage 4:** H.C. was required to independently self-monitor, and was rewarded if his recordings were within 50 per cent of those of the therapist. Initially accuracy was poor again, but this improved.
- **Stage 5:** H.C. was required to continue to independently self-monitor, but in addition, a programme of reward for increasingly lower rates of inappropriate requests was introduced. This brought about a reduction in the rate of problem behaviour. Importantly this change was maintained over a four-month follow-up period.

Another study by Knight *et al.* (2002) produced a similar improvement, first in self-monitoring and then in behaviour. What is less clear with these studies is the extent to which these patients might be considered to have improved general self-monitoring skills, or whether in fact they have essentially only improved in relation to these specific aspects of their behaviour. Evidence is not presented in relation to the former.

The studies described in the previous section all have as their explicit aim, improving problem-solving or goal management skills using a retraining approach. Some success has been reported. Is it reasonable to conclude therefore that these problem-solving or goal management skills have been restored to normal function as a result of these interventions? This is not at all certain. For example, for some individuals, slowed speed of processing may mean that dealing with a range of stimuli, making plans and holding several things in mind is difficult. If an attempt is made to do this, the impaired system cannot cope and fails. However, using a more formally applied, slowed-down approach to problem-solving, with an emphasis on managing working and long term memory limitations, may enable the process to proceed more effectively (if more slowly). If this is what is brought about by some of the retraining approaches, it might be said that 'normal' functioning has not been restored, but 'effective' functioning has nevertheless been achieved. From a clinical perspective, so long as people are more effective at dealing with problems in their life as they arise, and managing to complete important tasks, it perhaps matters less exactly *how* this is being achieved and more *whether* they are being achieved. Nevertheless it is clearly important that we develop a better understanding of just what is happening as a result of the interventions we undertake with our clients.

In the following section a number of approaches are described where interventions have been used that explicitly target some aspect of impaired problem-solving or goal management. However, in these interventions the aim was not so much to restore normal functioning, but to provide some means of compensating for a deficit that is present. In several of these studies, there is perhaps an issue as to whether the intervention is being applied at the level of the disability that arises from the impairment or at the level of the impairment itself. Nevertheless, in each there is a focus on addressing the specific impairment that is considered to underlie the disability, rather than simply focusing on the disability directly.

Impairment-focused compensatory approaches

Using the concept of 'goal neglect', Duncan (1986), like Luria (1966) previously, highlighted how people with frontal lobe lesions often fail to maintain goal-directed behaviour. Despite apparently being able to remember the intended goals, they appear to 'lose sight' of the main goals they are intending to achieve, with actions becoming somewhat stuck on a sub-goal or perhaps even appearing random. The emphasis in Robertson's Goal Management Training described earlier was on helping people to be more effective at encoding the goals and sub-goals and learning a mental checking routine that enables them to maintain task focus. Manly et al. (2002) described an alternative approach to helping people maintain task focus, examining the impact of external alerting. Performance of patients who had suffered traumatic brain injury on a multi-element task was tested under two conditions. The task used, the Hotel Test, is similar in format to the Modified Six Elements Test (Wilson et al. 1996). It involves the patient completing six different tasks, including a prospective remembering task, that are presented as tasks that might be given to an assistant hotel manager. The test is illustrated in Figure 20.2.

Like the Six Elements Test, not everything from all of the tasks can be completed in the 15 minutes allocated, and the main goal presented is that the testee is required to do at least something from all of the tasks. Two parallel versions were used in the two experimental conditions. In one condition, an external alert (a tone on an audio tape) was presented at random, relatively infrequent intervals. In the other condition no tone was presented. Subjects were told simply that from time to time they would hear a tone and that when they did, they should think about what they were doing. The study used

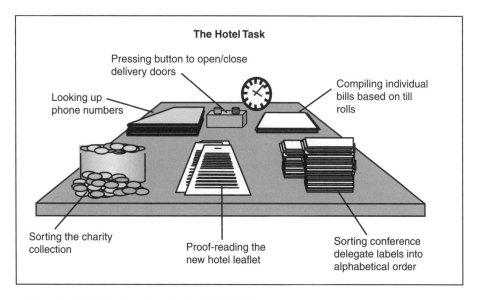

Figure 20.2 The Hotel Task used by Manly *et al.* (2002).

a counterbalanced, cross-over design. The results showed that participants performed more effectively during the bleeped condition, than the control condition. It was argued that the alerting tones improved the link between a well-represented goal and current behaviour. The tones did not specifically prompt task switching, but rather seemed to improve the ability to maintain the overall task goal actively in mind, and hence switch tasks more flexibly. Generalisation was not examined.

A more practically oriented examination of the impact of external alerts was provided in a study by Evans *et al.* (1998). NeuroPage is a paging-based reminding system that has been shown to be effective in improving functional performance in people with brain injury (Wilson *et al.* 1997, 2001). Evans *et al.* (1998) described the use of Neuropage with Patient R.P. who suffered a cerebro-vascular accident as a result of a ruptured aneurysm. Her main problem was that she had difficulty translating intention into action. She was also distractible and had difficulty completing tasks. Despite adequate memory and intelligence, R.P.'s combination of executive and attentional deficits had a significant impact on her day to day life. Although she could accurately say what she had to do, she had to be prompted to do many things by her husband, which put some considerable strain on their relationship. She was highly distractible. When she did manage to set off to do a task, she was frequently distracted by something else along the way and failed to return to the original task. In this respect she demonstrated significant goal neglect. A study of R.P.'s performance in carrying out a range of day to day tasks, using an ABAB single case experimental design, showed that NeuroPage was highly effective in helping R.P. to complete tasks she needed to do on time. This significantly reduced the stress on her husband. Evans *et al.* noted that there appeared to be two important aspects to the success of the paging system. The first was the presentation of an external text message that appeared to be important for R.P. and prompted behaviour in a way that an internal intention to act failed to do. This is consistent with Luria's view of the frontal lobes being involved in the control of behaviour by inner speech. The second aspect was the bleeping of the pager that provided an arousal boost to facilitate R.P.'s initiation of tasks and help her sustain attention to the main goal during the course of task completion. On the one hand, therefore, this intervention could be considered as being directly targeted at the disability i.e. prompting her to do the things she does not do otherwise. In the case of most people with memory impairment this is clearly the case. However in R.P.'s case, the intervention worked primarily because of a direct impact on the impairments she has (initiation and distractibility).

In their model of the problem-solving processes associated with the functioning of the supervisory attentional system, Shallice and Burgess (1996) highlighted the importance of the retrieval from memory of past experience. When faced with a novel task or problem, the strategy of recalling previous incidents of tackling similar problems in the past may help in the present situation. Dritchel *et al.* (1998) demonstrated that people with head injury often fail to refer to previous experiences in solving practical planning tasks. Hewitt *et al.* (2000) hypothesised that if patients were given a brief training relating to the retrieval of autobiographical memories, they may improve their ability to plan practical tasks. The training took the form of an illustration of the value of recalling specific autobiographical experiences from the past in practical problem-solving, a cue-card to prompt specific memory retrieval and practice at doing this in order to plan how to tackle a particular task. The performance of two groups of subjects was compared, one receiving the training and the other not. The results showed that the training group improved significantly more than the no-training group in terms of the number of specific memories recalled, the number of steps and the overall effectiveness of the plan produced in relation to a set of eight hypothetical practical demands (e.g. how would you organise a surprise birthday party, how would you find a new house). One limitation of this study is that there was no control for non-specific effects (e.g. motivation to perform for a therapist etc.) of the training. Furthermore, generalistion to other tasks or everyday life was not studied. Nevertheless, incorporating some form of training relating to retrieval of specific autobiographical memories may be helpful in a problem-solving training programme.

Fasotti *et al.* (2000) developed a compensatory strategy training that they call Time Pressure Management. The aim was to teach brain-injured patients a technique to help compensate for slow information processing. The strategy consisted of a general self-instruction ('Give myself enough time to do the task') followed by four specific steps:

1. Ask yourself if two or more things for which there is not enough time must be done at the same time? If yes, go to step 2, if not, do the task;
2. Make a short plan of which things can be done before the actual task begins;
3. Make an emergency plan describing what to do in case of overwhelming time pressure;
4. Use the plan and emergency plan regularly, monitor performance during the task.

This simple approach is essentially focused on teaching patients to be more planful and more consciously aware of their performance, with a particular emphasis on helping patients to become better managers of their environment. Fasotti *et al.* showed that use of the strategy helped patients improve performance on a practice task, though once again no evidence for generalisation to everyday life was provided.

Cicerone and Wood (1987) provide an example of the use of a self-instructional technique in a 20-year-old man with a severe head injury. He was described as functioning relatively independently, but impulsively interrupted conversations and generally appeared not to think before he did something. They used the Tower of London Test as a training task, asking the client to state each move he was about to make while attempting to solve the problem and then to state the move while he performed it. In stage two the patient was asked to repeat the first stage except to whisper rather than speak aloud. Finally in the third stage he was asked to 'talk to himself', (i.e. to think through what he was doing). This approach was successful in improving performance on the trained task, but more importantly, there was generalisation to two other untrained tasks. In addition, with some generalisation training, there were improvements in general social behaviour, rated by independent raters. The main change brought about by this simple self-instructional technique was that it helped the patient to slow his approach to the task in hand and, in effect, develop a habit of thinking through his actions rather than responding impulsively.

Conclusions

The question for this chapter was whether impairments of executive functioning can be effectively treated. The evidence presented would suggest that the answer to this question is a cautious 'yes'. Caution is required for several reasons. First, it is not yet clear exactly what underlies improvements in performance on tests or rating scales and we are a long way from being able to conclude that exercising the cognitive skills involved in problem-solving and goal management brings substantial improvement in the exercised skills. Second, very few of the studies present evidence of significant generalisation of training gains to everyday life. Mostly this is because this has not been assessed rather than there being evidence of no change. Obtaining this evidence is very difficult because of the nature of the behaviours in question. In many areas there is simply a lack of research studies. This is particularly evident in relation to whether pharmacological agents have a role to play in the rehabilitation of executive functioning. Several of the problem-solving training approaches described involve a 'broad-brush' approach, training problem-solving in its entirety. Others might be considered to be targeting specific elements of the process that may be impaired, or indeed targeting underlying cognitive skills, such as self-monitoring or attention, which are necessary for task completion. In the absence of assessment tools that allow us to pinpoint accurately specific processes that are impaired (see Crawford and Henry, Chapter 19, this volume), it is likely that the broad-brush approach is likely to be most useful in the average clinical setting. However, this should not stop our attempts to identify deficits more specifically, and then target interventions at those deficits, bearing in mind of course that the functional outcome for the individual is the most important goal of cognitive rehabilitation.

21 Rehabilitation of executive deficits:

Effective treatment of related disabilities

Andrew Worthington

Abstract

Executive skills are implicated in virtually all intelligent behaviour and are central to everyday adaptive living. Equally, executive dysfunction produces some of the most pervasive and debilitating forms of disability, threatening employment, family integrity and social relationships, and striking at the heart of personal autonomy. While significant progress has been made at a theoretical level, clinical approaches to the remediation of executive disorders remain largely atheoretical and pragmatic. Cognitive models can help therapists understand what to treat, and may even suggest how to treat, but our knowledge of how specific techniques work is poorer than is generally acknowledged. Furthermore, many diverse influences conspire to produce disability, demanding an eclectic approach to intervention. Outcome evaluation should focus on evidence of socially and personally meaningful change. On this basis there is now a growing literature suggesting that disability can be ameliorated by a variety of interventions for executive disorder. Although we are limited in our understanding of how such interventions might work, we are now starting to define some of the key parameters to effective intervention.

Introduction

Executive abilities are high-level cognitive processes implicated in virtually all intelligent behaviour. As a result of neurological injury or illness these processes can be severely disrupted, leading to pervasive disabilities affecting many everyday living skills. The effects of such disruption on an individual's competence and social relationships are evident at home, at leisure and in the workplace (Eslinger and Damasio 1985; Lhermitte 1986; Varney and Menefee 1993; Malloy *et al.* 1993; Brazzelli *et al.* 1994; Dimitrov *et al.* 1996; Petty *et al.* 1996; Crepeau *et al.* 1997; Goel and Grafman 2000; Nies 2002). Research has demonstrated what clinicians have long understood, that it is these disturbances of social conduct and adaptive behaviour following brain injury (especially frontal brain injury) that constitute the most significant obstacles to social reintegration (e.g. Mazaux *et al.* 1997).

This chapter will review the effectiveness of interventions for executive dysfunction in terms of the impact of rehabilitation procedures on everyday activities. The level of difficulty that a person has in carrying out tasks such as washing and dressing, preparing a meal, and driving a vehicle are all representative of some form of disability. The impact that these deficiencies have on the performance of social roles largely determines the degree of handicap that the individual experiences. The term disability is used throughout the chapter as defined by the World Health Organization (WHO 2001) as an umbrella term to encapsulate limitations in activity and restrictions in participation in a life situation, in this case imposed by a disorder of executive functioning. Further discussion of these terms can be found elsewhere in this volume (see Chapter 4) and in the *International Classification of Functioning, Disability and Health* (WHO 2001). The implication of this scheme for practitioners is that proper evaluation of rehabilitation procedures should include assessment of the range of activities that a person can perform and the extent to which their behaviour is accepted in the community.

Disability and disorders of executive function

Cognitive rehabilitation has come a long way since its initial focus on remediation or compensation for specific impairments (Diller and Gordon 1981). There is now a recognition that rehabilitation of cognitive dysfunction requires an eclectic approach to treatment (Ben-Yishay and Diller 1993; Sohlberg and Mateer 2001) and is itself part of a broader enterprise aimed at reducing social disadvantage after brain injury (Wood and Worthington 2001). This shift in perspective is to be welcomed but the development of treatment strategies for executive disorders is still in its infancy, largely due to the complexity of executive functions. It is obviously difficult to embark on rehabilitation without a clear idea of what the problems are, but executive dysfunction often eludes traditional means of psychological assessment. In response clinicians have favoured a more ecological approach to investigation and the use of behavioural observation measures. This, in turn, has facilitated greater awareness of disabilities consequent upon executive dysfunction. It is now recognised that disruption to specific executive processes produces particular patterns of behaviour which underlies certain types of disability.

Another difficulty in developing treatments for executive disorders is the ambiguous relationship between an intervention strategy and the target deficit. Without a clearer understanding of how treatment works it is difficult to predict what will work for whom. Robertson (1999) argued that cognitive rehabilitation can produce non-obvious treatments if it has a 'proper cognitive neuroscientific theoretical basis'. The reality, however, is that many current approaches to treatment leave unresolved important issues of recovery and mechanisms of efficacy. A greater understanding of how certain interventions might work is crucial to the development of cognitive rehabilitation, but scientific progress will take time to influence clinical practice. A theory of executive functioning is a laudable starting point for rehabilitation (Sohlberg *et al.* 1993), but cognitive models are often underspecified with respect to core processes that a therapist needs to identify for remediation, and crucial variables such as learning and motivation are often neglected. Furthermore, such models are unlikely to provide an adequate understanding of how disabilities develop from impairments.

Historically, the development of rehabilitation has been driven by economics as much as medicine, and much of it has been based on pragmatism and intuition. Even today most interventions are still undertaken without any conceptual rationale and with little empirical justification. Consequently, and however one might like to argue differently, cognitive models of executive function are presently neither necessary nor sufficient for effective rehabilitation. Indeed, for therapists one of the most important concerns is to understand the factors responsible for the origin and maintenance of a person's disabilities. Thus while effective treatment of an impairment of executive function may be crucial in the alleviation of a disability, it will rarely be adequate. Understanding how disabilities arise involves an appreciation of many more factors than the nature of a processing impairment. Problems and issues are uncovered over time, requiring some theoretical adeptness and familiarity with different approaches. It may be impossible to define the parameters of a problem until one begins to intervene. Consequently a broad theoretical perspective on treatment is necessary (Wilson 2002).

Evaluating rehabilitation for executive disorders

In all areas of modern medicine the need for treatment to be empirically grounded is well recognised. New treatments are expected to demonstrate their worth against criteria for evaluating the quality of evidence for therapeutic efficacy. The problem with such quality standards is not that they set out an unattainable level of evidence to which rehabilitation is unsuited (the randomised double-blind placebo-controlled trial). This at least has encouraged the development of controlled studies of specific techniques and rehabilitation programmes (e.g. Engelberts *et al.* 2002; Powell *et al.* 2002). The real problem with such schemes is that they focus attention on *how* scientific data should be acquired, rather than on *what* should be acquired. Crucially, when evaluating the impact of rehabilitation on disabilities, one has to consider whether purported gains reflect socially or functionally meaningful outcomes. Thus Chambless *et al.* (1998) suggested distinguishing between the *efficacy* of an intervention as demonstrated in carefully controlled conditions and its *effectiveness* in the world at large. This chapter will concentrate predominantly on the latter, addressing the question of whether treatments for executive dysfunction really have any impact on behaviour in the real world. To do this adequately one needs to establish a reference against which to judge the effectiveness of particular intervention techniques for ameliorating disability. Rather like the standards for rating the quality of evidence, these criteria represent an ideal, something to aim for rather than a readily achievable level that all research should presently be expected to meet. The criteria can be represented as a triad of concepts, incorporating assessment, intervention and outcome as follows:

1. Rehabilitation of executive function disorders should be informed by a conceptual analysis of the underlying disability. This will involve careful history-taking as well as behavioural observations and task-analysis in everyday activities. It will usually be necessary to utilise more than one conceptual framework in order to appreciate how a disability has arisen, and how it relates to an underlying impairment.
2. The goal of the intervention should follow rationally from the preceding analysis. The specific techniques employed to achieve this aim should have some empirically proven, or at least theoretically plausible, relation to the therapeutic goal.
3. Finally, the outcome should be measurable as a socially meaningful (as opposed to statistically significant) change and be of relevance to the patient.

Interventions for disorders of executive function

Intervention studies can be divided into two groups. The first type includes case reports, brief communications, single-case experimental studies and case series, all claiming to report the efficacy of specific techniques in response to certain manifestations of executive dysfunction. The advantage of such investigations is that they can provide a detailed insight into the therapeutic process, but often any generalisations about treatment effectiveness that can be drawn are limited.

The other type of treatment evaluation is the large-scale rehabilitation outcome study where the therapeutic programmes being evaluated include a significant focus on executive disorders. These would seem to offer useful information about the impact of rehabilitation on functional independence and disabilities as well as the wider applicability of particular forms of intervention. In the following section, the effectiveness of specific treatment techniques will be reviewed first followed by a brief summary of the relevant evidence from programme outcome studies.

Evidence base for the effectiveness of specific intervention techniques

Treatment approaches are variously classified according to the type of manipulation or strategy employed, the putative mechanism of action (Evans 2001) or type of disorder being targeted (Mateer 1999; Callahan 2001). For example, Sohlberg and Mateer (2001) distinguish environmental management, training in specific tasks and training in metacognitive skills. These classifications are widely and uncritically employed in treatment studies. While they may appear to illuminate the therapeutic process, their ambiguity and imprecision actually makes it all the more difficult to evaluate intervention methods. One major problem is that the categories within them are rather intuitive and are not necessarily mutually exclusive. In general, such schemes are not based upon theoretical analyses of how interventions work and consequently they have contributed little to our understanding of mechanisms of recovery. Furthermore, treatment outcomes do not respect these a priori distinctions. For example, an intervention purported to work by improving problem-solving skills may show no generalisation from the training task, raising the question of whether it should be considered instead as an example of task-specific training (cf. Cicerone and Giacino 1992). Conversely, task-specific routines sometimes show a degree of carry-over to other activities, suggesting that there has been some internalisation of strategy that implies a metacognitive aspect to the intervention (e.g. Burke *et al.* 1991). For ease of comprehension, in the following section rehabilitation procedures will be reviewed under four broad headings: environmental modification, other compensatory techniques, task-specific routines and metacognitive skills training. As the evidence will show, however, these broad categories are somewhat loosely conceived and appear to overlap.

Environmental modification

A long-standing response to executive disorder has been to simplify the executive loading of a task by modifying the task environment. Examples of modification of the physical environment include changing the layout of a room, removing sources of extraneous stimulation and rearranging the location of objects to enhance efficient task performance. For individuals with severe sequencing problems, for example, it is possible to facilitate the execution of steps in a task by ensuring that the relevant objects associated with each action are encountered in the order in which the actions are to be performed. When introduced effectively, improvements can be observed in participation in social interaction and activities (Fluharty and Glassman 2001). In practice this approach (sometimes described as antecedent control) is often used in combination with other interventions, which confounds evaluation of this strategy alone. Group studies are few but work on designing optimal therapeutic environments for people with brain injury suggests that it can be a key part of the therapeutic process (Hayden *et al.* 2000). Possible mechanisms of action underlying environmental manipulation include the automatic triggering of over-learned behaviours through the presence of specific environmental cues. Alternatively, the aim could be to focus residual discriminative attention upon salient aspects of a task in order to facilitate learning. Unfortunately the theoretical rationale behind such interventions is rarely made explicit. However, the means of evaluation tends to be at the level of disability rather than impairment, as the focus is usually upon improving performance in specific tasks. Anecdotally there is much to commend physical manipulations of the environment, but robust evidence of efficacy is wanting.

Manipulation of the social environment is a core aspect of most behavioural interventions for severe executive disorder. The underlying principle of this form of treatment is to promote new learning by modifying the contingencies of social reinforcement. There is an extensive literature on the use of such techniques for disturbances of self-regulation, including perseveration (Matthey 1996), impulsiveness (Rosenstein and Price 1994), social disinhibition (Lewis *et al*. 1988) and aggression (Manchester *et al*. 1997). In most cases, effective treatment of the underlying behaviour disorder has a direct effect upon disability. A typical result was reported by Alderman and Knight (1997). They employed a regimen of differential reinforcement of low rates of responding (DRL) to reduce disinhibited behaviour in three individuals, thereby increasing their participation in functional activities (see also Turner *et al*. 1990). Empirically-supported behavioural interventions are a core component of many rehabilitation programmes (Eames *et al*. 1996; Wood *et al*. 1999).

Compensatory strategies

Compensation for deficits operates on several biological and psychological levels and can be achieved through various means, including increased effort, modifying the task environment, adjusting expectations or learning a new skill (Dixon and Backman 1999). In a clinical context compensation usually means employing methods that target specific functional behaviours without attempting to address the underlying impairments. Evaluation of the impact of these interventions is by definition at the level of disability. Perhaps the most widely-used example of such compensation techniques for executive deficits is in the use of checklists and schedules, which have the advantage of being flexible and can be tailored to address specific activities. Rather surprisingly, despite their widespread use, there are few well-conducted studies of their effectiveness. Typically the reliability of the checklists is untested and raters are not blind to the intervention they are evaluating. Utilising a multiple-baseline design, Burke *et al*. (1991) reported several effective uses of task-based checklists in the workplace. Interestingly, in some cases generalisation of learning occurred over the intervention period, possibly due to internalisation of a strategy implicit in the checklist. This raises the possibility that the checklists (which incorporated written verbal prompts) had both task-based and compensatory aspects, and may also have involved crucial aspects of metacognition (see self-instruction techniques, below). Conversely, many patients employ compensatory strategies spontaneously, regardless of the type of intervention they receive (Dirette *et al*. 1999). Thus detailed examination of the research evidence reveals the pitfalls of categorising interventions based on mode of action given our current limited knowledge of how they work.

At this stage, perhaps a clearer way to understand mechanism of action is to keep the intervention simple. Minimising the processing demands of the intervention in this way reduces the potential for outcome to be confounded by a change in the representation of the stimulus as a result of cognitive re-processing. Auditory tones, for example, have been shown to improve 'real world' analogue tasks by a putative process of 'suspension of current activity [providing] a window in which evaluation of actions against the goal is more likely to occur' (Manly *et al*. 2002, p. 280). The tones themselves are unlikely to be subject to elaborate cognitive processing, merely acting as external prompts for the executive system. Initial research suggests that these benefits can be translated into meaningful behaviour change. A series of studies have been undertaken to demonstrate the effectiveness of an electronic pager (NeuroPage®) in compensating for deficits in prospective remembering (see Chapter 13). Evans, Emslie and Wilson (1998) reported a single case ABAB experimental design with R.P., a 50 year-old lady who showed an inability to carry out intended tasks because of her distractibility, poor planning and organisation. The targets for intervention were everyday activities for which she usually required much prompting from her husband, such as taking medication and watering plants. R.P. was given the NeuroPager for three months, during which time she was notably more accurate in taking her medication on time and in carrying out other selected tasks. Withdrawal of the pager was associated with a return to baseline levels of performance, suggesting that the pager had been an effective means of ameliorating the disability. Further evidence of the effectiveness of this form of external aid for executive deficits was reported by Wilson *et al.* (1997).

Task-specific training

The usefulness of focusing on task-specific skills in rehabilitation has been the subject of much debate, with arguments that it is more efficient and direct being balanced by views that it can lengthen rehabilitation with outcomes that do not generalise (Gordon 1990). Task-specific training (also known as functional skills training) is most appropriately undertaken in circumstances where there are particular tasks that a person needs to be able to carry out (e.g. in order to return to work), or where extensive deficits undermine training of generalisable metacognitive skills. Thus task-specific routines can be taught to people who exhibit severe dysexecutive impairment including perseveration, environmental dependency, aspontaneity or impulsiveness. Several examples of brief task-based interventions resulting in improved functional task performance were reported by Liu *et al.* (2002). Worthington *et al.* (1997) reported the use of a multi-component intervention including modelling, prompting and self-instruction for retraining the specific activity of walking in two patients who lacked spontaneity in mobilisation.

A very different example was reported by Adam *et al.* (2000). They described a lady with Alzheimer's disease who had difficulty knitting due to poor planning, self-monitoring and inhibitory skills. The intervention consisted of adaptations in the presentation of the knitting pattern together with online feedback whenever an error occurred. This was implemented for two hours each week for 13 weeks, resulting in significant improvements in knitting accuracy and the length of time spent knitting each day.

Environmental manipulation and behavioural procedures, such as shaping, chaining and differential reinforcement can all be used very effectively to augment task-specific training and help people re-acquire everyday living skills (Giles and Clark-Wilson 1999). External compensatory methods such as checklists and aspects of self-instruction can also be incorporated. The evidence suggests that task-specific specific prompts can be internalised over time (see Burke *et al.* 1991). However, it is debatable whether these additional elements are truly task specific, or whether they introduce a metacognitive aspect to the therapeutic process. Presently, this is an empirical rather than theoretical question, but it is a matter which few studies address.

Training in metacognitive skills

One of the most promising but challenging aspects of rehabilitation for executive deficits is in the domain of self-awareness or metacognitive skills training (Birnboim 1995). These methods include verbal self-instruction, self-monitoring and the teaching of problem-solving skills, all purporting to promote behavioural change by increasing self-awareness and control over regulatory processes (Sohlberg and Mateer 2001). Detailed discussion of these programmes is beyond the scope of this chapter (see Pressly 1993) but it is important to consider whether these methods have any impact on behaviour in the real world as opposed to the training context.

Self-instructional techniques

Self-instruction training (Meichenbaum 1974) covers a variety of methods intended to promote self-regulation of behaviour by linking language with action. With repeated practice overt statements are gradually internalised and behaviour is brought under control. Terminology is confusing here, and it would be helpful to distinguish between activities for which there is a task-specific set of instructions (which may usefully be known as self-instruction), from training of more general metacognitive processes which is more readily termed verbal mediation training (Wood and Worthington 2001).

Numerous case studies have illustrated the effectiveness of this type of approach (Burke *et al.* 1991; Fasotti *et al.* 2000). Burgess and Alderman (1990) reported the case of a 24-year-old man with marked fronto-temporal damage following a road traffic accident. His behaviour was characterised by abusive shouting and swearing during many routine activities such as washing and dressing. This was interpreted as an automatic, anxiety-enhanced response that went unmodified by executive control. The intervention consisted of two techniques. The patient was taught to repeat a set phrase during his showering routine that was intended to modify maladaptive cognitions associated with the disturbed behaviour. He was also shown how to use the shower controls, and develop a greater sense of mastery over his immediate environment. After just five hour-long sessions the behaviour disturbance had resolved significantly. The intervention was considered to have been effective by replacing the negative behavioural schema with an alternative thought schema which triggered a more appropriate behavioural response.

Sohlberg *et al.* (1988) used external cues to prompt self-questioning in a patient with poor social communication to increase his awareness of his behaviour. Cicerone and Giancino (1992) reported two similar cases, one whose social awareness appeared to benefit from training on an unrelated problem-solving task, and another who showed no spontaneous generalisation. These different outcome profiles raise questions about whether self-instruction training is truly a metacognitive strategy, as Cicerone and Giancino (1992) claim (see also Liu *et al.* 2002), or a task-specific technique. On the one hand, some patients do appear to be able to apply self-regulation strategies in novel situations. It could be argued that failure to show this effect merely reflects the extent of their executive dysfunction rather than an inherent aspect of the treatment. However, while training people on real-life tasks results in a reduction of specific disabilities, transfer of gains from the training context does not usually occur spontaneously without additional 'generalisation' training, involving practice on real-life tasks (see Cicerone and Wood (1987) and also von Cramon and Matthes-von Cramon (1994)). Task-specific interventions may be erroneously termed metacognitive with no evidence of spontaneous improvement in non-trained tasks.

A different but promising approach to self-regulation was described by Alderman *et al.* (1995) in a case study of Self-Monitoring Training (SMT). This is really a two-stage intervention that focuses first upon raising awareness (this is the metacognitive aspect) followed by a more traditional DRL regimen. Initial reports suggest that this technique may be effective in ameliorating disability associated with antisocial behaviours where they are exhibited with high frequency, but more evidence is awaited. The author has used this approach successfully with a 21-year-old woman who presented with a two-year history of behaviour disturbance secondary to recovery from acute herpes simplex encephalitis. The focus of intervention was her disinhibited social communication, particularly her tendency to stray off the topic, make overly-personal inappropriate comments and to interrupt others. Self-monitoring training was provided in twice-weekly thirty-minute sessions, and incidents of target behaviours during these sessions were recorded as she progressed through the treatment programme. Importantly, covert recording of her behaviour outside formal treatment sessions was also regularly made throughout the programme. The results (hitherto unpublished) are summarised in Figure 21.1. This shows that the programme was associated with a significant reduction in frequency of key behaviours in social interaction, in and out of formal treatment sessions, as therapy proceeded.

Problem-solving therapy

Problem solving training (PST) was developed specifically to address 'problem-solving disabilities' (von Cramon *et al.* 1991) by providing patients 'with techniques enabling them to reduce the

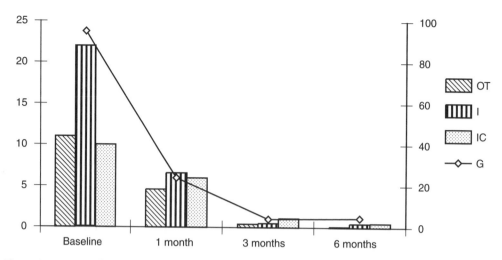

Figure 21.1 Example of a successful self-monitoring programme with generalisation of behaviour gains across settings. Key: I = interruptions; IC = inappropriate comments; OT = off the topic; G = generalisation probe (second axis).

complexity of a multistage problem by breaking it down to more manageable portions'. Its focus on real-life tasks makes it of interest to therapists. Early studies suggested that behavioural disabilities might be minimised by PST as a result of reduced concrete thinking and improved reasoning (von Cramon and Matthes-von Cramon 1990). Moreover this type of intervention can be delivered in a group format (Evans 2001), potentially increasing its application. Von Cramon and Matthes-von Cramon (1994) reported a detailed account of this approach exploring its efficacy in ameliorating disability. Their case involved a young physician with bilateral frontal damage in whom problem-solving therapy (utilising self-instruction) brought about task-related improvements in training contexts. The authors reported that two to three hours specific training using self-instruction each week for a period of twelve months improved his skills of histopathological diagnosis, and thereby his autopsy reports. They attributed this reduction of disability to the incorporation of new higher-level schemata in an attention-mediated contention scheduling process, allowing him to carry out routine thought processes. Crucially however, even after one year of intensive training, not only were his impairments unchanged but there was no transfer of problem-solving skills to non-trained novel situations, indicating that the amelioration of disability was context-specific. Without convincing evidence of generalisation, it may be premature to consider PST as a truly metacognitive technique. Certainly, the circumscribed impact of PST upon activity suggests that it is more appropriately considered to be an exercise in task-specific training. Moreover, a randomised controlled study by Rath *et al.* (2003) raises questions about the underlying mechanism of action of problem-solving skills training, which may work by teaching an elaborate set of compensatory techniques rather than by retraining metacognitive processes.

Goal management training

Goal management training is another problem-oriented approach that aims to address the disorganised behaviour often associated with executive dysfunction. The training procedure is structured around five steps, each corresponding to a stage of goal-directed behaviour. With the aid of a trainer's script, participants are taught to recognise and compensate for goal management failures, learning the five steps and practising on real-world tasks. In one study Levine *et al.* (2000) explored meal preparation in a patient with post-encephalitic executive deficits. They received five sessions of goal management training, the patient using a 'stop and think' prompt and a checklist. The result was a significant improvement in efficiency during meal preparation which was maintained at follow-up six months later. Although the intervention was clearly successful, it is doubtful whether GMT was crucial to the outcome, as interventions of this nature have long been used by therapists. In such a case perhaps the theoretical contribution of GMT was not in the choice of intervention but in suggesting why the intervention was effective.

The effectiveness of rehabilitation programmes for executive disorder

An additional source of evidence about the effectiveness of treatment for executive disorders is the literature on outcome from specific rehabilitation programmes. Brain injury, especially traumatic brain injury (TBI) with its characteristic anterior pathology producing a propensity for executive and behaviour disorders, offers potentially a rich vein of evidence for this purpose. In contrast to investigations of specific therapeutic techniques, many of which lack appropriate disability outcome measures, rehabilitation outcome studies seek to address more global measures of efficacy such as functional independence. Excellent summaries can be found in Cope (1995), High *et al.* (1995), Mazaux and Richer (1998), the National Institutes of Health consensus paper (NIH 1999) and Carney and du Coudray (Chapter 24, this volume). For the purposes of this review, however, it is important to consider whether the rehabilitation outcome literature adds anything specific to the evidence base for treatment of executive disorders, particularly at the level of disability.

At present there is little information available to address this question with any degree of precision. A review of rehabilitation outcomes by Bajo and Fleminger (2002) highlighted the inadequate consideration given to crucial treatment and patient-related variables. They identified 15 studies that looked at patient characteristics as predictors of outcome, and suggested that the presence of executive dysfunction may undermine therapeutic efforts. The real problem here is that the literature on generic outcomes has little to say about how executive dysfunction specifically may be treated and what impact this has on social functioning. Important treatment-related factors often omitted from studies include:

- Severity of brain injury
- Whether patients had executive deficits or disorders of self-regulation
- How long after injury the rehabilitation commenced
- Organisation of the rehabilitation programme (day attendance vs. residential, group vs. individual).
- Details of the treatment techniques employed
- Duration of rehabilitation.

Similarly, outcome variables are often limited to levels of impairment or provide only cursory assessment of residual disability. Outcome measurement should be related to specific activities and reintegration into the community (Wood and Worthington 1999). Depending on the focus of study the following should be considered:

- The type of accommodation to which people are discharged
- Degree of independence in everyday living skills (and continuing care needs)
- The extent to which it has been possible to return to competitive employment

- The meaningful constructive use of leisure time
- The nature of relationships within the family
- Participation in community life and civic institutions.

Unfortunately few programme outcome studies contain sufficient information to tell us much about how disabilities associated with executive dysfunction can be ameliorated. One randomised study suggested that inpatient rehabilitation is not necessarily more effective than a home-based programme (Salazar *et al.* 2000), at least in terms of return to work. However the eight-week duration of treatment may have been too brief to make an impact on severe dysexecutive problems in either setting. In a randomised controlled community study Powell *et al.* (2002) reported beneficial effects of multidisciplinary rehabilitation over written information in terms of self-organisation and psychological well-being, but not in terms of non-family social contact or employment, two key indicators of community integration. The interventions were individualised but outcome data are reported for the programme as a whole, so no conclusions can be drawn about treatment of executive disorders, although many patients may have been experiencing executive dysfunction.

More informative is the study by Wood *et al.* (1999) of a residential treatment programme designed for adults with disorders of self-regulation and executive function. Although no control group was utilised, there were significant improvements in both social functioning and independence which were also reflected in corresponding reductions in care costs. Improvements were noted even for persons treated five years or more post-injury, making it unlikely that these benefits would have accrued without formal rehabilitation. There is already much evidence that functional gains made in rehabilitation are reflected in discharge placements which have a direct bearing on long-term quality of life (Eames *et al.* 1996; Corrigan *et al.* 2001). What is required now is greater attention to the details of therapeutic programmes and the disabilities shown by persons receiving rehabilitation, if we are to learn more about who will benefit from what form of treatment and to what degree.

Conclusion

The amelioration of disabilities associated with executive dysfunction is one of the greatest challenges in cognitive rehabilitation. The impact of effective rehabilitation is undeniable, but to date the techniques and methods are poorly understood and many lack adequate empirical support. Cognitive theory may help us understand how treatments work (Seron *et al.* 1991; Shallice 2000) but only if there is a move from diagnostic models to theories of remediation (Caramazza and Hillis 1993; Baddeley 1993). The implications for rehabilitation of many current models of executive function are well reviewed by Burgess and Robertson (2002). Conceptualising disability, however, demands an altogether different approach (Johnston 1997) and currently there are few bridging paradigms (Condeluci 1992). Assessments identifying what to treat need to be augmented by assessments of how to treat. There are now some accepted approaches to management of executive dysfunction that are effective in ameliorating disability for some individuals. We know that the task-environment is crucial where attentional resources are limited or there is poor attentional control. Task-specific training can be an effective means of reducing a disability, but it can also be intensive and time-consuming. The use of task-specific interventions such as checklists and self-instructions may recruit metacognitive processes and help promote generalisation. The evidence that metacognitive strategies alone can reduce disabilities in novel contexts is weak. Such methods require additional generalisation training before skills are likely to be applied spontaneously to non-trained tasks.

This is the evidence at the present time, based upon twenty years of cognitive rehabilitation. How much progress will have been made in another twenty years rather depends on accumulation of the right kind of information. Current taxonomies of treatment are hardly scientific given how little is known about mechanisms of efficacy. There is a real need to consider why a technique might be (or might not be) effective, perhaps involving post-hoc testing of a priori assumptions about putative mechanisms of recovery. Given that the ultimate aim of rehabilitation is to enhance independence, due consideration should be given to relevant and sensitive measures of disability (in its broadest sense including participation) when designing and evaluating treatment. There is no doubt that moving patients through the system into rehabilitation is cost-effective (Ashley *et al.* 1990; McLaughlin and Peters 1993; Khan *et al.* 2002; Diller and Ben-Yishay 2003), but evidence that executive disorders can be treated in such a way that disability is reduced is only slowly emerging. As executive deficits underlie some of the most debilitating and costly brain injury sequelae, the need to establish a more substantive evidence base can hardly be more pressing.

Section 6

Cognitive rehabilitation theory

22 For a theory of cognitive rehabilitation

Progress in the decade of the brain

Argye E. Hillis

Abstract

A theory of cognitive rehabilitation should specify how change from a damaged state of cognitive processing can be modified into a normal, or more functional, state of cognitive processing. Such a theory should incorporate what is known about the cognitive representations and processes underlying normal cognition, how these are affected by brain damage, and how learning or modification of cognitive processing occurs. It is therefore argued that development of a useful theory of cognitive rehabilitation will require integrating advances from cognitive neuropsychology, experimental psychology, computational neuroscience, and molecular biology of the brain, as well as empirical evidence from various branches of rehabilitation. It is likely that such a theory will specify how behavioral rehabilitation strategies can be augmented by pharmacological agents.

Introduction

Rehabilitation of cognitive impairments is among the most challenging and rewarding endeavors of clinician-scientists. Hence, it is no wonder that seemingly everyone wants to 'get in on the act.' In the past two decades, cognitive rehabilitation has been the focus of investigators and therapists in a wide range of disciplines: speech-language pathology, occupational therapy, clinical psychology, neuropsychology, experimental psychology, neurology, neuroscience, linguistics, education, neuroimaging, computationalism, and others. This cross interaction has been productive. For example, many speech language pathologists treating aphasia or other cognitive impairments caused by focal brain damage have found it useful to consider cognitive neuropsychological models of the cognitive processes underlying the task to be treated (see Chapey 2001; Coltheart, Chapter Brunsdon and Nickess, Chapter 2 this volume; Hillis 2002; Riddoch and Humphreys 1994a; Seron and DeLoche 1989, for examples). Several authors have argued that these models provide an essential first step to rehabilitation, in terms of identifying the components of each task that are impaired, and the components that are spared, allowing the clinician to capitalize on the spared components and to focus treatment or facilitation on the damaged components (Beeson and Rapczak 2002; Hillis 1993, 1994, 1998; Riddoch and Humphreys 1994b; Wilson and Patterson 1990). The focus of this chapter concerns the next step: How do we move beyond the demonstrated success in determining 'what to treat' to the critical issues of 'when, how, and how much to treat'?

Caramazza and Hillis 1993 (see also Hillis 1993, 1998) have previously argued that the questions of when, how, and how much to treat cannot be answered on the basis of cognitive neuropsychological models. Such models have been developed to represent a theory of the normal cognitive processes that must be engaged in order to perform a task (e.g., reading a word). They are silent with respect to which of these cognitive processes are most subject to change, or how changes might be brought about. We did not offer a theory of rehabilitation, but did lay out some criteria for what a theory of rehabilitation would entail.

In response to Caramazza and Hillis (1993), Baddeley (1993) argued that at least some of the crucial aspects of a theory of rehabilitation could be provided by learning theory and by connectionist models. Baddeley pointed out rehabilitation requires re-learning, so that theories of learning and memory and connectionist models of learning may be relevant to rehabilitation.

I am in full agreement that learning theory and connectionism have much to offer toward developing a theory of rehabilitation of cognitive impairments resulting from brain damage. But below I will point out the limitations of each of these domains, and will propose that further advances toward a theory of rehabilitation will be provided by neuroscience. That is, I will argue that a theory that can direct clinicians as to when, how, and how much to treat will depend on advancements in knowledge about how the human brain works, how it is damaged by stroke, trauma, and disease, and how it recovers from these injuries. The biology of the brain will need to be integrated with our psychological and computational models of normal cognitive processes. First, I will discuss the contributions and limitations of such psychological and computational theories, and then turn to the potential contributions of biology of the brain.

Learning theory

Decades of experiments have provided a wealth of important principles about how people learn and retain new information: many of these principles have been based on the work of empiricists. We have learned much about operant and classical conditioning and shaping behaviors. Therapists incorporate random, intermittent reinforcement into their rehabilitation, based on evidence that these reinforcement schedules result in more durable training effects than constant reinforcement. Similarly, therapy is based on the principle that spaced practice is more effective than mass practice. There have also been recent illustrations of the effectiveness of 'errorless learning' (see Kessels and de Hann 2003 for review). Nevertheless, the limitations of these principles for cognitive rehabilitation are twofold. First, many of these principles are based on careful, well-documented, well-replicated observations, without concern as to the mechanisms of why they work (although we will return to issue of how and why they work, which has been elucidated by cellular level neuroscience). Without knowing the mechanisms, the principles cannot contribute much to a *theory* of rehabilitation. They only contribute to the *practice* of rehabilitation. Second, it is not clear that the damaged brain can always learn the same way as normal brains. For example, anoxic brain damage may cause substantial damage to the hippocampus and amygdala, structures that are crucial to learning new information. In such cases, intensive, spaced practice and appropriate reinforcement schedules, even in the appropriate modality, may not be sufficient for learning new facts. Also, brain injury may affect the chemistry of the brain in such a way that it can no longer respond to the rewards that would normally reinforce learning.

More recent learning theories have proposed mechanisms of laying down new memories, such as dependence on the phonological loop for learning through the auditory modality and dependence on the visual spatial sketchpad for learning visual information (Baddeley 1993). These theories recognize that brain damage can result in an inability to learn the way normal brains learn. Nevertheless, the constraints of such theories on rehabilitation are minimal (e.g., reliance on errorless learning, which might be chosen on the basis of other theories). Baddeley (1993) also suggests that in cases of impairment of the phonological loop, reliance on learning through the visual modality is crucial, while in cases of impairment of the visuospatial sketchpad reliance on learning through the auditory modality is essential. In other cases of impaired new learning, acquisition of new memories may depend on the use of episodic long term memory – e.g., use of visual imagery mnemonics to learn people's names (Wilson 1987) or reliance on implicit learning (Glisky *et al.* 1986). However, it is not clear how this approach differs from the cognitive neuropsychological approach of identifying the impaired and spared components of the cognitive processes underlying a task, and relying on the spared components (or focusing treatment on the impaired ones). Again, we see that cognitive models (in this case, of learning) help to identify what to treat more than how or when to treat.

Connectionism

Computational models come in two main forms: those that learn (change the strength of their connections in response to input; e.g., parallel distributed models of McClelland and colleagues), and those in which connections strengths or 'weights' are specified (e.g., Dell 1986). The former are based on principles of Hebb (see Hinton, McClelland and Rumelhart 1986, and Robertson, Chapter 23 this volume, for review). Hebbian learning has been summarized as, 'Cells that fire together wire together.' (author unknown; quoted from McClelland 2002). That is, the more often the firing of neuron A stimulates neuron B to fire, the more easily neuron A will be able to stimulate neuron B in the future. Connectionist models can capture this crucial feature of neurons – the more times a network is exposed to a particular stimulus, the stronger the connections that link the stimulus with the response become (and the more likely it becomes that the network will produce the same response to that stimulus in the future).

Furthermore, recent computational models have provided an account of the mechanisms of two complementary memory systems in the brain. It has long been recognized that the hippocampal system is crucial for laying down new information, but not for recall of remote memories, whereas the neocortex has the opposite role. A computational model described by McClelland and colleagues (1995) accounts for these two systems in the following way: new memories are laid down through changes in synapses in the hippocampal system, and these changes result in minor changes in the neocortex which support recent memories. Recent memories then decay, unless there is continued support from the hippocampal system. Continued support from the hippocampal system results in accumulated minor changes in the neocortex that eventually result in durable changes in synapses underlying remote memory. Computational models that have both rapid onset and fast decaying connections (like the rapid learning of new information by the hippocampal system) and gradual, interleaved, durable changes in connections (like the establishment of remote memories in the neocortex) that support one another can account for these learning systems.

Plaut (1996) also argued that connectionist models can not only simulate learning of new information and specific cognitive tasks (reading, naming), but can also reproduce some of the patterns of errors produced by neurologically impaired individuals when the network is 'damaged' (e.g., by adding noise, reducing connection weights, taking out a subset of connections, etc.). He went on to propose that connectionist models could be utilized in rehabilitation, and might provide a theory of rehabilitation. To illustrate, he reported that a network of his design learned a set of artificial associations more quickly when it was trained with atypical exemplars of a category than when it was trained with typical exemplars of the category.

This prediction was empirically tested by Kiran and Thompson (2002), who showed that four aphasic patients with impaired lexical-semantics learned to name pictures more reliably when atypical exemplars were trained (e.g., 'penguin' as an exemplar of birds) than when typical exemplars (e.g., robin) were trained via semantic features. One interesting observation made by the authors was that one patient actually produced more semantic errors (e.g., robin → cardinal) after training, suggesting the possibility that the patient simply learned to say a category of names in response to that category of pictures (e.g., any bird name in response to any picture of a bird), and by chance, sometimes selected the correct one. Furthermore, the difference in learning with atypical versus typical stimuli might have been due to the greater range of stimuli or semantic features employed when atypical stimuli were used than when typical stimuli were used. That is, there are more differences in features between penguins and chickens than between robins and sparrows. It is possible that utilizing equally similar atypical members (e.g. chickens and ducks and geese) and typical members would have yielded similar results.

Nevertheless, in this case it would appear that a connectionist model was useful in planning therapy. But the model did not really provide hints about how or when to treat, only a bit more detail on what to treat (atypical exemplars, or broader range of stimuli). However, another example described by McClelland and co-workers (McCandliss *et al.* 2002), indicates the possibility that such networks can shed light on how to treat as well.

McCandliss and colleagues (2002) described a connectionist model of learning to differentiate two very close phonemes, such as /r/ and /l/. They found that if the network was presented only with stimuli that are so close together that the stimuli elicit the same response, then the network could not learn the distinction. However, when the difference between stimuli was exaggerated, it could learn the distinction. Each error was followed by making the stimuli more distinct. After eight correct responses in a row, the distinction was made slightly more difficult. Finally, the network could make the difficult discrimination that it could not learn initially.

McCandliss and co-workers then tested this training model by teaching Japanese Americans to distinguish /r/ and /l/. The training was very intense (daily practice), comparable to the massive stimulation suggested by Hebbian learning. Results were mixed: the adults could learn just as the network had, beginning with exaggerated /r/ versus /l/ and progressing to incrementally harder distinctions (or regressing to easier ones with each error). And, as predicted, they did not learn the distinction when just intensively presented with the difficult (realistic) distinction. But what was unpredicted was that learning was considerably faster when the subjects were provided with feedback. In fact, they could learn the distinction just as quickly when only the difficult distinction was presented in intensive practice, as long as correct responses were followed by feedback.

Thus, connectionism provides some important insights into how people learn. It suggests that training should be intense (many repetitions of the stimuli are required), and nearly error free (to prevent incorrect connections from being strengthened). But it must allow enough errors or be sufficiently challenging to increase new connections.

The question remains: has connectionism provided the link between cognitive theory and the issue of when and how to treat? One key aspect of learning /r/ versus /l/ that was not predicted by the model was that learning was much faster once feedback was provided to the students. Furthermore, in the presence of feedback, learning was no faster when the exaggerated distinctions were presented first, compared to when the normal /l/ and /r/ sounds were presented first. This aspect of learning was not captured in the connectionist model; networks don't need feedback. But people do. McCandliss and colleagues report that the network could be modified to respond to feedback; nevertheless, the original network did not require it. Clearly, in some ways, people do not learn like computers do. We turn to crucial biological variables that distinguish network versus human learning, which may be the key to improving cognitive rehabilitation.

Biological theories: how computers are different from brains

Spatial organization In computers, information is stored or represented in nodes and connections between nodes. There is need for the nodes to be organized such that nodes representing two adjacent spaces, or two tones along a continuum, are spatially adjacent in the network. In contrast, there is compelling evidence that there is spatial organization of information in the brain (see Kandel *et al.* 1995, for review). There is retinotopic organization of visual cortex, such that two adjacent areas in the visual scene (or even an imagined scene) are represented in adjacent areas of cortex. Likewise, two similar tones are represented in auditory cortex closer to one another than are two dissimilar tones. That is, there is cochleotopic organization of human auditory cortex, although a network representing different tones would not need to have such localization. There is similar organization of the sensory cortex and motor cortex, representing the human body more or less in its physical shape. In fact, this localization of information in the brain may extend to higher levels of representation, such as multi-modality representations of concepts, such fruits or animals. At least, we know that focal brain damage can selectively impair access to semantic representations in one category (e.g., animals) but not in others (e.g., Goodglass and Budin 1988; Hart *et al.* 1985; Hillis and Caramazza 1991; McCarthy and Warrington 1988). There have been attempts to account for such selective impairments without assuming any categorical organization of the brain, but these accounts do not satisfactorily explain highly selective deficits (Caramazza and Shelton 1998). In any case, it is clear that the brain has much more localization of function than is 'necessary' according to connectionist theory. It is also clear that the localization is modifiable, either by lesions that disrupt the cortical map or by change in input to the cortical map, or by experience – intense practice, rehabilitation, etc. (see Jenkins and Merzenich 1987; Merzenich *et al.* 1983; Xerri *et al.* 1996).

Rate or intensity of stimulation Another feature of brains that is not captured by connectionist models is the fact that human learning depends on the rate of stimulus presentation. Recent studies at the cellular level have provided evidence that learning occurs in the brain (as in computers) by change in the strength of connections between neurons. In the brain, this change in connection strength depends on rapid firing of a neuron that elicits firing of a connected neuron. This rapid string of effective firing of a neuron by another results in a change in the 'threshold' of the connection between these two neurons, such that second neuron will fire more easily in response to the first neuron than it did before. This process, called long-term potentiation (or long-term depression, when the connection is inhibitory), is thought to be the basis for human learning. Connectionist models that entail Hebbian learning capture many aspects of this 'learning'. That is, connection strength is changed by massive presentation of a stimulus that causes one node to activate a connected node. However, in most connectionist models, the rate of presentation or 'activation' is not important (although networks with rapid decay, as well as slow decay, connections could simulate a requirement for rapid presentation). In the animal (human or non-human) brain, the rate of presentation is an essential feature in determining long-term potentiation (LTP) or long-term depression (LTD). The results from brain experiments suggest that frequent, as well as massive, practice would be most effective in learning.

This principle of intense practice is borne out in our every day experiences in learning. We do not expect a child to become a proficient violinist by playing the violin once a week, even if he or she does it for many years. Rather, lengthy, daily practice results in the most rapid and effective learning of the violin. Likewise, improvements in a sport are often observed most readily after a week or so of intense practice (e.g. spring training), rather than a few months of weekly or biweekly practice. As a final example, learning of a language occurs most rapidly and effectively when there is 'language immersion' (e.g., moving to a foreign country) rather than through taking classes a few times per week.

Rehabilitation of language, cognitive, or motor function probably also depends on the same principles. That is, there is evidence that relearning of a function, such as access to spoken word form representations for word retrieval, occurs most rapidly (and perhaps only) when training occurs daily, rather than a few times per week. To illustrate, a young woman, H.G., with severe impairment in accessing both semantic representations and spoken word form representations for speech, following severe left frontotemporal and parietal brain damage, was trained in oral naming of fabrics (so that she could attain her goal of working in a fabric shop). Training involved eliciting the correct name in response to a fabric, through a series of cues, designed to gradually foster more independent responses. This therapy was effective in improving her naming when it was provided in daily, two-hour sessions, but not when the same therapy was provided in twice per week two hour sessions, as shown in Figures 22.1 and 22.2 (described in Hillis 1998). H.G. rapidly improved in naming Sets A and B when treatment was initiated five days per week (Figure 22.1). However, she failed to learn Sets C and D, which were matched in word frequency and length to Sets A and B, when the same treatment was applied just twice per week (Figure 22.2).

Biochemical milieu in the brain Also unlike computers, change in connection strength in the brain depends on chemical milieu. For example, LTD and LTP depend on the presence of particular neuro-transmitters, which can be influenced by medications, reinforcement, motivation and other emotional states. Recent studies have shown that the presence of norepinephrine and acetylcholine together are essential for synaptic plasticity (LTD) (Kirkwood *et al.* 1999). Norepinephrine is released in states of

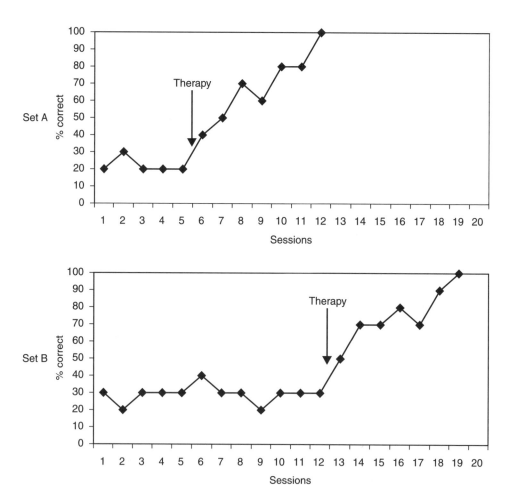

Figure 22.1 H.G.'s per cent naming of sequentially trained sets of fabrics when naming therapy was provided five days per week.

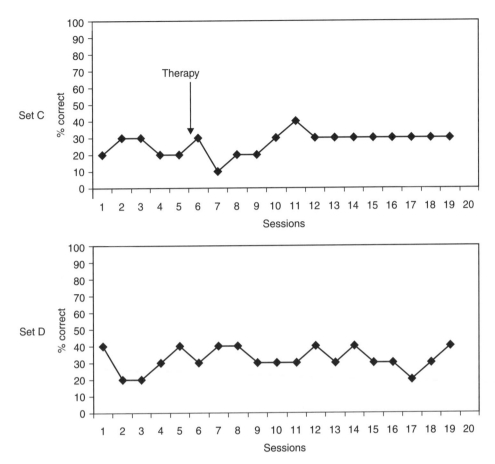

Figure 22.2 H.G.'s per cent correct naming of a set of trained fabrics (top) when therapy was provided twice per week. Set D was never trained (bottom) because the H.G. failed to meet criterion (≥ 80% correct for two sessions) on set C.

excitement or challenge, and in response to rewards. The essential role of norepinephrine can account for the remarkable effect of feedback during learning to discriminate /r/ versus /l/, as reported by McCandliss, McClelland and colleagues. This sort of feedback is not essential for learning in a connectionist network. Norepinephrine is also increased in response to certain medications, such as amphetamines. Recent studies, including small, double-blind randomized placebo-controlled trials, have demonstrated that administration of amphetamines along with language therapy resulted in more improvement in language in aphasic patients recovering from stroke, compared to language therapy alone (Walker-Batson 2000; Walker-Batson *et al.* 1991, 2001). Similar results have been reported for rehabilitation of motor skills after stroke (Walker-Batson *et al.* 1995).

The essential role of acetylcholine in synaptic plasticity is also borne out clinically. Neurons whose firing depends on acetylcholine degenerate in Alzheimer's disease (AD), a disease that severely affects memory and learning. Acetylcholine esterase inhibitors, which increase the amount of acetylcholine available to neurons, have been shown to improve cognition, or at least temporarily slow the rate of decline of cognition, in AD. These medications also may have a positive effect on recovery during language rehabilitation (Berthier *et al.* 2003).

Another medication that has been shown, at least in some studies (Albert *et al.* 1988; but see MacLennan *et al.* 1991), to improve outcome during language rehabilitation is bromocriptine, a dopamine agonist. Dopamine is a neurotransmitter that has an important role in the experience of reward. Serotonin, a neurotransmitter that has a role in the experience of punishment and emotional state, may also influence the effectiveness of rehabilitation. Medications that increase available serotonin (e.g., paroxetine) or norepinephrine (e.g., nortriptyline) are important in treatment of depression, and may improve outcome in rehabilitation (Gillen *et al.* 2001). It is not clear whether the positive influence on rehabilitation is solely through reduction of depression (and the concomitant increase in motivation), or whether these medications also directly affect synaptic plasticity and thus, learning. Wilson (1997) observed that feelings, emotional state, and social and behavioral consequences have important influences on rehabilitation; the influence of these key neurotransmitters on synaptic plasticity may explain why.

Medications can also have negative effects on crucial neurotransmitters and on rehabilitation outcome (see Goldstein 1998, for review). For example, reserpine (an older medication used to treat high blood pressure) reduces the release of norepinephrine and epinephrine, and can inhibit effectiveness of rehabilitation. Haloperidol and other neuroleptic medications that block dopamine receptors (having the opposite effect of bromocriptine), can negatively affect rehabilitation outcome as well (Small 2002).

There are other important differences between the brain and computers that are difficult to quantify. For example, concurrent activities of the brain, such as distraction with bodily needs or emotional needs, can greatly influence learning. Such influences may account for why two individuals with apparently the same deficits do not equally respond to the same therapy (Caramazza and Hillis 1993).

Stages of recovery Finally, the brain recovers from damage through various stages of recovery (Hillis and Heidler 2002). The first, acute stage during the first few days after onset stroke or brain injury, probably depends on tissue recovery, through restoration of blood flow to the brain, resolution of edema, restoration of membrane integrity, and normalization of ionic balance. For example, we (Hillis and Heidler 2002) found that all patients who had impaired word comprehension at Day 1 of stroke, and who recovered word comprehension by Day 3 of stroke, showed reperfusion (restored blood flow) to Wernicke's area by Day 3, as demonstrated by repeated magnetic resonance perfusion imaging. Patients who failed to recover word comprehension by Day 3 showed persistent hypoperfusion, or low blood flow, in Wernicke's area.

Intermediate recovery, starting days to weeks after stroke, and continuing for months or possibly years, involves variable degrees of reorganization of structure/function relationships. This reorganization can be shown by serial functional imaging (fMRI or PET scanning), which shows changes during recovery in areas of the brain that are 'activated' during a specific cognitive task (Cappa *et al.* 1997; Heiss *et al.* 1997, 1999; Karbe *et al.* 1995; Leff *et al.* 2002; Musso *et al.* 1999; Ohyama *et al.* 1996; Thiel *et al.* 2001; Thompson 2000; Thulborn *et al.* 1999; Warburton *et al.* 1999; Weiller *et al.* 1995; Weiller 2000). Reorganization has also been demonstrated through single cell recording experiments in monkeys, who show changes in cortical maps of motor and sensory function, demonstrated by individual neurons' responses to stimulation, after peripheral or central lesions (e.g., Merzenich *et al.* 1983). This reorganization depends on relearning through synaptic plasticity (LTP and LTD), as influenced by the availability of neurotransmitters during intense practice or stimulation. The availability of neurotransmitters, in turn, depends crucially on the correct chemical milieu, such as medications, and on the individual's mood and responses to reinforcements.

In the chronic stage (months to many years after brain lesion), recovery of cognitive skills may depend on learning new ways of carrying out the task. For example, patient S.J.D. (Hillis and Caramazza 1995) was unable to write verbs, although she could say verbs and could write both nouns and verbs at five years after her stroke involving the entire perisylvian language cortex. S.J.D. learned to write verbs by self-cuing the written form by converting the first sound of the oral form of the verb to a letter. This self-cuing strategy involved relearning of sound-to-print conversion rules. On the other hand, H.G. (Hillis 1998) was unable to *say* content words, although she had unimpaired articulation and other motor speech skills and was able to *write* content words spontaneously (the modality effect opposite to S.J.D.'s). She needed to relearn print-to-sound conversion rules in order to convert from the written to the spoken form of the content word. However, converting the first few letters did not result in effective self-cuing, analogous to S.J.D.'s self-cuing. Instead, she needed to relearn the pronunciation of each individual content word. To illustrate, H.G. pronounced the word *one* as 'own', and the abbreviation *Mrs.* as [mers]. These words had to be misspelled for her as the 'regularized' version of the word in order to elicit the correct pronunciation. That is, she had to learn that *one* is pronounced like *wun*, and Mrs as *missuz*. The relearning by both S.J.D. and H.G. would also have required new synapses, established through LTP and LTD, and would thus have been influenced by intensity of training and the neurochemical mileu.

It is very likely that different interventions are required for different stages of rehabilitation. That is, in the acute stage (the first few days after stroke or brain injury) medical and surgical interventions to restore blood flow (e.g., thrombolytics, revascularization, induced blood pressure elevation) in stroke, and perhaps neuroprotective medications in both stroke and traumatic brain injury, may be most effective in restoring tissue viability. In the intermediate stage, weeks after stroke, intense practice, perhaps combined with appropriate medications, may be best for inducing reorganization. In the chronic stage, behavioral approaches such as shaping and conditioning with appropriate rewards (+/− medications to increase the effectiveness of the reward system) may be most effective in teaching compensatory strategies and laying down new pathways to access previously established cognitive processes.

Conclusions

We are just beginning to have the elements with which a theory of rehabilitation can be built. These elements include, at the very least:

1. A model of the cognitive processes underlying the task to be relearned, and of the processes required to relearn it (relying on advances in cognitive neuropsychology and computational science);
2. A hypothesis about the network of neural structures and mechanisms underlying these cognitive processes (relying on advances in neuroimaging, single cell recording in primates, and other components of cognitive neuroscience);
3. A proposal about how change in these neural elements, such as synaptic plasticity, takes place (relying on recent advances in basic neuroscience), and
4. An informed theory of how neuroplasticity is influenced by medications and reinforcements (relying on recent advances in neuroscience, integrated with clinical neurology, physiatry, and psychiatry).

It is likely that the actual strategies of therapy that arise from such a theory will not differ substantially from those that have been discovered empirically in behavioral and cognitive approaches, although the intensity of treatment and combined use of cognitive rehabilitation and pharmacotherapy might be ramped up. Moreover, such a theory would shed light on why and how and when rehabilitation is most effective, and would thus allow clinicians to apply their strategies in the most effective times and frequencies, and to the most appropriate individuals.

23 The neural basis for a theory of cognitive rehabilitation

Ian H. Robertson

Abstract

In the chapters of this book it can be seen that some cognitive functions in some people can benefit from certain types of cognitive rehabilitation. The aim of this chapter is to address the question of how these effects might be mediated in the brain, with a view to establishing a theoretical framework for cognitive rehabilitation. Such a framework, we can hope, would enable us to improve cognitive rehabilitation strategies in the future and better synchronise them with the pharmacological and other related methods that will become increasingly available over the next decade.

Rehabilitation can harm as well as help: the need for theoretical models linking behaviour and biology

Implicit in the chapter's stated aim is the need to fill a major gap – both theoretical and practical – in our understanding of how cognitive rehabilitation works. This gap arises because the bulk of the research into recovery of function following brain damage has been carried out at the neurophysiological level of analysis. This is fine so long as treatments are focused also on this level of analysis, as is the case for pharmacological therapies. For the time being, however, by far the major type of treatment for brain damage is not pharmacological, but is behavioural – namely rehabilitation. It is assumed that this behavioural treatment will impact on the underlying neurophysiological processes of recovery, but what is missing is a theoretical framework within which these behaviourally-mediated treatments can be embedded, tested and improved. Such a framework must clearly be linked coherently to underlying neurophysiological processes, but must also yield a conceptual structure within which rehabilitationists can embed their work.

The question might arise as to why we should bother trying to link these two levels of analysis: should we not let the neurophysiologists and molecular biologists develop their biological treatments, and let the rehabilitationists develop purely behavioural frameworks within which to embed their therapies? This is not ideal, since the action of each type of therapy may be enhanced, limited or even reversed by processes in the other. To give one example, increasing the use of a limb impaired by sensori-motor cortex lesion in rats, given too early post-lesion can have detrimental effects on motor recovery, possibly via stimulation-induced neurotoxicity (Kozlowski, James, and Schallert 1996).

Under other conditions and timescales, however, motor stimulation can not only improve functional recovery, but can also 'rescue' neurons in the penumbra surrounding the lesion site that would otherwise die without such stimulation (Nudo, Wise, SiFuentes, and Milliken 1996). Understanding what rehabilitation given when will produce positive, neutral or negative results will only be possible through the building of theoretical bridges across these two levels of analysis – the cognitive/behavioural on the one hand, and the neurophysiological on the other.

Biological treatments must link to behavioural models of rehabilitation

Behavioural factors also limit biological interventions: one study (Mayer *et al.* 1992) showed that rats with striatal lesions given neural transplants only benefited from the transplants when they were given the opportunity for perceptuo-motor learning: in the absence of such behavioural 'driving' of the neural tissue, the necessary connectivity did not develop sufficiently to produce behavioural improvement, a conclusion strengthened by a more recent study (Dobrossy *et al.* 2000) of the effects of enriched environments on intrastriatal dopamine grafts.

Even the expression of genes linked to single-gene disorders such as Huntingdon's Disease is strongly influenced by environment. In one study (vanDellen *et al.* 2000), male Huntington's disease (HD) R6/1 mice were allocated to either a normal or a stimulating environment. All mice were in groups in standard cages, but the 'environmentally enriched' groups also contained cardboard, paper and plastic objects, changed every two days, from the age of four weeks. To define the onset of disease, motor coordination was tested every week in a 'turning task': the results clearly showed a very significant slowing of the disease onset in the enriched group. Furthermore, the peristriatal cerebral volume was 13 per cent larger in the environmentally enriched HD mice than in the non-enriched HD group. To give a further example of this, experience-dependent cortical plasticity seems to depend on the participant paying active attention to the stimulation/activity: where attention is deployed to some other stream of stimulation, such change is attenuated or absent (Iguchi *et al.* 2001; Recanzone *et al.* 1993). This suggests that the cognitive process of active attention is a critical ingredient for mediating the cellular and synaptic changes that occur in response to stimulation/activity, emphasizing the critical importance of the interaction between these two levels of analysis in understanding the processes of rehabilitation and recovery.

In other words, just as behavioural interventions must adjust to the limitations and dynamics of the brain's synaptic, cellular and molecular processes, so biological interventions must take into account the role of cognitive and behavioural factors in influencing biological systems. One important question that has arisen repeatedly in discussing cognitive rehabilitation concerns the role of compensatory versus restitutive processes.

Restitution versus compensation

The great neuropsychologist Luria argued strongly for a compensatory process known as 'functional reorganization' or 'functional adaptation' as the main mechanism underlying recovery of function following brain damage. His view was shaped by the assumption prevalent in his day that CNS cells do not regenerate: hence recovery of neuropsychological functions is achieved largely by the reorganization of surviving neural circuits to achieve the given behaviour in a different way. We know now, however, that neurons do indeed regenerate, in humans as well as other mammals (Eriksson *et al.* 1998; Gould *et al.* 1999).

Nevertheless, compensation is one important type of mechanism underlying recovery of function (Bäckman and Dixon 1992; Wilson 2002). In this chapter I concentrate on the possibility of rehabilitation-induced plastic reorganization of lesioned brain systems. An important caveat is required, however. Conceptually attractive as this distinction between compensation and restitution may be, there can be significant difficulties in making it. To demonstrate that restitution and not compensation has occurred faces the problem that though one may be able to show that a recovered behaviour appears identical to that shown by normal subjects, one can never exclude the possibility that a difference does exist and that the correct experimental manipulation to demonstrate this difference has simply not been found. In short, proving that restitution and not compensation has occurred using behavioural methods demands the logically impossible proof of the null hypothesis. The demonstration that restitution has occurred must therefore depend on physical measures of brain structure and function, showing that neuroanatomical structures known to be involved in the impaired function are activated when the relevant behaviour is produced.

Heuristically, however, the distinction between compensation and restitution has proved useful: in pragmatic clinical terms it is also hard to avoid. Faced with someone who cannot move her arm, for instance, does one devote limited rehabilitation resources to trying to get her to move that arm, or to developing compensatory strategies to allow her to live as normal a life as possible while avoiding the use of that arm? Faced with someone showing severe expressive dysphasia, do we as rehabilitationists try to train him to produce spoken words or do we teach him alternative means of communication? Confronted with 'dysexecutive' problems, do we focus our efforts on structuring the environment to support more organized behaviour, or do we struggle to retrain at least some internally-mediated attentional control skills? These are real dilemmas for clinical practice and policy, and they support the need to maintain – for the time being at least – this distinction between compensation and restitution. This is particularly the case if – as shall be shown later – some attempts at compensation may actually have *negative* effects on brain function and outcome.

Hebbian learning and plasticity

It is appropriate that a psychologist – Donald Hebb – should have articulated a neurophysiological principle that is central to the building of theoretical bridges between the behavioural/cognitive and neurophysiological levels of analysis (Hebb 1949). The concept of 'learning' derives from the cognitive/behavioural level of analysis, and Hebb linked this specifically to a neurophysiological process whereby the synchronous firing of pre- and post-synaptic cells leads to inter-neuron linkages through changes in synaptic strengths: in other words, 'cells that fire together, wire together'.

Hebbian Learning as a concept has stood the test of time – albeit with subtle refinements of the theory (Bi and Poo 2001), and has generated an enormous amount of research in the domain of neurophysiology. Murre and I laid out a number of assumptions about the role of Hebbian learning in recovery of function following brain damage (Robertson and Murre 1999), which can be summarized as follows:

1. The brain is capable of a large degree of 'self-repair' through synaptic turnover and may in fact continuously be engaged in this, even in the absence of overt damage. This synaptic turnover is to some extent experience-dependent and is a key mechanism underlying both learning and recovery of function following brain damage.

2. Recovery processes following brain damage share common mechanisms with normal learning and experience-dependent plasticity processes.

3. Variations in experience, and inputs available to damaged neural circuits will shape synaptic interconnections, and hence influence recovery.

4. An analysis of the determinants of normal short- and long-term plasticity in the undamaged CNS will yield useful guides to the key variables determining whether and how recovery of function can be guided and shaped by rehabilitation methods.

These principles suggest, for instance, that neurons which have been disconnected by a lesion may become reconnected if they are activated at the same time. Simultaneous activation will take place if both neurons are separately connected to a circuit whose neurons themselves are functionally interconnected. When this net of neurons is activated, the two neurons which are disconnected from each other are simultaneously activated. With several repetitions of this, these two neurons thus may become reconnected. Hebbian learning provides a model for how neural circuits which are partially lesioned may regain the original pattern of connections and hence the cortical functions which they subserve may be regained. This may be one of the mechanisms by which certain types of rehabilitation enhance recovery of function.

A rehabilitation triage?

Any clinician will be able to think of individuals who appear to have recovered without rehabilitation after brain lesions, and others who show little or very incomplete recovery even over tens of years. A third category of individual might be recalled – those who show some recovery, but only with the help of rehabilitation. Murre and I used a connectionist model (Robertson and Murre 1999) to demonstrate that while networks with a small number of lost connections could 'repair' themselves via normal synaptic turnover according to Hebbian principles, networks that lost more than a critical number of neurons suffered catastrophic loss of connectivity.

An intermediate loss of connections could be recovered, however, through a process we called 'guided recovery' – patterned external input that induced coactivation of disconnected 'neurons', resulting in reconnection through Hebbian principles (Robertson and Murre 1999). Our prediction was that the triage category would be determined by three factors:

1. Total size of the lesioned neural circuit;
2. Degree of connectivity within the network; and
3. Size of lesion.

This triage of course has only descriptive and not explanatory value. The focus of this chapter is on the second layer of the notional triage – that is guided recovery – focusing on how to provide inputs to lesioned networks that foster plastic reorganization and recovery.

Guided recovery

How do we provide the input necessary for 'rescuing' these stage 2 lesions? One way is simply to try to provide additional forms of the type of stimulation that the lesioned circuit would be exposed to normally, or engage in repeated practice of the motor or cognitive functions it normally subserves.

General stimulation

Environmental enrichment – non-specific social and behavioural stimulation has in animal research led to such changes in synaptic connectivity (Will and Kelche 1992). More specific stimulation such as repeated practice of skilled movements has also produced both improved function and rescue of neurons that would otherwise die, as mentioned earlier (Nudo *et al.* 1996). Jaap Murre and I showed that completion and reconnection in a lesioned neural network will normally occur more fully if a greater number of coactivations of the to-be-connected nodes takes place (Robertson and Murre 1999). Hence usually, non-specific environmental stimulation can be expected to facilitate synaptic connectivity by increasing the probability of reconnection through Hebbian learning mechanisms.

Under some circumstances, however, we found that such non-specific stimulation may foster faulty or maladaptive connections. This would tend to occur if the stimulations tend to produce a greater coactivation of part of the lesioned circuit with some other neural circuit than it does with other parts of the partially disconnected lesioned circuit.

The strange phenomenon of phantom limb mapping onto the face (Ramachandran *et al.* 1992) may also be a result of such maladaptive reorganization – in this case of somatosensory representations in the cortex. It has also been suggested that tinnitus after acquired deafness might arise through similar plastic changes in synaptic weights within the central auditory system, resulting in the false auditory sensations of tinnitus (Jastreboff 1990).

Patients usually themselves make attempts to generate such stimulation and activity in an attempt to try to recover the lost function. One case study of optic aphasia (Beauvois 1982) revealed a patient trying to compensate for the deficit by repeated subvocal rehearsals. Instead of helping re-establish the lost function, however, this attempt at general stimulation actually seemed to interfere with recovery: when the researcher – with the patient's consent of course – placed soft tape across the lips in order to discourage this implicit verbalization, the optic aphasia improved considerably!

More recently research on non-fluent aphasia suggested that activation of areas in the undamaged right hemisphere homologous to damaged left hemisphere regions might actually interfere with language output. To test this, the researchers applied repetitive slow wave transcranial magnetic stimulation (rTMS) at a frequency known to produce inhibition of function to two of these right hemisphere regions. They then examined the effects on naming ability (Naesser *et al.* 2002). They found that rTMS of area 45 in the right frontal lobe improved subsequent naming ability, while the same rTMS applied to the motor cortex did not.

There is therefore evidence that restitution of function in damaged circuits may at times be hindered by compensatory adjustments which improve function in the short term, while at the same time hindering reactivation of the damaged circuits themselves. General stimulation and general attempts to activate damaged neural networks may produced unforeseen negative consequences. Hence the need for better planned and patterned stimulation to these networks, the second type of guided recovery.

Bottom-up specific stimulation

The discussion above would suggest that, where possible, stimulation should be targeted such as to foster adaptive connections within the lesioned circuit. Such inputs can be considered in terms of 'bottom-up' versus 'top-down' types of guided, targeted stimulation: we will consider the former type first.

An example of this was where voluntary EMG activity in hand extensor and flexor muscles was used to trigger electrical stimulation of these muscles, resulting in improved movements (Hummelsheim *et al.* 1996). As voluntary force levels improved, the threshold of EMG activity required to trigger stimulation was gradually increased. This training produced enduring improvements in a number of hand and arm function measures, and it is likely that the specific bottom-up stimulation of the lesioned sensorimotor cortex facilitated long term potentiation and hence synaptic reconnection in these circuits, as has been demonstrated in animals (Asanuma and Keller 1991).

To give another example, Taub and colleagues have demonstrated the effects of specific motor stimulation on patients who have suffered unilateral strokes leading to partial hemiplegia of one upper limb (Miltner *et al.* 1999; Taub *et al.* 1993). They showed that it was possible to improve function in the hemiparetic limb by (a) discouraging patients from using the limb on the unaffected side of the body and (b) encouraging use of the partially hemiparetic limb. With just a two-week period of such training, a significant improvement in motor function lasting up to two years was observed in the hemiparetic limb. These were also patients who were long past the period where maximum motor recovery takes place. These positive effects were predicated on a specific pattern of stimulation – activation of one limb combined with de-activation of the other – which would likely not have occurred if the motor stimulation had been non-specific and fostered activity in both limbs.

Though there were elements of 'top-down' input in this training procedure, insofar as the movements of the hemiparetic limb were generated voluntarily, we conceive this as a largely 'bottom-up' phenomenon, insofar as the restitutive effectiveness of this training is contingent on the repeated activation of the impaired sensori-motor circuits, leading, it is hypothesized, to plastic reorganization of the cortical sensori-motor circuits (Taub and Wolf 1997).

Related evidence for the effectiveness of bottom-up stimulation in fostering recovery of function comes from a study of gait rehabilitation in nonambulatory hemiparetic stroke patients (Hesse et al. 1995). Seven patients who could not walk were partially supported with a modified parachute harness and were encouraged to walk on a treadmill. Very significant improvements in walking were found, with three participants walking independently after the end of training, and three more requiring only verbal supervision.

Related findings have emerged in the study of rehabilitation of unilateral left neglect – a visuospatial attentional disorder leading to impaired perception of and responses to stimuli on the left side of space. Robertson and colleagues carried out a series experiments examining the therapeutic effects of left arm activation (Robertson et al. 1992) on unilateral neglect. We showed that only when a left limb was moved on the left side of space, temporary improvements in perception of left sided stimuli was achieved. These temporary improvements could, via the use of a procedure known as Limb Activation Training, be translated into clinically significant long-term effects, particularly on left-sided motor function, as a recent randomized controlled trial shows (Robertson et al. 2002). Furthermore, acute neglect patients receiving this minimally labour-intensive additional treatment are discharged from hospital on average 28 days earlier than patients who do not receive it (Kalra et al. 1997).

Schindler and his colleagues in Munich have shown that doing something quite implausible – applying a standard electro-mechanical vibrator to the left neck muscles of patients while they engage in visual search exercises – produces marked and enduring clinical and real-life benefits (Schindler et al. 2002). This bottom-up stimulation-based treatment arose out of basic research into the brain mechanisms of sensory integration and higher-level perception. Neck vibration was used because of its known effects on the body's normal co-ordinate frame of reference according to which sensory inputs and motor outputs are integrated. In neglect, not only is this egocentric reference frame biased to the right, but also the neck vibration can temporarily correct this imbalance. What we see in the Munich paper is that, when combined with systematic visual search training, and when systematically applied for 15 therapy sessions over 3 weeks, temporary effects become long lasting and hence therapeutically important.

Similarly impressive results in neglect rehabilitation have been obtained with another new, cognitive neuroscience-derived treatment – prism adaptation training (Frassinetti et al. 2002). Here, neglect patients learn to adapt make perceptuo-motor adapatations to prisms that laterally shift the visual field, and this produces significant changes in both the impairment (unilateral neglect) itself, as well as in functional activities.

The concept of bottom-up stimulation is, at first sight, less straightforwardly applicable to problems of attentional control partly associated with frontal lobe lesions. This appears to be the case because of the fundamental architecture of the brain, whereby most sensory input is directed primarily to posterior brain regions. What, then, might constitute a 'bottom-up' input for a lesioned prefrontal cortex?

One mechanism might be through increased arousal in a bottom-up way, via the mesencephalic reticular formation and the thalamic relay nuclei (Heilman *et al.* 1987). Furthermore, this mid-brain alerting system can also be activated in a 'top-down' fashion, particularly from the right dorsolateral prefrontal cortex (Heilman *et al.* 1987; Kinomura *et al.* 1996; Posner 1993). This type of system would be needed in tasks where the external environment provides no intrinsically arousing stimulation, but where nevertheless an alert readiness to respond must be maintained endogenously.

We have demonstrated this principle in a quasi-therapeutic paradigm: when a phasically alerting exogenous auditory cue is periodically presented during the course of a complex activity requiring executive control, executive control is significantly improved, indicating a possible bottom-up effect of an alerting cue on sustained attention (Manly *et al.* 2002). Similarly, natural circadian fluctuations in arousal have also been shown to alter executive/attentional performance in a bottom-up way (Manly *et al.* 2002b). Though these effects are temporary, they do show the possibility of modulating attentional control in a bottom-up way, using external, alerting stimuli. We are currently evaluating clinical methods based on this principle, where we will test the prediction that more enduring effects of this type of bottom-up stimulation on attentional control may be found.

Top-down specific stimulation

There is abundant evidence that attention can 'gate' the processing of information in primary as well as secondary sensory areas of the brain, and it is assumed that attentional circuits – argued to be based in part at least in the frontal lobes – are the source of such gating (Desimone and Duncan 1995). Attention can modulate synaptic activity in posterior circuits of the brain (Büchel and Friston 1997), influences synaptic connectivity in animals (Recanzone *et al.* 1993) and modulates experience-dependent plasticity in humans (Iguchi *et al.* 2001).

If this is true, then recovery of function in a wide range of neural circuits in the brain should be influenced by the integrity of the attentional systems of the brain. Put another way, the better the functioning of the attentional circuits of the brain (partly, but not exclusively, based in the prefrontal cortex), the greater should be the chance of recovery of more posterior cognitive, sensory and motor functions in brain lesioned patients, or conversely, an impaired frontal cortex will impair such recovery.

If, however, top-down input from attentional circuits can foster connectivity in the non-damaged brain, then such input should also be able to foster reconnection and repair in the damaged brain. Is there, however, any evidence from human clinical research to indicate that top-down attentional processes influence recovery of function following brain lesion? We have shown that motor recovery following stroke over a two-year period was significantly predicted by measures of sustained attention taken two months after right hemisphere stroke (Robertson *et al.* 1997).

If attentional systems can act as one source of patterned input to lesioned circuits and hence contribute in some way to repair and reconnection in these circuits, are there any rehabilitation studies which demonstrate such an effect? There is relatively little data on this yet, and none which show directly neural effects of top-down attentional modulation of neural repair. Nevertheless, there is some recent behavioural evidence which is supportive of this hypothesis. Furthermore, training aimed at enhancing sustained attention led to significant improvements not only in sustained attention, but also in unilateral neglect in one study (Robertson *et al.* 1995), a phenomenon also demonstrated using exogenous alerting stimuli to initiate temporary improvements in unilateral neglect (Robertson *et al.* 1998b).

Inhibitory processes

Marcel Kinsbourne proposed that the two hemispheres of the brain are in competition (Kinsbourne 1993): if this is the case, then damage to one hemisphere should reduce its inhibitory influence on the other. There are many demonstrations of this: for instance, repetitive transcranial magnetic stimulation that inhibited the parietal cortex of one hemisphere in normal subjects caused an increase in sensitivity to ipsilateral cutaneous stimuli (Seyal *et al.* 1995). The authors argued that this is because the TMS transiently inhibits the parietal cortex, thus freeing the contralateral parietal cortex from competitive inhibition. As a result, ipsilateral cutaneous stimuli which are processed by this disinhibited contralateral parietal cortex are more strongly represented and hence have a lower threshold for perception.

Evidence indeed exists that damaged circuits in the brain suffer further loss of function because of inhibitory competition from undamaged circuits, particularly – but not uniquely – interhemispherically across the corpus callosum. As mentioned earlier (Naesser *et al.* 2002), attempts at compensation by brain damaged patients may result in deterioration in performance, and this deterioration may reverse if the brain regions involved in the compensation are temporarily inhibited using repetitive TMS.

Following on from the studies of limb activation on unilateral neglect described above, a further study (Robertson and North 1994) showed that the beneficial effects of single left limb activation in left hemispace could be eliminated if the right limb was simultaneously moved. This result was interpreted in terms of competition between the two hemispheres. Whereas a single left movement in left hemispace activated representations of both personal and peripersonal space, resulting in an improved ability to attend to contralesional stimuli because of this combined activation, bilateral movements activated competitor circuits in the undamaged left hemisphere. As a result of this competition, the activation in the right hemisphere was competitively extinguished, it was argued. This finding has been replicated in both single-case and group studies (Ladavas *et al.* 1997; Mattingley *et al.* 1998).

Arousal

There is considerable evidence to suggest that noradrenergic and cholinergic neurotransmitter systems may have a 'permissive' function in neuronal plasticity (Will and Kelche 1992). In one study dextroamphetamine potentiated the effect of language rehabilitation to produce improved outcome in aphasia (Walker-Batson *et al.* 2001). Conversely, common clinically-used drugs which depress noradrenergic activity have been shown to retard recovery from hemiplegia (Goldstein *et al.* 1990).

Implications for clinical rehabilitation

Some cautious but potentially important conclusions can be drawn from the review so far. They can be summarized in simple terms as follows. Following damage to the brain, a proportion of individuals will recover relatively normal function spontaneously through Hebbian learning-based self-repair processes. In this 'autonomous recovery' group, only significant extraneous factors may impede this self repair. One such factor could include abnormally low neuromodulator availability (for instance caused by drug administration which lowers levels of plasticity-enhancing neuromodulators in the brain). But in most cases, circumscribed lesions which affect only a relatively small proportion of cells and connections in circuits subserving a particular function should be restitutable through spontaneous self-repair processes. One caveat to this conclusion is that 'bottleneck' lesions that destroy a pathway connecting two distinct processors may have a large effect, even though the lesion is small (Levine *et al.* 1998).

A critical question for the framework proposed here is how one can avoid circularity in defining in advance which individuals belong to which category in the triage. Present clinical methods do not allow us easily and directly to measure the extent of remaining connectivity in lesioned circuits, though earlier in this paper we did review considerable biological evidence that restitution of function often appears feasible if a rump of 10–20 per cent of undamaged cells and connections remain (Sabel 1997). However, the presence of residual behavioural function apparent under certain circumstances may represent a reasonable clinical basis for assessing which individuals may potentially fall into the 'rescuable' part of the triage, where guided recovery of primary functioning may be possible.

Using transcranial magnetic stimulation, it is possible to assess the degree of residual motor function in the acute stages following unilateral stroke; such residual function detected early post-stroke predicts long-term recovery of motor function (Heald *et al.* 1993). A further example of this principle comes from the work of Taub and colleagues described above. They showed motor recovery in the hemiplegic limbs of chronically hemiparetic victims of stroke, using a combination of deactivation of the unimpaired limb with encouragement to move the affected limb. The individuals selected for this study had to have some degree of movement in the affected limb. Specifically, patients had to be able to extend at least 10 degrees at the metacarpophalangeal and interphalangeal joints and 20 degrees at the wrist.

As a clinical yardstick therefore, it would seem appropriate to suggest that restitution-oriented attempts at guided recovery of intrinsic functions, as opposed to compensatory approaches, may be attempted where some residual capacity in the affected function can be detected. Residual function may however be masked due to low levels of alertness/arousal, poor awareness of deficits, inhibition by competitor circuits or inadequate ability to deploy attention to the relevant behaviours, as discussed earlier in this paper. The assessment as to whether residual functioning exists therefore requires these variables to be monitored, and where possible manipulated, in order to determine whether residual function can be unmasked.

At the moment, standardized assessment measures in neuropsychology and rehabilitation do not tend to take into account such variables when assessing particular functions. Yet, to take the example of the arousal/sustained attention complex, dramatic changes in the manifestation of unilateral neglect can be induced by modifying levels of alertness (Robertson *et al.* 1998b). Standard assessment procedures for unilateral neglect do not take such findings into account, and hence the assessment of the degree of residual function is difficult to carry out using existing methods.

Sterzi and colleagues (1993) have found that there is significantly greater incidence of apparently primary visual field, tactile sensation, limb position sense difficulties and motor problems in patients who have suffered right hemisphere strokes compared to carefully matched patients who have suffered left hemisphere strokes. The authors argue that this can only be attributable to a subtle bias of attention towards the right side of the body, leading to impaired performance on sensory, proprioceptive and motor tasks on the left side which masquerade as primary deficits in these areas. This has also been dramatically confirmed with vestibular stimulation approaches to unilateral neglect, where improvements in hemianesthesia, limb position sense and distorted body image can be obtained purely by methods which activate the vestibular system of the impaired hemisphere (Cappa *et al.* 1987). These findings show clearly that in these particular cases, the apparently primary sensory and motor problems were actually attentional in origin.

Timescale of rehabilitation

It follows from the framework proposed in this paper that the timing of rehabilitation may be critical. If networks can decay, they may do so quickly following a lesion. The provision of patterned input, along with the discouragement of responses which might foster faulty connections, should be provided – theoretically at least – as soon as medical stability is achieved. The work of Nudo and colleagues (Nudo *et al.* 1996) reviewed earlier, showed for instance that a lesion may result – possibly through deafferentation of neighbouring regions – in additional loss of synaptic connectivity and behavioural capacity over and above what is caused by the lesion itself. Such additional loss of function could be prevented by the timely input of behavioural stimulation to 'rescue' the at-risk networks. In other words, for certain circuits, there may conceivably be a critical period within which the appropriate patterned stimulation must be given if the networks are to survive. It seems very likely that similar processes may occur in humans, and hence the timing as well as the nature of rehabilitative input becomes critical. A reasonable working principle would be that this input should be provided as soon as it is medically feasible. Though the timely and intensive application of patterned stimulation to accelerate self-repair of networks may be of crucial importance, this need not necessarily imply an increase in total rehabilitation time, but rather the more timely deployment of the resources available; this may require a flexibility of rehabilitation input, intensively for short but carefully-timed intervals of treatment. Again, however, this is a hypothesis and not a fact. We hope that in advancing this hypothesis, rehabilitation research can be oriented to this and other related questions, thus helping to develop theoretically-based rehabilitation.

Attention and arousal

A further limitation on the duration of treatment concerns the attentional capacities of the individual. As we showed earlier in the paper, it is known that plastic neural reorganization does not occur passively, but instead requires that active attention be paid to the relevant behaviours during stimulation. It follows therefore that if attention can only effectively be deployed for periods of seconds or minutes, then rehabilitation input should ideally be confined to such 'attentional windows' – with more frequent, brief, sessions of therapy offered, rather than bureaucratically-determined sessions lasting up to one hour.

Arousal – the generalized state of alertness which is linked to diurnal variations in wakefulness – may also have to be at optimal levels for successful guided recovery and plastic reorganization to take place. This is also supported by our connectionist model (Murre and Robertson 1995), where arousal must be at a certain minimum level for representations to recover, and hence patterned input may not be indicated until appropriate levels of arousal are achieved. This may require the combination of pharmacological interventions with behavioural training in some cases, and preliminary studies using such an approach have produced promising results, as we outlined earlier in the paper. Conversely, the importance of neuromodulator levels in the brain means that much more attention should be paid to the choice of drugs given to patients during recovery from brain damage.

Generalizability of therapeutic effects

Rehabilitation effects rest on many of the same neural processes as underlie normal learning. The failure of learning to generalize from one setting to another is not necessarily a mark of failure of the process of learning. There are circumstances where learning is context-dependent, and hence if one wishes to see learning generalize to other settings, then one must repeat the training within that context. This is often true for compensatory scanning in unilateral neglect, for instance. In one study, patients with unilateral left neglect were trained to scan to their left for obstacles that were marked by bright-coloured markers. Even when these markers were removed, the patients successfully learned to avoid the previously-marked obstacles. When these patients returned home, however, there was no generalization of the leftward scanning strategies they had learned in hospital, and the scanning habit had to be retrained in the home setting (Lennon 1994).

Learning, however, need not always be so closely tied to context. In limb activation treatments for unilateral neglect, for instance, relatively enduring effects of this training have been found without the need for training to be repeated in every different context within which the patient operates (Robertson *et al.* 1998, 2002). In this case, latent attentional and perceptual function in the damaged right hemisphere are being inhibited by competitor activity from the undamaged left hemisphere. Activating the left limb can temporarily overcome that inhibition. But how is this temporary activation translated into enduring improvements in everyday life? Our hypothesis is that there the hemiparetic limb is underused because of lack of attention to that side of the body caused by the left neglect. This lack of use contributes to the under-activation of the damaged right hemisphere. With repeated activation of the left limb (as opposed to short-term activation for experimental purposes), attention to the left side of the body is improved, because of the 'revived' latent activation in the right hemisphere. And because attention to the left side of the body is improved, the patient is more likely to use that side of the body, resulting of course in further activation in the damaged right hemisphere. This, we argued, causes Hebbian learning, reinforcing the activation pattern and making it easier to reproduce it with repeated activation. Thus we have – hypothetically at least – a virtuous, self-strengthening circle of induced activation, leading to improved attention, leading to more activation, leading to greater attention, and so on. This type of learning – with associated reduction in inhibition – is of course married to a context, but this is a context that patients carry with them – their own bodies.

Conclusion

Recent progress in neuroscience provides us with an opportunity to try to place the rehabilitation of brain damage on a scientific basis. New evidence about experience-dependent plasticity of the adult brain allows us cautious optimism about the possibility of restitution of brain function following damage. This endeavour, however, will require strong interactions between basic and clinical research: basic cognitive scientists must become intimately involved in supplying the necessary information to help make decisions about (a) whether potentially restitutable residual capacity exists in specified lesioned circuits and (b) what the inputs should be to maximize this restitution. This is central to the development of what must inevitably become a properly scientifically-based approach to rehabilitation.

Section 7

Pathology-based outcomes

24 Cognitive rehabilitation outcomes for traumatic brain injury

Nancy Carney and Hugo du Coudray

Abstract

In 1998, the Evidence-Based Practice Center (EPC) of Oregon Health and Science University (OHSU) conducted a systematic review of the scientific literature about the effectiveness of cognitive rehabilitation for the treatment of traumatic brain injury (TBI) in adults. The review was part of a larger report, funded by the Agency for Healthcare Research and Quality (AHRQ), in which the evidence for the effectiveness of rehabilitation interventions for TBI at various phases of recovery was summarized (Chesnut et al. 1999). In this chapter, we summarize the process and findings about cognitive rehabilitation from that report, as well as the findings from an update conducted to review the literature from 1998 to 2002.

Original evidence report

Causal pathway and categorization of outcomes

With the assistance of a panel of technical experts, including a neuropsychologist, a speech and language pathologist, a survivor of brain injury, a case manager, physicians, etc., we defined important health outcomes, and distinguished those from intermediate measures of improvement, generally used in clinical settings, that may or may not associate with improved abilities in everyday environments. Health outcomes specified by the panel were:

- Activities of daily living
- Long-term measures of disability
- Long-term measures of impairment
- Independence, relationships, family life, satisfaction
- Long-term financial burden.

We constructed a causal pathway to illustrate the relationships between interventions, intermediate tests, and outcomes (see Figure 24.1). An intervention is a treatment, or the introduction of a stimulus, thought to influence one or more behaviors. An intermediate measure is a test of the influence of the intervention, usually in a clinical setting. By contrast, an outcome measure is a test of the influence of the intervention in a real-life setting. As illustrated in Figure 24.1, a test such as the Paced Auditory

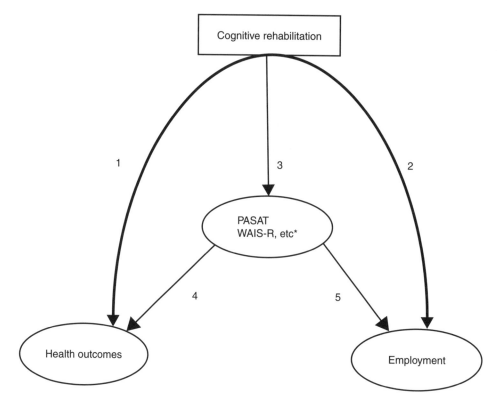

Figure 24.1 Casual pathway for cognitive rehabilitation. * PASAT – Paved auditory serial additional task; WAIS-R – Wechsler adult intelligence scale revised.

Serial Addition Task (PASAT), administered by a neuropsychologist during a clinical evaluation, is an intermediate test of the intervention of cognitive rehabilitation. Outcome measures might be the extent to which the person is able to remember to take medications, take the bus across town, or maintain employment. Arcs 1 and 2 of Figure 24.1 represent the direct effect of cognitive rehabilitation on health outcomes and employment. In the context of a systematic review, 'direct' evidence comes from comparative studies that examine the effect of cognitive rehabilitation on measures of these outcomes. 'Indirect' evidence refers to a causal chain that relies on intermediate measures. In Figure 24.1, the first link in this chain is between the intervention and intermediate measures of improvement (arc 3). The next links in the causal chain correspond to the question, 'Do intermediate measures used to assess the effect of cognitive rehabilitation predict improvement in real-life function (arc 4) and employment (arc 5)?' In evaluating the studies that contribute to this body of evidence, we focused on measures of the important outcomes specified for us by our technical panel. Thus we do not report all outcome measures for all studies included in the review.

Method

We conducted an electronic search of MEDLINE from 1966 to the present for randomized controlled trials (RCTs) and 1976 to 1997 for other types of literature; HealthSTAR from 1995 to 1997; CINAHL from 1982 to 1997; PsychINFO from 1984 to 1997 and the Cochrane Library. In general, we sought RCTs, non-randomized comparative trials, and prospective observational studies, excluding non-traumatic brain injury, mild brain injury, pediatric samples, pharmacological interventions, case reports, retrospective reports, and trials with fewer than five participants (see Chesnut *et al.* 1999 for detailed inclusion parameters). Two researchers, blinded to each other's results, read 600 abstracts and identified 114 potential references. An additional 20 were located from reference lists of review articles and peer recommendations. Thirty-two publications met the inclusion criteria and were abstracted for evidence, as follows:

- Eleven randomized controlled trials: five measuring health outcomes (Helfenstein and Wechsier 1982; Neistadt 1992; Novack *et al.* 1996; Ruff and Niemann 1990; Schmitter-Edgecombe *et al.* 1995), and six measuring intermediate outcomes (Kerner and Acker 1985; Niemann *et al.* 1990; Ruff *et al.* 1989; Ryan and Ruff 1988; Thomas-Stonell *et al.* 1994; Twum and Parente 1994).
- Four comparative studies: one measuring employment outcomes (Prigatano *et al.* 1984) and three measuring intermediate outcomes (Batchelor *et al.* 1988; Gray *et al.* 1992; Wood and Fussey 1987).
- Eight studies of the relationship between intermediate tests and employment (Brooks *et al.* 1987; Cicerone *et al.* 1996; Ezrachi *et al.* 1991; Fabiano and Crewe 1995; Fraser *et al.* 1988; Girard *et al.* 1996; Ip *et al.* 1995; Najenson *et al.* 1980).
- Nine observational studies: one measuring health outcomes (Wilson *et al.* 1997), and eight measuring intermediate outcomes (Cicerone and Giacino 1992; Deacon and Campbell 1991; Glisky *et al.* 1986; Goldstein *et al.* 1988; Middleton *et al.* 1991; Ponsford and Kinsella 1988; Ruff *et al.* 1994; Scherzer 1986).

Summary of results

A complete review of the results as well as evidence tables for all included publications can be found in Carney *et al.* (1999). The following summarizes only the studies that demonstrated clear treatment effects.

One small RCT (Schmitter-Edgecombe *et al.* 1995) and one observational study (Wilson *et al.* 1997) provide direct evidence of the effect of compensatory cognitive devices (notebooks, wristwatch alarms, programmed reminder device) on the reduction of everyday memory failures for persons with TBI (arc 1 of the causal pathway). A second RCT (Helfenstein and Wechsier 1982) provides evidence that compensatory cognitive rehabilitation reduces anxiety, and improves self-concept and interpersonal relationships for persons with TBI. However, the durability of the effects at follow-up intervals was not consistently demonstrated.

Three RCTs (Kerner and Acker 1985; Thomas-Stonell *et al.* 1994; Twum and Parente 1994) and two non-randomized comparative studies (Gray *et al.* 1992; Wood and Fussey 1987) provide limited evidence that practice and computer-aided cognitive rehabilitation improve performance on intermediate, laboratory-based measures of immediate recall (arc 3 of the causal pathway). However, there were no studies addressing the association between intermediate tests and health outcomes (arc 4 of the causal pathway), and the results of the studies about the association between intermediate tests and employment were equivocal (arc 5 of the causal pathway). Therefore, these studies only provide information about the effect of the specific cognitive rehabilitation treatment on intermediate measures, and do not tell us if the treatment improves a person's ability to function in everyday circumstances.

Limitations of the research

Classification of outcomes

There is no standard or agreed set of outcome measures for cognitive rehabilitation that can be used across clinics to evaluate both patient progress and program effectiveness. Of the studies in the original review, there were 91 different intermediate measures of outcome (see Table 24.1).

Table 24.1 Summary of results of intermediate measures of cognitive function (please see text for explanation)

Cognitive domain and associated tests	Number of tests found to have a positive effect or association			Number of tests done without a positive effect or association			Proportion of positive effects found	
	RCTs (a)	Comparative studies (b)	Correlational studies (c)	RCTs (d)	Comparative studies (e)	Correlational studies (f)	RCTs and comparative $\dfrac{a+b}{a+b+d+e}$	Correlation Studies $\dfrac{c}{c+f}$
Attention and orientation								
Digits	0	1	1	3	3	3	.14	.25
Mental Control	0	0	0	1	0	0	0	0
Trails A and B	0	0	3	1	1	1	0	.75
PASAT	0	1	2	2	1	0	.25	1.0
Test d2	0	0	0	1	1	0	0	0
Continuous Test of Attent.	0	0	1	0	0	0	0	1.0
Divided Attention	0	0	0	1	1	0	0	0
Ruff 2 and 7	0	0	0	1	1	0	0	0
Letter Cancellation	0	0	0	0	0	0	0	0
Time Estimation	0	1	0	0	0	0	1.0	0
Attention to Task	0	1	0	0	0	0	1.0	0
Attention Rating Scale	0	0	0	0	0	0	0	0
WMS Attent./Concentr.	0	0	0	0	0	2	0	0
Digit Symbol	0	0	1	2	1	1	0	.50
Ruff-Light Trail	0	0	0	0	0	0	0	0
Tactual Performance	0	1	1	0	0	0	1.0	1.0
Choice Reaction Time	0	0	0	0	1	0	0	0
Simple Reaction Time	0	0	0	0	0	0	0	0
Vigilance	0	0	0	0	1	0	0	0
Totals	**0**	**5**	**9**	**12**	**11**	**7**	**0.18**	**0.56**
Memory								
WMS General	0	0	0	0	0	2	0	0
WMS Verbal	0	0	0	0	0	2	0	0
WMS Visual	0	0	2	2	1	0	0	1.0
WMS Delayed Recall	0	0	1	0	0	1	0	.5
WMS Memory Quotient	0	1	0	0	0	0	1.0	0
WMS Logical Memory	0	0	2	3	2	0	0	1.0
WMS Paired Associates	0	0	1	0	1	0	0	1.0

Rivermead Beh. Mem. Test	0	0	1	0	0	0	0
Everyday Memory Quest.	0	0	1	0	0	0	0
Calif. Verb. Learn. Test	0	1	0	1	1	0	1.0
Rey Complex Figure	0	1	1	0	0	0	0
Rey Audit. Verb. Learn.	0	0	1	1	0	0	0
Block Span Learning	0	0	1	0	0	0	0
Benton Vis. Memory Test	0	0	1	0	0	0	0
Taylor Complex Figure	0	1	1	1	0	0	1.0
Buschke Select. Remind.	0	0	0	1	0	0	0
Recalling Sentences	1	0	0	0	0	1.0	0
Totals	**1**	**8**	**12**	**7**	**6**	**0.10**	**0.57**

Verbal and language

WAIS-R Information	0	0	0	0	1	0	0
WAIS-R Vocabulary	0	1	0	1	0	0	1.0
Language Competence	1	0	0	0	2	1.0	0
Word Fluency	0	0	0	1	1	0	0
Mill Hill Vocabulary	0	0	0	0	1	0	0
Token Test	0	0	0	0	0	0	0
Totals	**1**	**0**	**1**	**2**	**5**	**0.33**	**0.17**

Construction

Parquetry Block Design	1	0	0	0	0	1.0	0
WAIS-R Block Design	2	1	0	0	1	0.67	1.0
Object Assembly	0	0	0	1	1	0	0
Rey Complex Figure Copy	0	1	0	0	0	0	1.0
Totals	**2**	**2**	**1**	**1**	**1**	**0.60**	**0.67**

Concept Formation and Reasoning

WAIS-R Similarities	0	0	0	0	1	0	0
WAIS-R Picture Arrangem.	0	1	0	1	0	0	1.0
WAIS-R Picture Complet.	0	0	0	0	1	1.0	0
WAIS-R Arithmetic	1	1	0	0	1	1.0	1.0
Making Inferences	0	0	0	0	0	0	0

Continued

Table 24.1 Summary of results of intermediate measures of cognitive function (please see text for explanation)—cont'd

Cognitive domain and associated tests	Number of tests found to have a positive effect or association			Number of tests done without a positive effect or association			Proportion of positive effects found	
	RCTs (a)	Comparative studies (b)	Correlational studies (c)	RCTs (d)	Comparative studies (e)	Correlational studies (f)	RCTs and comparative $\frac{a+b}{a+b+d+e}$	Correlation Studies $\frac{c}{c+f}$
Raven's Progress. Matrices	0	1	0	0	0	0	1.0	0
Category Test	0	0	1	0	0	2	0	0.33
Wisconsin Card Sorting	0	0	0	0	1	1	0	0
Comprehension	0	0	1	0	1	0	0	1.0
Totals	**0**	**3**	**4**	**1**	**3**	**5**	**0.43**	**0.44**
Executive Functions and Motor Performance								
WISC-R Mazes	0	0	1	0	0	1	0	0.50
Austin Maze	0	0	0	0	1	0	0	0
Hals. Reit. Finger Tapping	0	0	0	0	2	1	0	0
Grooved Pegboard	0	0	1	0	0	0	0	1.0
Grip Strength	0	0	0	0	0	1	0	0
Totals	**0**	**0**	**2**	**0**	**3**	**3**	**0**	**0.44**
Batteries and global tests								
WAIS-R Full Scale I.Q.	0	0	1	0	0	1	0	0.5
WAIS-R Verbal I.Q.	0	0	1	0	2	1	0	0.5
WAIS-R Performance I.Q.	0	1	3	0	1	1	0.33	0.75
Russell Neur Av. Imp. Rat.	0	0	0	1	0	0	0	0
San Diego Neuro. Test Bat.	0	0	0	0	0	0	0	0
Wide Range Achiev. Test	0	0	0	0	0	1	0	0
Hals. Reit. Impair. Index	0	0	1	0	0	0	0	1.0
Totals	**0**	**1**	**6**	**1**	**4**	**4**	**0.17**	**0.60**

Miscellaneous and clinic-specific tests

Adolescent Word Test A	1	0	0	0	0	0	1.0	1.0
Adolescent Word Test B	0	0	0	1	0	0	0	1.0
Adolescent Word Test C	1	0	0	0	0	0	1.0	1.0
Adolescent Word Test D	0	0	0	1	0	0	0	1.0
Picture Vocabulary Test	1	0	0	0	0	0	1.0	1.0
Word Association Subtest	1	0	0	0	0	0	1.0	1.0
Understanding Metaphors	0	0	0	1	0	0	0	1.0
Peabody Picture Vocabulary	0	0	0	1	0	0	0	1.0
Ambiguous Sentences	1	0	0	0	0	0	1.0	1.0
Listening to Paragraphs	0	0	0	1	1	0	0	1.0
Neale Analysis of Reading	0	0	0	0	1	0	0	1.0
Pursuit Rotor	0	0	0	1	0	0	0	1.0
Sentence Assembly	0	0	0	0	0	0	0	1.0
Recreating Sentences	0	0	0	0	0	0	0	1.0
Single Reaction Time	0	0	0	1	0	0	0	1.0
Choice Reaction Time	0	0	0	1	0	0	0	1.0
NYUMT Acq. Rec. Scaled	1	0	0	1	0	0	1.0	1.0
NYUMT Acq. Rec. Stand.	0	0	0	0	0	0	1.0	1.0
Memory Index Scaled	1	0	0	1	0	0	1.0	1.0
Memory Index Standard	1	0	0	0	0	0	1.0	1.0
VerPa	1	0	0	0	0	0	1.0	1.0
VisPa	1	0	0	0	0	0	1.0	1.0
TeachWare Screen. Module	1	0	0	0	0	0	1.0	1.0
Name Writing	0	0	1	0	0	0	0	1.0
Totals	**11**	**0**	**1**	**10**	**2**	**0**	**0.48**	**1.0**
Grand Totals	14	12	33	37	33	31	0.27	0.52

Note: Tests were placed into categories consistent with taxonomy provided by Lezak (1995).

Potential bias in clinic-specific tests

Table 24.1 summarizes the results of the studies that used laboratory tests of cognition to measure treatment effects. Tests are organized within six cognitive domains, as defined by Lezak (1995), as well as a category for test batteries, and one for miscellaneous tests and those developed by a clinic for the purpose of program evaluation (clinic-specific tests). Note that the category with the highest proportion of positive effects is clinic-specific tests, suggesting that a study conducted in a practice setting that has generated a unique protocol for program evaluation is more likely to show a positive result of its treatment.

Duration of intervention

Many of the interventions in the published studies provide minimal treatment hours that do not accurately reflect the years of work usually involved in the rehabilitation of moderate to severe brain injury.

Spontaneous recovery and stimulation

Either through insufficient follow-up time, or by use of comparison groups with major baseline differences from treatment groups, the effect of spontaneous recovery is not clearly distinguished in these studies. In general, the studies in this review that did not show an effect of the treatment compared one form of cognitive rehabilitation with another form – that is, compared two treatments – rather than comparing a group that received a treatment with a group that received nothing. Statistically significant treatment effects were not observed when one kind of remediation was compared with another, *given equal levels of stimulation for both groups*. The contributions to the recovery process of spontaneous recovery, general stimulation, and cognitive rehabilitation must be tested with strong research designs capable of distinguishing the effects.

Review update – 1998 to 2002

Method

We conducted an electronic search of MEDLINE, PsychINFO, CINAHL, and the Cochrane Controlled Trials Register to capture literature from 1998 to 2002[1]. We sought RCTs, non-randomized comparative trials, and systematic reviews. Publications in which samples included non-trauma brain injury and did not distinguish data for those patients from data for patients with TBI were excluded. Maintaining the exclusion criteria from the original review, we also did not include in the update (1) observational studies, and (2) studies in which the comparison group consisted of non-injured people.

Of 1,904 abstracts, and 24 additional references provided by peers, nine publications met the inclusion criteria and were abstracted for evidence, as follows:

- Seven randomized controlled trials: three that included follow-up evaluations (Fasotti *et al.* 2000; McMillan *et al.* 2002; Salazar *et al.* 2000), and four that did not include follow-up evaluations (Dirette and Hinojosa 1999; Eakman and Nelson 2001; Levine *et al.* 2000; Wilson *et al.* 2001).
- Two comparative studies (Grealy *et al.* 1999; Parente and Stapleton 1999).

---

[1]Electronic search did not include the entire publication year of 2002.

Summary of results

The following summarizes results from the RCTs. Refer to Evidence Table 24.3 for information regarding the comparative studies.

Randomized trials with post-treatment follow-up

Three RCTs with post-treatment follow-up evaluations (Fasotti *et al.* 2000; McMillan *et al.* 2002; Salazar *et al.* 2000) compared forms of cognitive rehabilitation with alternative methods or no-treatment control groups (see Evidence Table 24.1). One targeted speed of information processing with time pressure management, one targeted attention with a training embedded in relaxation exercises, and a third targeted overall function and return to work with comprehensive, multidisciplinary, in-hospital rehabilitation. Treatment time varied from two hours total, to months of daily rehabilitation. Follow-up ranged from 6 to 12 months. As can be seen in Evidence Table 24.1, studies varied in populations, sample size, chronicity, severity, and patient characteristics. Of 252 participants in these studies, 116 received the intervention, 88 an alternative intervention, and 48 were no-treatment controls. Outcome measures included batteries of neuropsychological tests, reproduction or task execution scores, and return to work. Treatment effects were observed in two of the studies (Fasotti *et al.* 2000; McMillan *et al.* 2002). There were no treatment effects observed for the entire sample in the trial that tested the effect of inpatient rehabilitation versus home-based rehabilitation on return to work (Salazar *et al.* 2000). However, a subgroup analysis of the more severely injured patients showed a significant effect of the inpatient program compared to the home-based program.

In one of these trials (Fasotti *et al.* 2000), although treatment group patients were observed to incorporate more of their training strategies into the process of performing their tasks, *they did not actually perform better* on the tasks than the comparison group. Treatment time was minimal, and the comparison group was provided equal treatment time with concentration training, suggesting that a general stimulation effect was present in both conditions. In a second trial providing about four hours of treatment time (McMillan *et al.* 2002), the treatment group (attention training) and second intervention group (physical exercise) scored significantly higher than no-intervention controls on only one of 11 outcome measures: self-reported cognitive failures. There were insufficient data to calculate the magnitude of effect in these publications. As with the studies in the original review, little can be concluded about the effectiveness of these interventions without applying them for longer periods of time and testing their effect in everyday circumstances.

Salazar *et al.* (2000) found no difference in outcomes between comprehensive inpatient rehabilitation and family-provided care. In this case, the control condition is potentially an especially powerful intervention. The patients were returned to their homes rather than detained in a hospital. Family caregivers were given training and regular, personalized follow-up. Recent innovative rehabilitation programs are being designed and tested that capitalize on the potential power of being cared for by the family (Braga in press; Sohlberg *et al.* 1998; Ylvisaker and Feeny 1998). Thus, the lack of difference in outcomes may not reflect a lack of effectiveness for the targeted rehabilitation, but may simply emphasize that there is more than one 'ideal' way to care for patients with TBI.

The patients in this sample had relatively short mean length of coma, implying they are not representative of TBI patients in general. In addition, both groups had very high recovery rates. Either both interventions were extremely effective, or the base rate of recovery was so high that it put a floor under the failure rate for the entire study, making the outcomes equal as a result of the artifact of a uniform high recovery for all patients.

For the sub-group analysis, the sample was categorized for severity based on the length of unconsciousness (>1 hour or <1 hour). Of the 75 patients unconscious for more than 1 hour, 28 of 35 in the

Evidence Table 24.1 Randomized controlled trials of cognitive rehabilitation for traumatic brain injury – with follow-up evaluation

Source	Target deficit	Treatment	Setting/population	Sample	Chronicity	Severity measures
Fasotti 2000	Speed of information processing	Time pressure management (TPM)	Patients admitted to rehabilitation center of Hoensbroek (The Netherlands)	N = 22 (15 male) Severe closed head injury Mean PTA for treatment and control groups = 64 days	At least 3 months Mean for treatment group = 9.8 months, control group = 8.3 months	Russell's criteria, 1971
McMillan 2002	Attention	Attentional control training (ACT)	Patients recruited from neurosurgical unit at Atkinson Morley's Hospital and from St. George's Hospital, London	N = 110 (of original sample of 130, 71% male) Median GCS, Mean PTA days = 9, 36 (ACT group), 10, 21 (PE group), 9, 30 (control group)	Between 3 months and 1 year	Glasgow Coma Scale and PTA
Salazar 2000	Overall function to enable return to work	Comprehensive cognitive rehabilitation	273 consecutive admissions to Walter Reed Army Medical Center from January, 1992 to February, 1997	N = 120 (113 male) All severe.	Mean for hospital group = 38 days, home group = 39 days.	Axonal shear, cerebral contusions, PTA, and unconsciousness.

Evidence Table 24.1 Randomized controlled trials of cognitive rehabilitation for traumatic brain injury – with follow-up evaluation—cont'd

Source	Randomization/concealment	Blinding	Exclusions/attrition	Baseline differences between groups
Fasotti 2000	Method/concealment not specified. Separate distribution of 16 patients with chronicity > 6 months and 6 with chronicity 3 to 6 months.	Pre, post, and 6 month follow-up evaluations performed by person blind to group allocation	Recruited patients with evidence of slow speed of information processing, WAIS IQ > 75, who explicitly expressed interest in study. Exclusions: severe intellectual, aphasic, agnostic, or personality disorders.	None on demographics or neurological variables.
McMillan 2002	Method/concealment not specified.	Assessments conducted by person blind to group allocation	Recruited patients presenting attention problems on neuropsychological testing or who reported problems; fully oriented × 3; living at home; aware of cognitive problems. Exclusions: previous TBI or neurological disease, history of drug or alcohol abuse, significant language problems. Of 145 patients recruited, 130 completed treatment, and 110 had 1 year follow-up. Total attrition = 24%	None between group who dropped from study and group who remained on demographics and pre-treatment measures. Treatment groups scored significantly higher than controls on Cognitive Failures Questionnaire at pre-treatment.
Salazar 2000	Blocked randomization performed using variable-sized blocks. Randomization for first 40 subjects weighted at 2 to 1 in favor of the in-hospital group.	Not reported	Inclusion criteria: Adm. GCS < 13, or PTA > 24 hours, or positive image. Injury within 3 months of randomization. Minimum Rancho Level 7. Active duty military member. Home setting with at least 1 adult. Independent ambulation. No prior severe TBI or other disability. Of 167 eligible, 47 refused, and 7 withdrew. Total attrition = 32%.	None between group who refused and 120 who were randomized on demographics, injury severity, and clinical status at study entry. None between groups on demographics, age, sex, military rank, education, race, type and severity of injury, and if alcohol-related. Significantly fewer MVAs, more assaults, and fewer patients unconscious for > 1 hour for in-hospital group.

Continued

Evidence Table 24.1 Randomized controlled trials of cognitive rehabilitation for traumatic brain injury – with follow-up evaluation—cont'd

Source	Duration of intervention	Follow-up interval	Group allocation	Intervention/treatment group	Comparison group/2nd treatment group
Fasotti 2000	2 – 3 weeks maximum 3 sessions per week 1 hour per session possible range of 2 to 9 hours	6 months	n = 12 experimental group n = 10 control group	Presentation of nine videotaped short stories of two types: Story – topics likely to be encountered in daily life. Computer – use of computer programs. Time pressure management provided in 3 stages: awareness of errors and deficits, acceptance and acquisition of TPM strategy. TPM training.	Concentration training of verbal suggestions, 2 to 5 hours per week for 3 to 4 weeks.
McMillan 2002	Five 45 minute sessions over 4 weeks 3 hours 45 minutes total	1 year	n = 37 ACT group n = 35 PE group n = 38 control group	ACT – Attentional training embedded in relaxation training – patient learns to control attention by extended periods of breathing concentration.	PE – Physical exercise and audio-tapes Control – no intervention
Salazar 2000	Varied among patients	1 year	n = 67 hospital group n = 53 home group	In-Hospital Rehabilitation: Interdisciplinary cognitive rehabilitation, combined group and individual therapies, modeled after Prigatano milieu-oriented approach.	Home Rehabilitation: TBI education, individual counseling from psychiatric nurse. Provided educational materials and strategies. Trained in home exercises. Weekly 30-minute telephone calls from nurse.

Evidence Table 24.1 Randomized controlled trials of cognitive rehabilitation for traumatic brain injury – with follow-up evaluation—cont'd

Source	Measures	Analysis	Results
Fasotti 2000	Story task: Patient asked what he/she remembered – reproduction score (calculated by dividing reproduced items by 41 [total possible] and multiplying by 100). Computer task: Number of steps (maximum 41) reached in execution of computer task. Behavioral observations: 1 point each for five preventive steps used by patient.	Multivariate repeated measures analysis of variance	Story and Computer Task Performance: No significant group differences. Behavioral observations: Treatment group scores significantly higher than control on number of preventive steps taken to perform computer task. Treatment group scores significantly higher than control on number of time pressure managing steps for story and computer tasks at post-test, and on computer tasks at 6 month follow-up. Insufficient data to calculate magnitude of effect.
McMillan 2002	Test of Everyday Attention, Adult Memory and Information Processing Battery, Paced Auditory Serial Addition Test, Trail Making Test, Sunderland Memory Questionnaire, Cognitive Failures Questionnaire, Hospital Anxiety and Depression Questionnaire, General health Questionnaire, Rivermead Post-Concussional Symptoms Symptoms Questionnaire, postal survey at 6 months.	Analysis of variance Analysis of covariance (pre-training scores and reported practice time as covariates)	ACT group and PE group had significantly greater decrease in self-reported cognitive failures than control group. Insufficient data to calculate magnitude of effect.
Salazar 2000	Primary outcome measure: return to work and fitness for military duty at 1 year post-treatment. Multidisciplinary Tests and additional psychosocial outcomes, [cognitive, psychiatric, and neurological outcomes and quality of life] 8 weeks after randomization, and at 6, 12, and 24 months.	Fisher Exact t-tests 95% confidence interval Intent-to-treat	No significant differences in return to work (90% hospital group, 94% home group), fitness for active duty, quality of life, verbal and visual memory or attention, or general measures of cognitive or psychiatric function. For sub-group analysis of patients unconscious > a hour, number needed to treat calculated from proportions that returned to work in both groups = 4.5.

Evidence Table 24.2 Randomized controlled trials of cognitive rehabilitation for traumatic brain injury – no follow-up evaluation

Source	Target deficit	Treatment	Setting/population	Sample	Chronicity	Severity measures
Dirette 1999	Visual processing	Computer-aided Internal compensatory strategies	Adult volunteers Regular attendees of cognitive program New York University	N = 30 (22 male) Convenience sample avg. age 38 years Mild, moderate, and severe	2 to 12 months, avg. 5 months	Length of coma, CT scan, and GCS
Eakman 2001	Memory	Hands-on occupational therapy	Nine rehabilitation centers	N = 30 (all male) avg. age 29.6 years Mean Rancho = 7.2 Mean Weschler summed score = 25.1	avg. 53.5 months	Rancho and Weschler Memory Scale
Levine 2000	Disorganized behavior	Goal management training (GMT)	94 consecutive admissions to major trauma center	N = 30 (14 male) n = 24 GOS Good Recovery n = 6 GOS Moderate Recovery	3 to 4 years	GCS and PTA
Wilson 2001*	Memory for everyday tasks	Individualized computerized paging system	Referrals from clinical psychologists, occupational therapists, speech and language pathologists, psychiatrists, and patient organizations	N = 63	6 months to 32 years **	Not specified

Evidence Table 24.2 Randomized controlled trials of cognitive rehabilitation for traumatic brain injury – no follow-up evaluation—cont'd

Source	Randomization/concealment	Blinding	Exclusions/attrition	Baseline differences between groups	Duration of intervention
Dirette 1999	Matched on severity, gender, age, and chronicity, then randomized. Method/concealment not specified.	Data collectors blind to subjects' group allocation	Screened for no deficits in basic visual system, intact motor skills	None reported	6 weeks 1 hour per week First and last week testing only 4 intervention hours total
Eakman 2001	Method/concealment not specified.	Research assistant performing scoring blind to group allocation	Screened for ability to follow simple instructions, motor function, 30 minute attention	None on age, chronicity, Rancho, and baseline Weschler Memory Scales.	One session
Levine 2000	Method/concealment not specified.	Not specified	Exclusions: serious medical illness, death, psychiatric illness, substance abuse, and refusal. No focal neurological syndromes; no linguistic or amnestic disorders. Post-exclusion attrition not specified. Total loss = 68%	None on severity, age, and education. GMT group significantly slower than MST on Stroop interference procedure.	One 1 hour session
Wilson 2001	Method/concealment not specified. Randomization restricted; some patients not randomly assigned due to schedule or inpatient status (9 from entire sample; number of those that were in the TBI sample not specified).	Not specified	For the entire sample (TBI and other etiologies), 32.5% attrition.	None on demographics, neuropsychological tests, average number of messages sent per day. No difference between groups in task achievement at baseline.	7 weeks Paging system used throughout the day

Continued

Evidence Table 24.2 Randomized controlled trials of cognitive rehabilitation for traumatic brain injury – no follow-up evaluation—cont'd

Source	Follow-up interval	Group allocation	Intervention/treatment group	Comparison group/2nd treatment group
Dirette 1999	Post-test 1 week after final intervention session	5 subjects each in 6 conditions: experimental/ control by mild, moderate, and severe	Computer-aided instruction in 3 internal compensatory strategies: verbalizing, chunking, and pacing.	Four 45-minute weekly sessions Remedial computer activities
Eakman 2001	Immediate – no follow-up	15 per group	Training in meatball preparation. 10-step note card instructions, each followed by hands-on (HO) task manipulation.	Verbal instruction only (VO). Presentation of note-card instructions.
Levine 2000	Immediate – no follow-up	15 per group	Goal Management Training (GMT) Verbal definitions of goal management, concrete examples, illustrative activities. Workbook and paper/pencil exercises. Final activity (setting up an answering machine) partitioned into sub-goals and performed by subject.	Motor Skills Training (MST). Training in reading and tracing mirror-reversed text and designs.
Wilson 2001	None	Not reported for subset of patients with TBI	Computer paging system sends reminders individualized according to each patient's needs.	No intervention

Evidence Table 24.2 Randomized controlled trials of cognitive rehabilitation for traumatic brain injury – no follow-up evaluation—cont'd

Source	Measures	Analysis	Results
Dirette 1999	*Pre/Post Measures*: Speed and accuracy on two data entry tasks (Lotus and address typing) and a computerized reading program *Weekly visual processing measures*: PASAT and 'Matching Accuracy Test' segments of The Brain Game program	Repeated measures ANOVAs	No significant difference between groups; no main effects or interactions among 3 severity levels.
Eakman 2001	Verbal report of 10 steps in meatball preparation. Best total score = 38.	Mann-Whitney U test; one-tailed.	HO mean score = 11.8 VO mean score = 2.3 HO median score = 11 VO median score = 2 HO scores significantly higher than VO (p < .001)
Levine 2000	Three clinic-specific measures, administered at pre- (Everyday Tasks 1) and post-training (Everyday Tasks 2): *Proofreading* (time to read instructions, time to complete task, # of errors) *Grouping* (time to read instructions, time to complete task, # of errors) *Room Layout* (time to answer questions, # correct answers) Neuropsychological tests administered at pre-training: Stroop interference procedure, Trails A and B, WAIS-R Digit Symbol subtest	2 (GMT, MST) × 2 (pre/post-training) mixed-design ANOVAs	Accuracy: *Proofreading*: For GMT, no significant difference between pre- and post-test accuracy. For MST, significantly more errors in post- than pre-test (p < .01). [Authors' interpretation is that post-test task was more difficult than pre-test task, and lack of decline for GMT indicates a treatment effect.] *Grouping*: For MST, no significant difference between pre- and post-test accuracy. For GMT, significantly fewer errors in post- than pre-test (p < .01). *Room Layout*: No significant group differences. Speed: *Proofreading*: GMT took significantly more time to perform task at post- than pre-test. No significant difference in time for MST. [Authors' interpretation is that taking more time indicates increased care and attention.] *Room Layout and Grouping*: No significant group differences.
Wilson 2001	Each patient received reminders for tasks that were individually relevant. Outcome measure was successful task achievement.	Odds ratio Chi square Task achievement measured during last 2 weeks of 7 week intervention period.	*First Phase*: (Group A had pager, Group B did not) Group A task achievement = 71.8%; Group B = 49.05% (Group A significantly better) *Second Phase*: (Group B had pager, Group A did not) Group A task achievement = 67.23%; Group B = 73.62% (Group B significantly better)

*Publication combined data from various brain pathologies. Author provided data on the sub-set with TBI, reported in this table.
**Data from entire sample that combined data from various brain pathologies
There were insufficient data in these trials to calculate the magnitude of the effect, when one was observed.

Evidence Table 24.3 Comparative studies of cognitive rehabilitation for traumatic brain injury

Source	Target deficit	Treatment	Setting/population	Sample	Chronicity	Severity measures
Grealy 1999	Cognitive Function	Virtual Reality Exercise	Brain injury rehabilitation unit in Edinburgh, Scotland	Treatment group – 13 consecutive admissions who met criteria and volunteered (8 males) Control group – 320 previous TBI patients matched for age, severity, and chronicity	Ranged from 1.7 to 178.6 weeks	GCS
Parente 1999	Employment potential	Group Cognitive Skills Training	In- and out-patients of Maryland Rehabilitation Center	Treatment group – 33 patients recruited from referrals to Division of Rehabilitation Services. Control group – 64 patients comparable to treatment group, selected from database of 568 patients with TBI.	Not specified	Not specified

Evidence Table 24.3 Comparative studies of cognitive rehabilitation for traumatic brain injury—cont'd

Source	Allocation Method	Blinding	Exclusions/Attrition	Baseline differences between groups	Duration of intervention
Grealy, 1999	Treatment group patients were consecutive admissions who volunteered and who met criteria. Control group data collected from database of 320 patients admitted to same hospital in previous 2 years. Matched 1 treatment group patient to 25 control group patients on age, severity, and chronicity.	Pre-intervention scores obtained by independent assessor blind to nature of study.	Inclusion criteria: Ambulatory, good sitting balance, no perceptual disabilities preventing monitor viewing. Exclusions: Unable to score on the Digit Span (forward and backward) or Digit Symbol. Unable to carry out simple instructions. Insufficient language skills to be able to express verbal learning.	Not specified	Not specified
Parente, 1999			Prior to referral, patients were screened to determine functional limitations and employment potential. One person dropped out during first year.	Clients in both groups received equal amounts of services other than the intervention. No differences in age, educational level, prior marital status, gender, and prior vocational training.	Ranged from 2 months to one year, average 4 months.

Continued

Evidence Table 24.3 Comparative studies of cognitive rehabilitation for traumatic brain injury—cont'd

Source	Follow-up Interval	Intervention/Treatment Group	Comparison Group/2nd Treatment Group
Grealy, 1999	None	Patient rode an exercise bicycle while viewing a virtual environment. Steered a course or participated in a race. Sessions ranged in number from 13 to 18.	Retrospective chart review. Treatments not specified.
Parente, 1999	1 year	Cognitive skills training (training modules for problem solving, concentration/attention, decision making, remembering names and faces, study skills, functional mnemonics, prosthetic memory devices, social cognition, organizational skills, imagery rehearsal, organization, goal-setting, non-verbal perception, and test-taking strategies), computer training, prosthetic aid training, interviewing skills training. Employs "clients teaching clients".	Retrospective chart review of clients in various training programs during same year.

Evidence Table 24.3 Comparative studies of cognitive rehabilitation for traumatic brain injury—cont'd

Source	Measures	Analysis	Results
Grealy, 1999	*Attention and Information Processing* Digit Symbol Trails A and B *Learning and Memory Functions* Auditory Verbal Learning Visual Learning Logical Memory Complex Figure	Mean scores calculated for each group of 25 control patients. Scores of each treatment group patient expressed in standard deviations from the control mean. Compared each patient's performance relative to control group means before and after intervention. Repeated measures ANOVAs	Significant improvement on Digit Symbol. Significant improvement on Verbal and Visual Learning for trials 1 to 5 and the delayed trial, but not for interrupted trial. No improvement on Logical Memory and Complex Figure.
Parente, 1999	1 year	Method not specified. Statistical comparisons not reported.	*Return to Work*: At 1 year, 13 clients completed group services training. Ten of 13 were working at time of publication (76% employment rate). Employment rate for control group during same time period was 58%. *Job Longetivity*: No comparison with control group. All treatment group clients who became employed were still employed at time of publication. *Performance in Training*: No comparison with control group

inpatient rehabilitation group returned to work (80 per cent) versus 23 of 40 in the home-based reha-bilitation group (58 per cent). To estimate the magnitude of the effect of the inpatient program, we calculated the number needed to treat (NNT = 1/Control Group Proportion – Treatment Group Proportion). For this subgroup, the NNT was 4.5. That is, one patient returned to work for every four to five who were treated by inpatient rehabilitation versus home-based rehabilitation. These findings suggest that inpatient rehabilitation may be more effective than a home-based program for the more severely injured TBI patients.

Randomized trials without post-treatment follow-up

Four RCTs with minimal or no post-treatment follow-up evaluation (Dirette *et al.* 1999; Eakman *et al.* 2001; Levine *et al.* 2000; Wilson *et al.* 2001) compared the effect of computer-aided instruction, hands-on training, practice, and compensatory devices with the effect of alternative methods or no treatment on various measures (see Evidence Table 24.2). They targeted memory, visual processing, and disorganized behavior. In two studies total treatment time was one session, and a third provided four hours of treatment. In the study for which the intervention was a compensatory device (Wilson *et al.* 2001) the intervention, a paging device, was used all day for seven weeks.

When performance on data entry tasks and visual processing measures was compared between patients who received computer aided training for internal compensatory strategies and those who received an equal amount of time in remedial computer activities, no significant differences were observed. At the conclusion of one session of training in meatball preparation, patients who received hands-on instruction performed significantly better than those who received only verbal instruction in reporting the preparation steps. Outcomes were mixed in the study that compared Goal Management Training with Motor Skills Training on tests of speed and accuracy.

Significant treatment effects were observed in the crossover trial that provided a personalized paging system to patients with TBI. During a two-week baseline, Group A (Phase I – pager for first seven weeks) and Group B (Phase II – pager for second seven weeks) had no significant differences in task achievement. When measured during the last two weeks of Phase I, Group A performed significantly better than Group B; when measured during the last two weeks of Phase II, Group B performed significantly better than Group A.

The data provided in these publications did not allow for an estimation of the magnitude of effect, when one was observed.

Limitations and strengths of the research

Key limitations in research design observed in the original review are also seen in the body of litera-ture reviewed for the update. The field still lacks a standardized classification of outcomes, which limits the ability to compare and pool data. It is not surprising that interventions lasting only hours do not produce treatment effects in patients who require years, and sometimes a lifetime, of rehabili-tation. And the question of the effects of stimulation and spontaneous recovery remains unanswered. As in the original review, in the update we observe equal improvement when comparing equal amounts of sophisticated treatment with simple stimulation.

The literature search for the update showed that well-controlled studies are now being performed at a higher rate, especially randomized controlled trials. We also found the first meta-analysis of research on cognitive rehabilitation (Loya 2000). These developments indicate substantial progress in the field since the original evidence report (Chesnut *et al.* 1999).

As discussed, the results of the randomized trial that compared comprehensive inpatient rehabilitation with family-provided care (Salazar *et al.* 2000) generate several new hypotheses for future research. It is possible that one model is more effective for severe TBI patients while the other is for milder injuries.

The development of the observational study about compensatory devices from the original review (Wilson *et al.* 1997) into a randomized trial (Wilson *et al.* 2001) is clear progress, and provides important information to providers, patients, and family, given the significant treatment effect. At this time, the strongest evidence from the scientific literature for the positive influence of cognitive rehabilitation on important health outcomes is demonstrated in the application of compensatory cognitive devices and strategies.

25 Outcome of cognitive rehabilitation in clinical stroke services

Nadina Lincoln

Abstract

Cognitive rehabilitation can be effective for people with stroke. The aim of this chapter is to evaluate the evidence for the effectiveness of cognitive rehabilitation in the context of different clinical services and resources.

Introduction

The aim of this chapter is to bring together some of the separate components of cognitive rehabilitation for people with stroke described in previous chapters and to highlight issues of particular relevance to people with stroke. Stroke is a common problem affecting 1.5–2 people per 1,000 per year. An average hospital in the UK will admit 300–500 stroke patients a year. These people tend to have multiple pathologies and the stroke results in both physical and cognitive impairments. Thus any rehabilitation strategy likely to have an impact on clinical services will need to be relevant for elderly people with multiple problems. Patients mainly have unilateral hemisphere lesions which lead typically to problems with language, visuospatial abilities, unilateral inattention and apraxia. The main focus of cognitive rehabilitation after stroke is on these cognitive domains. Patients also have problems with attention, memory, executive abilities and visual agnosia (Tatemichi *et al.* 1994; Desmond *et al.* 1996).

The emphasis of this review will be on the effectiveness of the cognitive rehabilitation services provided. It is clear from previous contributors that there are examples of effective interventions for patients with cognitive deficits arising due to stroke. Cognitive rehabilitation can be effective with individual stroke patients (Robertson *et al.* 1998; Wilson 1999; Riddoch and Humphries 1994; Coltheart, Brunsdon and Nickels, Chapter 2 this volume). However the question is whether the clinical services provided for stroke patients with cognitive impairment improve outcome in the majority of people with that cognitive impairment. An important consideration for cognitive rehabilitation practice is whether the interventions shown to be effective in single case experimental design studies or randomised trials, as conducted by researchers with well-controlled studies in highly selected participants, are equally effective when applied as part of a complex rehabilitation programme with a heterogeneous group of participants.

This is an important question. We know that cognitive problems can affect the time patients spend in rehabilitation, their level of independence in activities of daily living and whether they are discharged home or to residential accommodation (Mercier *et al.* 2001; Heruti *et al.* 2002; Patel *et al.* 2002; Paolucci *et al.* 2001).

The assumption is that if cognitive impairment can be reduced then the functional outcome may be improved. While this seems self-evident it may not be the case. The severity of the cognitive impairments may simply reflect the size or site of the lesion, or they may be simply markers of severity and reducing the marker will not substantially affect the outcome. Thus it is important that the effectiveness of cognitive rehabilitation is assessed on both measures of cognitive impairment and of their effect on functional abilities in daily life.

If cognitive rehabilitation does improve outcome this will have important implications for the development of clinical services. Cognitive impairments affect many people with stroke. Aphasia affects about 30 per cent (Wade *et al.* 1986, Pedersen *et al.* 1995). Estimates of visuospatial impairment are more variable but are probably of the order of 30 per cent (Bowen *et al.* 1999). Apraxia in a mild form is probably very common (Sunderland *et al.* 1999) though whether this is of clinical relevance has not been established. More marked apraxia may occur in a few. Similarly estimates of memory impairment are high (Stewart *et al.* 1996, Tinson and Lincoln 1987) though the impact of these is also uncertain.

It has been recognised that cognitive impairment should be assessed early after stroke (Royal College of Physicians 2002). This has led to a wide range of screening measures. While the Mini Mental State Examination (MMSE) is widely used in clinical practice, its limitations have been recognised (Grace *et al.* 1995). Other more specific measures have been put forward, such as the Frenchay Aphasia Screening Test and Sheffield Screening Test for Acquired Language Disorders (Al-Khawaja *et al.* 1996) for aphasia, Rey figure (Lincoln *et al.* 1998) and Ravens Coloured Progressive Matrices (Blake *et al.* 2002) for visuospatial problems, star cancellation (Marsh and Kersel 1993) for unilateral inattention and bean spooning for apraxia (Sunderland *et al.* 1999). The Middlesex Elderly Assessment of Mental State (MEAMS) (Golding 1989) is also used clinically but has limited sensitivity after stroke (Cartoni and Lincoln in press). However, the limitation of such routine screening is that it may not lead directly to a cognitive rehabilitation programme.

It is also evident that without routine screening many cognitive problems will be missed. Ruchinskas (2002) obtained ratings from 20 physiotherapists and 8 occupational therapists on the presence of cognitive impairment in 102 elderly patients admitted to hospital. There was low correspondence between the ratings of therapists and cognitive impairment as assessed on the MMSE. Thus therapists missed many cognitive problems. It is also possible that some patients had cognitive impairments not detected by the MMSE, and these also would have been missed. Cognitive rehabilitation will not be effective if cognitive impairments are not detected.

There may also be some benefits from simply providing a cognitive assessment on its own. McKinney *et al.* (2002) evaluated the effect of a cognitive screening assessment for stroke patients admitted to hospital. Patients were randomly allocated either to receive routine care, which essentially comprised no cognitive assessment or cognitive rehabilitation, or an assessment group, who received a brief cognitive assessment. Information from this assessment was summarised in written form and also conveyed verbally to therapists, nurses, patients and carers. Although there were no significant differences in outcome between the groups on measures of independence in activities of daily living (Barthel, EADL), mood (GHQ28 for both patient and carer) or satisfaction, there was a trend to reduced carer strain (p <0.06) in the cognitive assessment group. Results are shown in Figure 25.1. The limitations of this study are that there was no formal intervention for the cognitive problems once they had been identified. The psychologists were working across a variety of sites and therefore had little opportunity for educating staff about the impairments identified. Wade (2002) pointed out that as they were not working in established multidisciplinary teams their effectiveness may have been reduced, and suggested that evaluating this component of a service in isolation may have reduced the chances of identifying an effective intervention. Thus, although these gains were probably minimal in the context of a comprehensive rehabilitation programme, they do suggest some benefit of even a minimal assessment process.

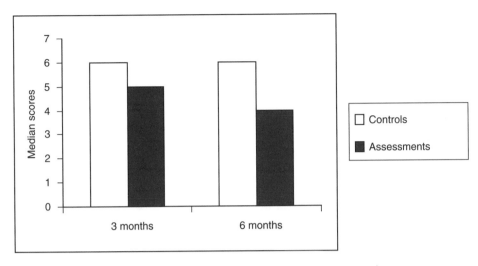

Figure 25.1 Effect of cognitive assessment on carer strain (McKinney *et al.* 2002).

In clinical practice in the UK much of the intervention for cognitive problems takes the form of advice to therapists and nurses as to the best way to deliver their own intervention, according to the nature of the problems identified. Thus physiotherapists are encouraged to use demonstration for patients with language problems and verbal instruction for those with visuospatial problems. Specific strategies may also be suggested on the basis of cognitive impairments, for example, patients with apraxia may have significant difficulty complying with physiotherapists' instructions to perform specific exercises. They may perform far better if given functional activities to perform. A major component of the treatment of unilateral inattention may be the prompts given by nursing staff and therapists to scan the visual field and to adopt systematic search strategies. There has been little formal evaluation of the effectiveness of such advice. Lincoln *et al.* (1997) reported the effects of a stroke rehabilitation unit on cognitive outcomes. Patients were randomly allocated to receive rehabilitation on a specialist stroke rehabilitation unit or on conventional medical and health care of the elderly wards. As part of the outcome evaluation they were assessed on the Rey figure copy 3, 6 and 12 months after the stroke. The therapists and nurses routinely encouraged strategies to compensate for neglect (Edmans *et al.* 2001) as part of their rehabilitation programme. There were significant differences on the Rey figure copy between stroke unit patients and those receiving rehabilitation on general medical and health care of the elderly wards, suggesting that rehabilitation on a stroke unit may have reduced cognitive impairment.

More specific investigations of the relation between cognitive abilities and functional performance may also indicate strategies that can be applied by all members of the rehabilitation team. Walker *et al.* (2004) examined in detail the relation between cognitive impairment and dressing ability, as assessed by video analysis of patients putting on a polo shirt. They found that patients with right hemisphere lesions tended to fail to select the correct sleeve and failed to cover the paretic shoulder, whereas those with left hemisphere lesions dressed the non-paretic arm first and showed disorganised dressing strategies. However, although it was likely that the deficits observed were due to the cognitive impairments, neglect and apraxia, the correspondence with tests of these abilities (line cancellation and Kimura box) was only moderate. Single case experimental design studies are in progress to ascertain whether interventions targeted at the specific components of the dressing sequence in relation to the specific cognitive impairments can improve patients' ability to learn to dress. These specific strategies are not currently used. A survey by Walker *et al.* (2003) of techniques used by occupational therapists to teach dressing skills found that occupational therapists did not report using different strategies to take account of cognitive impairments.

Most evaluations that indicate that cognitive rehabilitation can be effective after stroke have used single case experimental design studies to evaluate effectiveness. This has limitations in terms of evaluating the specific input of cognitive rehabilitation services. The patients treated may not be representative of the majority of stroke patients; they tend to be younger and have fewer co-morbid problems. Intensive therapy for aphasia can be effective (see Basso, Chapter 16, this volume). Group treatment for perceptual problems can benefit individuals (Towle et al. 1990), but examination of those who failed to complete treatment or for whom it was ineffective indicates that while a few may benefit, many may not. Conflicting evidence exists for the effectiveness of the same procedure in different individuals. For example Prada and Tallis (1995) found sensory stimulation to reduce neglect but Yates et al. (2000) did not. This suggests that selection criteria need to be well defined in advance, so that it would be possible to apply them to a clinical group. Many of the successful interventions reported in the literature are on individual cases with no indication of how that individual case was selected. Unsuccessful attempts at cognitive rehabilitation are not likely to be submitted for publication.

The evaluation of clinical services generally requires randomised controlled trials. These have the advantage that the inclusion and exclusion criteria are usually well defined in advance, the intervention is standardised in a way that it can be applicable to a wide range of patients, the outcome can be assessed blind to the intervention and the effect of services is applicable to a sufficiently wide range of patients to yield information that is relevant to the organisation of clinical services.

Recent reviews have identified trials of cognitive rehabilitation, many of which are relevant to stroke rehabilitation services. Cicerone et al. (2000) conducted a comprehensive review of cognitive rehabilitation, identifying 655 published articles. The general message from this review was that support exists for the remediation of language and perception impairments after right and left hemisphere stroke. This was based on an appraisal of the methodological quality of the studies reported and consideration of the specification of the intervention. Other reviews (Robey 1998; Holland et al. 1996; Manly 2002; Pierce and Buxbaum 2002) yield similar conclusions, despite variations in the studies that are included.

More formal analyses of controlled clinical trials and randomised controlled trials have been conducted through the Cochrane Collaboration. Four reviews of cognitive rehabilitation in stroke have been published (Majid et al. 2001; Lincoln et al. 2001; Bowen et al. 2002; Greener et al. 1999). The results of meta-analysis are generally consistent with the non-statistical reviews.

Cognitive rehabilitation for attention problems, memory problems and aphasia after stroke have been reviewed and trials with positive outcomes identified. However, formal analysis has been limited by the lack of common outcome measures and insufficient studies. Bowen et al. (2002) conducted a meta-analysis of the treatment of spatial neglect: this included 15 trials with 400 patients. The results indicated that treatment of inattention reduces cognitive impairment, as assessed on measures of cancellation. Results are shown in Figure 25.2. However, there was insufficient evidence to support or refute the effect of treatment on disability or discharge destination. Results are shown in Figure 25.3. The effects of treatment on impairment measures did persist beyond the end of treatment.

The advantage of meta-analysis is that it provides a more general conclusion applicable to clinical services. Several small trials showing no benefit of treatment may be combined together to show the benefits of intervention. However there are also limitations. In these reviews there were generally only a few trials that met the selection criteria. The methodological quality of many of the trials was unsatisfactory. Few used concealed random allocation with blind assessment of outcome. The results are less convincing when only those trials that meet the most stringent methodological criteria, are included. For example Bowen et al. (2002) no longer found a significant effect of intervention when only those trials which were methodologically the most rigorous were included. This may be due to reduced power or it could be due to observer bias in trials with unblended assessment of outcome.

A major problem with conducting the reviews was the lack of consistency of outcome measures used. In the review of treatments for spatial neglect (Bowen et al. 2002) most trials used a cancellation

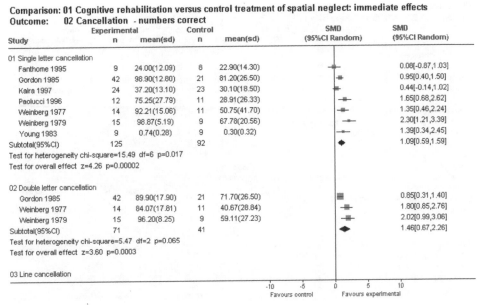

Figure 25.2 Cognitive rehabilitation for spatial neglect following stroke.

measure and this was used in the analysis. Very few trials assessed the effect of the intervention on daily life activities. Thus we remain in the situation of having evidence to indicate that scanning training reduces errors in letter cancellation but no indication of what impact this has on rehabilitation outcome, activity or participation. Can intensive practice of scanning tasks be justified unless we know whether it is of any functional relevance? Cicerone et al. (2000) concluded there was evidence to show that cognitive rehabilitation was effective, but that conclusion was based largely on measures of impairment and the evidence of effects on disability was limited.

Trials of cognitive rehabilitation are complex and expensive and it is likely that effect sizes will be small. It is therefore likely that some form of meta-analysis will be required to ascertain effectiveness for a group of patients. Efforts are therefore needed to standardise outcome measures, both at the level of impairment and of disability. Several appropriate outcome measures exist for impairments after stroke, the goal is to ensure that trials use comparable ones.

Disability tends to be measured using scales of independence in activities of daily living, such as the Barthel Index (Wade and Collin 1988) and Functional Independence Measure (Turner-Stokes et al. 1999). While independence in ADL is a reasonable goal, it may be more appropriate to measure cognitive

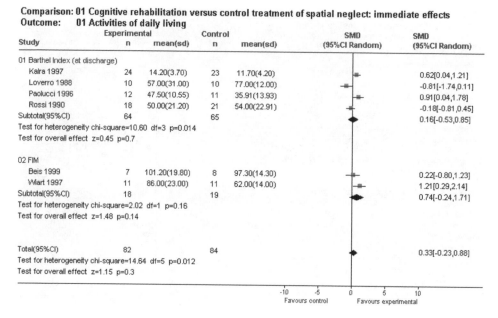

Figure 25.3 Cognitive rehabilitation for spatial neglect following stroke.

activities in daily life, as an outcome of cognitive rehabilitation. Measures of functional communication exist as outcome measures for trials of language rehabilitation (Walker 1992). There have been attempts to assess the effect of unilateral inattention on daily life (Towle and Lincoln 1991; Azouvi *et al.* 1996) but these have rarely been used in trials. Attentional rating scales have been developed (Ponsford and Kinsella 1991) but only used to assess outcome in a few studies. Evidence for the effectiveness of cognitive rehabilitation would be more convincing if the outcome could be demonstrated using these functional measures rather than impairment measures. The reliability of these measures may not be as good as that of ADL measures, and it is recognised that those with severe impairment may be unaware of the extent of their deficits. The scales may require modification to increase their reliability or carers may provide proxy reports in situations where the accuracy of patients' answers is a problem. Measures of cognitive abilities with greater ecological validity than traditional psychometric tests have been designed. For example the behavioural subtests of the Behavioural Inattention Test (Wilson *et al.* 1987) may reflect the effects of interventions for spatial neglect more accurately that impairment measures, such as letter cancellation or line bisection.

One additional issue rarely considered in reviews of treatment effectiveness is the control group against which the intervention group is being compared. We generally assess cognitive rehabilitation in comparison with a 'no intervention' or 'routine care' comparison. However, clinical practice may vary considerably both between centres and between countries. The routine care may be what determines the likelihood of obtaining an effective treatment itself.

The other international issue is the nature of the interventions evaluated. Many reviews indicate consideration of the country in the analysis of results. For example, most of the effective language rehabilitation studies come from the US or Italy; the effective visual inattention studies are mainly from the US, problem-solving and attention studies come from Germany. This could reflect the routine care, but it also raises the question of whether the treatments found to be effective are relevant to other contexts. Despite the evidence for the effectiveness of scanning training, it is rarely provided in clinical practice in the UK. It may be that intensive treatment is needed and most stroke rehabilitation in the UK is community-based. What may be appropriate at home may be different from in hospital. We know there is considerable variation in rehabilitation practice in different centres. For example observational studies have shown that in the UK stroke patients spend 50 per cent of their day sitting doing nothing (Lincoln *et al.* 1996; Tinson 1989), whereas those in Belgium and Switzerland have more active programmes (De Weerdt *et al.* 2000). Specific training programmes may be more effective when little is going on because baseline recovery rates are lower. Alternatively it could be that adding in a specific intervention is only appropriate if there is already an intensive schedule of rehabilitation activities. This will only be ascertained when there are more trials of the specific interventions in a variety of settings and contexts.

The effectiveness of cognitive rehabilitation after stroke therefore remains uncertain. We have evidence that it can be effective with individual highly selected stroke patients (largely from single case experimental design studies). We know it can be effective for certain cognitive impairments (letter cancellation). It can be effective when provided intensively (language rehabilitation for 10 hours a week). It can be effective when provided in certain centres. However, in order to plan services more specific information is needed relevant to the many contexts in which stroke patients are treated.

26 Cognitive rehabilitation in early-stage dementia

Evidence, practice and future directions

Linda Clare

Abstract

Rehabilitation approaches aiming to optimize well-being and manage disability provide an appropriate framework for the care of people with dementia. There is a long-standing tradition of cognition-focused intervention in this area, and recent work has applied the principles of cognitive rehabilitation, primarily to assist people in the early stages of dementias such as Alzheimer's disease. Drawing on theoretical and empirical literature, a set of criteria is presented against which cognition-focused interventions may be evaluated. Three distinct types of cognition-focused intervention for people with early-stage Alzheimer's disease are identified and described: cognitive stimulation, cognitive training, and cognitive rehabilitation. Each of these approaches is considered in relation to the evaluation criteria, and the evidence base for each is critically reviewed. Evidence for effectiveness of cognitive training is very weak, but both cognitive stimulation and cognitive rehabilitation hold promise, with cognitive rehabilitation approximating most closely to the parameters set out in the evaluation criteria. It is argued, therefore, that cognitive rehabilitation addressing individual, personally-relevant goals and assessed in terms of impact on disability offers the most beneficial way forward, and that advice to practitioners should be amended to reflect this finding.

Introduction

Central to the concept of rehabilitation is the aim of helping people to achieve an optimal level of well-being. This is encapsulated in the definition of rehabilitation provided by McLellan (1991), who describes the core activity of rehabilitation as 'enabling people who are disabled by injury or disease to achieve their optimum physical, psychological, social and vocational well-being'. This aim is relevant to people at different life-stages, old as well as young, and to people with different kinds of difficulties, whether acute or chronic, stable or progressive, although specific goals will need to vary according to the particular situation of each individual. In the case of people with progressive impairments, the goals of rehabilitation will need to change over time as the impairments become more extensive, but the concept of optimising well-being remains relevant throughout. Indeed, Cohen and Eisdorfer (1986) proposed that rehabilitation was the most appropriate conceptual framework within which to approach the care of people with dementia. More recently, researchers have started to describe the application of cognitive rehabilitation for people with dementia (Clare and Woods 2001).

Since 'dementia' is a broad category, and the needs of people with different forms of dementia will vary considerably, especially in the mild stages, the present chapter will concentrate on early-stage Alzheimer's disease (AD). The intention is to consider the focus of cognitive rehabilitation in early-stage AD, to present a rationale for its application, to review the evidence currently available, and to highlight future directions for this important area of practice.

The focus of cognitive rehabilitation in early-stage AD

The impact of dementia is most usefully viewed in terms of a disability model. The World Health Organization model of disability (World Health Organization 1980, 1998; see also Chapter 4), summarized in Figure 26.1, distinguishes between organic impairment, limitations on activity (disability) and restrictions on participation (handicap). While activity limitation and participation restriction are related to impairment, they are also influenced by the personal, social and environmental context.

Rehabilitation in dementia care has tended to focus mainly on enabling the person to engage in desired activities and interactions as best they can within his or her own context, in order to enhance well-being for the individual and for his or her supporters or caregivers. Reducing underlying impairment has not usually been a primary goal. Instead, the emphasis has been on tackling 'excess disability' (Reifler and Larson 1990) – activity limitation and participation restriction that is considered out of proportion to the underlying organic impairment. This has also been the case with cognitive rehabilitation in early-stage AD, where the aim has been to work together with the person, and where appropriate with his or her family, to find ways of dealing with the difficulties arising from the cognitive impairments. However, outcome measurement, while clearly needing to target those areas expected to be altered by the intervention, has often been conducted at the level of impairment, using alterations in performance on neuropsychological tests as the criterion by which efficacy is judged.

Recent formulations aimed at understanding dementia support the focus on disability to a large degree, but also point to more far-reaching predictions. Kitwood's dialectical model of dementia

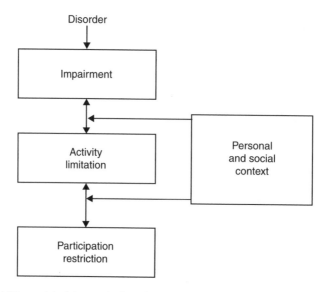

Figure 26.1 Disability model of dementia (based on WHO 1980, 1998).

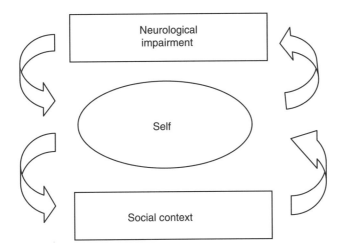

Figure 26.2 Kitwood's dialectical model of dementia (based on Kitwood 1997).

(Kitwood 1997), summarized in Figure 26.2, proposes that the behavioural manifestations of dementia for each individual are the result of a dialectical process in which neurological impairment and social context (social psychology) engage in a continual interplay. In this formulation, social psychology can affect neurological state just as neurological state can affect social psychology. Thus, the effects of a 'malignant social psychology' could result in acceleration of neurological impairment as well as increased activity limitation and participation restriction, while enhancements in care, such as an enriched environment or more rewarding interactions with caregivers, could delay the progression of impairments as well as reducing excess disability (Karlsson *et al.* 1988; Sixsmith *et al.* 1993). This implies the need for a person-centred approach and for careful attention to contextual factors in developing a rehabilitation plan.

With the advent of new pharmacological treatments that can help to delay progression, and the prospect of further developments in this arena, interest in the impact of rehabilitation at the level of impairment is likely to increase. The question arises as to whether cognitive rehabilitation could contribute to delaying or preventing the progression of impairments, and leading on from this, whether it could contribute to preventing or delaying the onset of impairments in those at risk. Further research is needed to delineate the extent of the possibilities that cognitive rehabilitation offers in this respect, and to explore how this approach might be most effectively combined with interventions at the biological level.

Rationale for cognitive rehabilitation in early-stage AD

In considering the needs of the person with early-stage dementia, there is a wide range of factors to take into account; Table 26.1 gives an overview of key elements to consider within a biopsychosocial framework. Of these, cognitive functioning is just one. It is, however, a very important and significant one, since impairment in memory and other cognitive functions is a defining feature of AD, and problems with memory in particular tend to be a major focus of concern in terms of their impact on everyday life during the early stages. Theoretical models and experimental evidence from neuropsychology and cognitive psychology provide a strong rationale for the relevance of interventions directed at memory difficulties in early-stage AD, as well as a number of clear recommendations regarding the kinds of interventions likely to be effective.

Table 26.1 A biopsychosocial approach to intervention in early-stage dementia

Biological aspects	Psychological aspects	Social aspects
Genetic vulnerability and family history	Cognitive functioning	Social networks and communication
Reversible causes of impairment	Emotional reactions and needs	Needs of family and primary caregiver
Brain changes and neurological signs	Life history and past experience	Care practices of professional helpers
Physical, sensory and mobility problems	Personality and coping resources	Social and financial circumstances
Pain	Activities of daily living	Physical environment
Medication effects and interactions	Richness of environment and level of stimulation	Representations of dementia; discrimination and stigma

Taking a systems model of long-term memory (Squire and Knowlton 1995), the evidence indicates that in early-stage AD memory is usually severely impaired (Brandt and Rich 1995) while semantic and procedural memory functioning is relatively spared (Salmon and Fennema-Notestine 1996; Salmon *et al.* 1992). Consideration of the processes involved in acquisition of new memories indicates that the main difficulty for people with early-stage AD arises at the encoding stage, with long-term storage remaining relatively unaffected, as evidenced by normal rates of forgetting (Christensen *et al.* 1998; Kopelman 1992). This suggests that interventions may usefully attempt to build on those subsystems found to be intact, such as procedural memory, while compensatory methods may be employed to reduce demands on impaired aspects of memory. Where acquisition of new long-term memories is required, there needs to be a focus on ensuring successful encoding.

The impairment in episodic memory in early-stage AD relates to damage in the medial temporal lobe areas, and specifically the structures of the hippocampal complex, which are critical for the establishment and consolidation of new episodic memories (Glisky 1998). Semantic memory becomes affected at a later stage when pathology extends beyond the hippocampal complex into the temporal neocortex (Hodges and Patterson 1995), disrupting the ability to form links with existing stored knowledge. It has been suggested that other brain areas may be able to take over this integrative function if appropriate strategies are provided at encoding (Glisky 1998). This, again, suggests that a focus on successful encoding is appropriate where the goal is the acquisition of new long-term memories. Since learning would be expected to be less efficient in this context, the importance of allowing sufficient time and exposure for new learning to occur is highlighted. Clearly, too, any attempts to facilitate acquisition of new long-term memories should be limited to information that is important and personally meaningful to the individual.

Alongside memory, executive function is typically affected at an early stage in the progression of AD (Greene *et al.* 1995; Morris 1996; Perry and Hodges 1999), and difficulties in allocation of attentional resources lead to impairments in dual-task performance (Baddeley *et al.* 1991). This has significant implications for memory functioning, as impaired executive function affects strategic aspects of encoding and retrieval (Glisky 1998), giving rise to problems in effortful search of memory and in linking episodic memories with their source and temporal context. It follows that people with early-stage AD can be expected to have particular difficulty with some aspects of retrieval and also with implementing strategies to help themselves remember (Bäckman 1992), and interventions need to incorporate ways of helping to compensate for this.

This rationale is supported by experimental evidence demonstrating that new learning is possible in early-stage AD. People with AD can change their behaviour in response to altered environmental contingencies (Burgess *et al.* 1992; Camp *et al.* 1993). They can learn or re-learn skills and procedural routines (Salmon *et al.* 1992), and they can learn new verbal information (Little *et al.* 1986). Clearly, improvements in memory functioning can be demonstrated. Bäckman (1992) emphasises, however, that this requires the provision of appropriate cognitive support at both encoding and retrieval. It is not reasonable to expect the person with early-stage AD to learn under the same conditions as someone without AD; extra support and adaptation of the learning environment is crucial.

Experimental and clinical studies provide some guidance as to the kinds of support for learning that are likely to be helpful. These include: the twin guiding principles of effortful processing (Bird and Luszcz 1993) and errorless learning (Clare *et al.* 1999, 2000, 2002, 2003b); enriched encoding through targeting of multiple sensory modalities (Karlsson *et al.* 1989); cueing methods (Glisky *et al.* 1986; Thoene and Glisky 1995) with compatibility of cues at encoding and retrieval (Herlitz and Viitanen 1991) and where possible self-generation of cues (Lipinska *et al.* 1994); spaced retrieval (Camp 1989; Camp *et al.* 2000); and simplified verbal and visual mnemonic strategies (Bäckman *et al.* 1991; Bird and Luszcz 1993; Clare *et al.* 1999; Hill *et al.* 1987; Clare *et al.* 2003b). Bäckman (1992) also notes that there is likely to be a need for ongoing input after the end of an intervention if gains are to be maintained.

Thus, there is a strong rationale for applying cognitive rehabilitation in early-stage AD, and the literature provides clear guidance as regards both the overall approach to be taken and the specific techniques to be adopted. It is possible, therefore, to delineate a set of theoretically- and empirically-derived criteria that should underlie the development of cognition-based interventions in early-stage AD. Within this framework, interventions should:

- Be based on a person-centred plan and take into account the personal, social and environmental context of the individual.
- Incorporate tasks that are directly relevant to everyday life and meaningful to the individual.
- Present tasks in a way that is adapted to the specific needs of people with early-stage AD, and allow sufficient time and opportunity for exposure or practice.
- Have a clearly-defined focus (whether impairment, activity limitation or participation restriction), and ensure that effectiveness is evaluated using outcome measures appropriate to the chosen focus.
- Adopt an approach based on the implications of neuropsychological models outlining impaired and preserved skills in early-stage AD.
- Use techniques of demonstrated value or with a clear rationale based on empirical evidence.
- Include ongoing input to promote maintenance of gains.

The existing literature on cognition-based interventions in early-stage AD will now be considered in relation to these criteria.

Evidence for effectiveness of cognition-based interventions in AD

Reflecting the centrality of cognitive impairments in conceptualisations of dementia, there has been a long-standing tradition of interventions targeting cognitive functioning. Within this literature, three main strands can be discerned: reality orientation or general cognitive stimulation, cognitive training, and cognitive rehabilitation. Each of these will be considered in turn, focusing on definitions, conceptual bases, modes of delivery, and evidence from outcome studies, and will be related to the criteria set out above. Interventions focusing primarily on giving advice and information to caregivers will not be included here.

Reality orientation and general cognitive stimulation

The earliest developments in this field were largely separate from concurrent developments in brain injury rehabilitation, drawing instead on new initiatives in the psychosocial rehabilitation of long-term residents of psychiatric institutions. The groundbreaking adaptation of Reality Orientation (RO) therapy for people with dementia served a valuable purpose in demonstrating for the first time the possibilities for psychological work with people experiencing progressive cognitive impairments. While the aims of RO include the provision of a supportive, accepting atmosphere in which direct confrontation or correction is avoided, there has been a widespread misapplication of the concept with frequent use of a confrontational approach, which has attracted considerable criticism (Woods 2002). Nevertheless, RO remains influential in dementia care today.

RO therapy aims to increase orientation to the here-and-now and to improve cognitive and behavioural functioning through cognition-based activities, social interaction and discussion, combined with the use of cues and prompts to assist remembering (Woods 1996). It is typically offered by means of group sessions, although in residential or day care settings cues and prompts may be generalised throughout the environment and used by staff at any time. The prototypical exemplar would be the presence of a 'reality orientation board' in a dayroom or social area. While RO has most often been used with people who have moderate to advanced dementia in formal care settings (e.g. Spector *et al.* 2003), there are strong similarities with the general cognitive stimulation methods that have been successfully applied in recent years with people who have early-stage AD (Breuil *et al.* 1994), and Woods (2002) has proposed that RO be subsumed under the category of 'cognitive stimulation', since this term seems to more accurately capture the essence of the approach.

Interventions targeting both early- and later-stage AD were included in the most recent Cochrane systematic review of RO (Spector *et al.* 1998). This identified six randomised controlled trials that could be included in a meta-analysis. Results of the meta-analysis indicated that RO could produce significant improvements on measures of cognition, although these were not evident in all included studies, and provided weaker evidence for a positive effect on behaviour. There are a number of difficulties, however, with interpreting the evidence from RO and cognitive stimulation studies (Bird 2000). RO interventions incorporate a number of different elements, and this varies between studies, so it is not possible to establish clearly which are the 'active' ingredients. Often the actual interventions are poorly described, which limits the clinical usefulness of the reports. Furthermore, the finding from one study that a social activity control group, given equal amounts of group time and therapist attention, made equal improvements to the RO group suggests that cognitive stimulation per se may not be the crucial component, yet the majority of studies have not included a control group of this kind.

In terms of criteria for evaluating cognitive approaches, cognitive stimulation or RO presents a number of strengths. It offers the scope to ensure that content is relevant to everyday life, and the usual extension of cues and prompts throughout the setting addresses the issue of generalisation to some degree, although of course this does not apply where cognitive stimulation groups are conducted on an outpatient basis for people with early-stage AD. Presentation of tasks would be expected to take place at an appropriate pace, although it is acknowledged that this might not always be the case in practice. In addition, the need for ongoing input in order to maintain any treatment gains is clearly acknowledged in this literature. However, there are also significant limitations. First, the emphasis on group intervention means that both the overall approach and the specific content are unlikely to be particularly individually-tailored to participants' needs; thus, the method cannot be assumed to be person-centred in concept or application, and the group training format allows for limited consideration of individual context. Indeed, the Cochrane review of RO (Spector *et al.* 1998) advocates the development of more individualised methods. Second, the focus of intervention and its relationship to measures of outcome is not clearly defined. Outcome has primarily been evaluated through measures of impairment in the form of cognitive test scores, although some studies also incorporate measures of psychosocial functioning. Finally, cognitive stimulation and RO lack a strong foundation in theoretical models from neuropsychology and have been limited in the extent to which they employ empirically-validated learning methods. Overall, therefore, cognitive stimulation or reality orientation methods appear to have some value for people with dementia, but they show limitations in relation to several of the key requirements for effective cognition-based interventions.

Cognitive training

Cognitive training (sometimes termed 'cognitive retraining' or 'cognitive remediation') involves guided practice on a range of standard tasks relating to one or more domains of cognitive functioning, such as memory, language or attention. In some cases tasks are offered at varying levels of difficulty to allow some adjustment for individual ability. Tasks may also be personalised to some degree; for example, a standard task involving learning of face–name associations may utilise face–name pairs derived from the individual's network. Cognitive training may be offered in one of a range of possible formats, including group training, one-to-one sessions, training guided by the family carer in the home setting, or computer-delivered training.

Some studies have reported limited effects of cognitive training, calling into question the relevance and usefulness of this approach (e.g. Zarit et al. 1982), while others have reported at least some significant effects. One comprehensive review (Gatz et al. 1998) supported the latter conclusion, arguing that 'memory and cognitive retraining programs based on carefully selected technique are probably efficacious procedures for slowing the decay of skills in demented patients'.

However, a Cochrane systematic review of randomised controlled trials (RCTs) of cognitive training (Clare et al. 2003a) was less positive (Clare 2003; Clare and Woods, 2004). Literature searches identified six RCTs that could be included. Three studies provided training in group or individual therapy sessions (De Vreese et al. 1998; Davis et al. 2001; Koltai et al. 2001), two used daily home practice directed by the carer (Quayhagen et al. 1995, 2000), and one (Heiss et al. 1994) offered computerised cognitive training over a six-month period. Four of the studies (Quayhagen et al. 2000, Quayhagen et al. 1995; De Vreese et al. 1998; Davis et al. 2001) reported some significant effects either on the specific areas targeted or on general measures of cognitive function, although these tended to be very circumscribed. The other studies (Heiss et al. 1994; Koltai et al. 2001) reported no significant benefits of training. Within the Cochrane meta-analysis framework, in which a fixed effects model was applied in calculating weighted mean differences and 95 per cent confidence intervals, the six studies, taken individually, all failed to demonstrate any significant differences between cognitive training and comparison conditions on any outcome measure. As the studies used diverse methods, comparison conditions, and outcome measures, few direct cross-study comparisons could be made. It was possible, however, to explore the impact of training on global measures of dementia severity (three studies), memory test scores (five studies), verbal fluency scores (three studies), self-ratings of depression (two studies), and behaviour ratings (two studies). In no cases did the observed effects reach statistical significance.

These non-significant findings must, of course, be interpreted in the context of methodological limitations (Clare 2003; Clare and Woods, 2004) that may impact on the conclusions. The issues identified included limited statistical power due to small sample sizes, insufficient duration and intensity of intervention, comparison with other active treatments rather than placebo, repetition of neuropsychological tests as outcome measures over short intervals rendering the results liable to practice effects, and selection of outcome measures that reflect impairment rather than disability, and therefore fail to capture some changes that do occur as a result of intervention. In view of the limitations in the existing evidence, it would appear that further rigorous RCTs might provide a more definitive evaluation of the efficacy of cognitive training approaches.

In relation to the criteria adopted here for evaluating cognitive approaches, cognitive training interventions have the advantage that they are typically clearly related to neuropsychological models of impaired and preserved functioning, and they often draw on experimentally-validated techniques, although the kinds of tasks used appear to vary considerably in their relevance to everyday life. Brief interventions in particular may not be sufficiently intensive to produce optimum benefits, but there is often a lack of any ongoing input that could help to maintain treatment gains. Although some tasks can be personalised to a degree, the cognitive training approach is not strongly person-centred, and is likely to allow little room for adjustment to individual needs or for attention to emotional reactions or social issues. There is some attention to context in that caregivers are involved as co-therapists, and in some studies the outcomes for caregivers are also considered. However, there may also be potential difficulties inherent in this, particularly where family relationships are strained or particular skill in dealing with difficult emotional reactions is required, and this clearly requires consideration. Finally, the focus of intervention in cognitive training studies is not always clearly defined, and outcome measures tend to focus on impairment rather than disability. Overall, therefore, the evidence for the effectiveness of cognitive training approaches is weak, and existing applications have significant limitations in respect of a number of key criteria for cognition-based interventions.

Cognitive rehabilitation

Cognitive rehabilitation involves a collaboration between client, family member (where appropriate) and professional aimed at devising and carrying out an individually-planned intervention that addresses negotiated, personally meaningful goals which are directly relevant to specific aspects of cognitive functioning as these impact on everyday life. Such interventions are typically conducted on an individual rather than a group basis, and outcome evaluation primarily reflects performance on the specific goals addressed by the intervention rather than scores on cognitive tests. Extensive literature searches currently yield no RCTs that have adopted this approach for people with AD, so it is only possible to offer a preliminary assessment of efficacy based primarily on studies employing rigorous single-case experimental designs.

With respect to memory functioning in AD, the specific goals of individualised cognitive rehabilitation interventions can be considered in terms of three categories: developing compensatory strategies through the use of memory aids, optimising procedural memory functioning through skills training, and facilitating residual long-term memory performance through provision of appropriate support for learning and recall.

Several studies have demonstrated that people with AD can learn to use a compensatory memory aid for various purposes. For example, Bourgeois (1990, 1991, 1992) used memory wallets as a means of enhancing conversational engagement. Another study (Clare *et al.* 2000) used a calendar and memory board to improve orientation and reduce the need for repetitive questioning of the caregiver. Both sets of studies demonstrated that gains could be maintained over a significant period.

Attempts to optimise procedural memory functioning focus on maintaining or restoring the ability to carry out selected activities of daily living independently. Josephsson *et al.* (1993) developed individualised skills training programmes, using tasks that were part of the person's everyday routine and that the person was strongly motivated to carry out, and achieved improvements for three out of four participants.

Methods such as expanding rehearsal, vanishing cues, semantic elaboration and simple visual mnemonic strategies have been used to facilitate learning or relearning of relevant information (Clare *et al.* 1999, 2000, 2002; Clare *et al.* 2003b). Expanding rehearsal has proved particularly successful in teaching face–name associations, names of everyday objects and memory for object locations, as well as enhancing prospective memory functioning (Abrahams and Camp 1993; Camp 1989, 2000;

McKitrick and Camp 1993). There is some evidence that treatment gains can be maintained for considerable periods (Clare *et al.* 2001), which is especially significant in the context of a progressive disorder.

The use of a single case approach naturally directs attention to individual variability in response to intervention. Within the context of a cognitive rehabilitation approach, researchers have recently begun to investigate what factors may be related to successful outcome. One such factor is awareness of impairments, which has recently been shown in retrospective (Koltai *et al.* 2001) and prospective (Clare *et al.* 2004) studies to be associated with outcome of cognitive rehabilitation, such that people with higher levels of explicit awareness of their memory problems tend to be more successful with regard to learning outcomes, while those who do not express explicit awareness or do so only to a very limited extent are less likely to do well with this approach. Clearly it will be important to develop a better understanding of factors that may be predictive of particular outcomes in order to allow clinicians to select the most appropriate form of intervention for a given individual.

An overview of individualised cognitive rehabilitation interventions shows that they draw on theoretical models from neuropsychology and make use of experimentally-validated methods designed to support learning in people with AD. They have a clear focus on disability, and outcome evaluation reflects this focus by placing the main emphasis on changes in performance in relation to the specific goals of intervention. Studies in this area have also attempted to assess the longer-term effects of intervention. Because these interventions are individually tailored, there is scope for flexible adaptation to individual needs and contexts, and goals and tasks are relevant and meaningful. Such interventions have the scope to form part of a person-centred approach within dementia care. In addition to the work with people who have early-stage AD described here, the methods of individualised cognitive rehabilitation have been adapted and applied for use with people who have more advanced AD living in residential care settings (Bird 2000, 2001), with the aim of enhancing adaptive behaviour. On the basis of this overview, it can be argued that these individualised cognitive rehabilitation interventions should offer the most appropriate way forward. A recent comprehensive review (De Vreese *et al.* 2001) noted that 'the available evidence shows that … memory rehabilitation in mild to moderate AD patients can indeed be clinically effective or pragmatically useful.' However, further evidence is needed regarding the effectiveness of individualised cognitive rehabilitation in early-stage AD.

Cognitive rehabilitation in dementia: the way forward

There is a growing body of evidence to support the value of some forms of cognition-based intervention for people with early-stage AD. To date, practice guidelines have tended to pay little attention to the possibilities offered by cognition-based interventions (e.g. Small *et al.* 1997; Doody *et al.* 2001), but advice to practitioners will need to change in order to reflect the available findings. There is a strong theoretical and empirically-derived rationale for the application of cognitive rehabilitation, and it has been argued here that an approach based on individually designed and individually targeted interventions tackling meaningful and relevant goals and situated within the context of a person-centred approach to care is likely to prove most beneficial. This is likely to apply equally to people with forms of dementia other than AD.

This review of the evidence indicates a number of ways in which the quality and appropriateness of cognitive rehabilitation interventions for people with dementia might be enhanced. A developing understanding of the processes involved in change at both biological and behavioural levels may allow a clearer focus in terms of impairment or disability, along with improved selection of outcome measures, and may in time provide further insights into the possibilities for slowing or preventing progression. Additionally, clarification of the parameters of successful intervention, in terms of intensity, duration, ongoing input to ensure maintenance, and factors that impact on outcome, will assist in developing more appropriate methods and targeting those individuals who are likely to benefit.

The existing evidence provides a valuable basis for the further development of cognitive rehabilitation approaches for people with dementia, although a fully articulated framework remains to be elaborated. It is clear, however, that there are grounds for a modest degree of optimism as regards the possibilities offered by cognitive rehabilitation for people with dementia, and that further research in this area is warranted.

References

Abrahams, J. P. and Camp, C. J. (1993). Maintenance and generalisation of object naming training in anomia associated with degenerative dementia. *Clinical Gerontologist*, **12**, 57–72.

Adam, S. Van der Linden, M. Juillerat, A.-C., and Salmon, E. (2000). The cognitive management of daily life activities in patients with mild to moderate Alzheimer's disease in a day center: a case report. *Neuropsychological Rehabilitation*, **10**, 485–509.

Adams, J. H., Graham, D. I., and Jennet, B. (2000). The neuropathology of the vegetative state after acute brain insult. *Brain*, **123**, 1327–38.

Aftonomos, L. B., Steele, R. D., Appelbaum, J. S., and Harris, V. M. (2001). Relationships between impairment-level assessments and functional-level assessments in aphasia: Findings from LCC treatment programmes. *Aphasiology*, **15**, 951–64.

Albert, M. L., Bachman, D. L., Morgan, A., and Helms-Estabrooks, N. (1988). Pharmacotherapy in aphasia. *Neurology*, **38**, 877–79.

Alderman, N. (1996). Central executive deficit and response to operant conditioning methods. *Neuropsychological Rehabilitation*, **6**, 161–86.

Alderman, N. and Burgess, P. W. (2003). Assessment and rehabilitation of the dysexecutive syndrome. In *Handbook of Neurological Rehabilitation* (eds R. Greenwood, T. M. McMillan, M. P. Barnes and C. D. Ward), 2nd edn. pp. 77–101. Hove: Psychology Press.

Alderman, N. and Knight, C. (1997). The effectiveness of DRL in the management and treatment of severe behaviour disorders following severe brain injury. *Brain Injury*, **11**, 79–101.

Alderman, N., Fry, R. K., and Youngson, H. A. (1995). Improvement of self-monitoring skills, reduction of behaviour disturbance and the dysexecutive syndrome: comparison of response cost and a new programme of self-monitoring training. *Neuropsychological Rehabilitation*, **5**, 193–221.

Alderman, N., Knight, C., and Burgess, P. W. (2003). Ecological validity of a simplified version of the Multiple Errands Test. *Journal of the International Neuropsychological Society*, **9**, 31–44.

Al-Khawaja, I., Wade, D. T., and Collin, C. F. (1996). Bedside screening for aphasia: a comparison of two methods. *Journal of Neurology*, **243**, 201–24.

Allport, D. A. (1985). Distributed memory, modular subsystems and dysphasia. In *Current perspectives in dysphasia* (ed. R. Epstein) pp. 32–60. Edinburgh: Churchill Livingstone.

Allport, D. A. (1987). Selection for action: Some behavioural and neurophysiological considerations of attention and action. In *Perspectives on perception and action* (eds H. Heuer and A. F. Sanders), pp. 395–419. Hillsdale, NJ: Lawrence Erlbaum Associates.

Allport, D. A. (1993). Attention and control: Have we been asking the wrong questions? A critical review of twenty-five years. In *Attention and performance XIV* (eds D. E. Meyer and S. Kornblum), pp. 183–218. Cambridge, MA: MIT Press.

Allport, D. A. and Funnell, E. (1981). Components of the mental lexicon. *Philosophical Transactions of the Royal Society of London*, B **295**, 397–410.

Alzheimer, A. (1907). Ueber eine eigenartige Erkrankung der Hirnrinde. *Allgemeine Zeitschrift für Psychiatrie*, **64**, 146–8.

American Psychological Association (2001). *Publication manual of the American Psychological Association*. Washington, DC: American Psychological Association.

Armstrong, E. (1993). Aphasia rehabilitation: a sociolinguistic perspective. In *Aphasia treatment: World perspectives* (eds A. Holland and M. Forbes). San Diego, CA: Singular Publishing group.

Armstrong, E. (2000). Aphasic discourse analysis: the story so far. *Aphasiology*, **14**, 875–92.

Armstrong, E. (2002). Variation in the discourse of non-brain-damaged speakers on a clinical task. *Aphasiology*, **16**, 647–58.

Asanuma, H., and Keller, A. (1991). Neuronal mechanisms of motor learning in mammals. *Neuroreport*, **2**, 217–24.

Ashley, M. J., Hrych, D. K., and Lehr, R. P. (1990). Cost/benefit analysis for post-acute rehabilitation of the traumatically brain injured patient. *Journal of Insurance Medicine*, **22**, 156–61.

Aten, J., Caligiuri, M. P., and Holland, A. L. (1982). The efficacy of functional communication therapy for chronic aphasic patients. *Journal of Speech and Hearing Disorders*, **47**, 93–6.

Auerbach, S. H., Allard, A., Naeser, M. A., Alexander, M. P., and Albert, M. L. (1982). Pure word deafness: analysis of a case with bilateral lesions and a defect at the prephonemic level. *Brain*, **105**, 271–300.

Axelrod, B. N., Goldman, R. S., Heaton, R. K., Curtiss, G., Thompson, L. L., Chelune, G. J., and Kay, G. G. (1996). Discriminability of the Wisconsin Card Sorting Test using the standardization sample. *Journal of Clinical and Experimental Neuropsychology*, **18**, 338–42.

Azouvi, P., Marchal, F., Samuel, C. *et al.* (1996). Functional consequences and awareness of unilateral neglect: a study of an evaluation scale. *Neuropsychological Rehabilitation*, **6**, 133–50.

Bäckman, L. (1989). Varieties of memory compensation by older adults in episodic remembering. In *Everyday cognition in adulthood and late life* (eds L. W. Poon, D. C. Rubin and B. A. Wilson), pp. 509–44. New York: Cambridge University Press.

Bäckman, L. (1992). Memory training and memory improvement in Alzheimer's disease: rules and exceptions. *Acta Neurologica Scandinavica*, Supplement, **139**, 84–89.

Bäckman, L. and Dixon, R. A. (1992). Psychological compensation: A theoretical framework. *Psychological Bulletin*, **112**, 259–83.

Bäckman, L., Josephsson, S., Herlitz, A., Stigsdotter, A., and Viitanen, M. (1991). The generalisability of training gains in dementia: effects of an imagery-based mnemonic on face-name retention duration. *Psychology and Aging*, **6**, 489–92.

Baddeley, A. (1993). A theory of rehabilitation without a model of learning is a vehicle without an engine: A comment on Caramazza and Hillis. *Neuropsychological Rehabilitation*, **3**, 235–44.

Baddeley, A. D. (1986). *Working memory*. Oxford: Clarendon Press.

Baddeley, A. D. (2000). The episodic buffer: a new component of working memory? *Trends in Cognitive Science*, **4**, 417–23.

Baddeley, A. (2002). Is working memory still working? *European Psychologist*, **7**, 85–97.

Baddeley, A. D. and Della Sala, S. (1998). Working memory and executive control. In *The Prefrontal Cortex: Executive and Cognitive Functions* (eds A. C. Roberts, T. W. Robbins and L. Weiskrantz), pp. 9–21. Oxford: Oxford University Press.

Baddeley, A. D. and Wilson, B. A. (1994). When implicit learning fails: Amnesia and the problem of error elimination. *Neuropsychologia*, **32**, 53–68.

Baddeley, A., Emslie, H., and Nimmo Smith, I. (1994). *Doors and People*. Bury St Edmunds: Thames Valley Test Company.

Baddeley, A., Della Sala, S., Papagno, C., and Spinnler, H. (1997). Dual-task performance in dysexecutive and nondysexecutive patients with a frontal lesion. *Neuropsychology*, **11**, 187–94.

Baddeley, A. D., Lewis, V., Eldridge, M., and Thomson, N. (1984). Attention and retrieval from long-term memory. *Journal of Experimental Psychology: General*, **113**, 518–40.

Baddeley, A. D., Bressi, S., Della Sala, S., Logie, R., and Spinnler, H. (1991). The decline of working memory in Alzheimer's disease. *Brain*, **114**, 2521–42.

Badgaiyan, R. D. (2000). Neuroanatomical organization of perceptual memory: an fMRI study of picture priming. *Human Brain Mapping*, **10**, 197–203.

Bajo, A. and Fleminger, S. (2002). Brain injury rehabilitation: what works for whom and when? *Brain Injury*, **16**, 385–95.

Bartlett, F. and John, E. R. (1973). Equipotentiality quantified: the anatomical distribution of the engram. *Science*, **181**, 764–7.

Basso, A. (1987). Approaches to neuropsychological rehabilitation: language disorders. In *Neuropsychological rehabilitation* (eds M. J. Meier, A. L. Benton and L. Diller), pp. 294–314. London: Churchill Livingstone.

Basso, A. (1992). Prognostic factors in aphasia. *Aphasiology*, **6**, 337–48.

Basso, A. (2003). *Aphasia and its therapy*. New York: Oxford University Press.

Basso, A. and Caporali, A. (2001). Aphasia therapy or the importance of being earnest. *Aphasiology*, **15**, 307–32.

Basso, A. and Marangolo, P. (2000). Cognitive neuropsychological rehabilitation: The emperor's new clothes? *Neuropsychological Rehabilitation*, **10**, 219–29.

Basso, A., Capitani, E., and Vignolo, L. A. (1979). Influence of rehabilitation of language skills in aphasic patients: a controlled study. *Archives of Neurology*, **36**, 190–6.

Basso, A., Faglioni, P., and Vignolo, L. A. (1975) Etude controlée de la rééducation du langage dans l'aphasie: comparaison entre aphasiques traités et non-traités. *Revue Neurologique*, **131**, 607–14.

Batchelor, J., Shores, E. A., Marosszeky, J. E., Sandanam, J., and Lovarini, M. (1988). Cognitive rehabilitation of severely closed-head-injured patients using computer-assisted and noncomputerized treatment techniques. *Journal of Head Trauma Rehabilitation*, **3**, 78–85.

Bates, E. (1976). *Language in Context*. New York: Academic Press.

Beauvois, M. F. (1982). Optic aphasia: A process of interaction between vision and language. *Philosophical Transactions of the Royal Society of London*, B **298**, 35–47.

Bechterew, W. von (1900). Demonstration eines Gehirns mit Zerstörung der vorderen und inneren Theile der Hirnrinde beider Schläfenlappen. *Neurologisches Zentralblatt*, **19**, 990–1.

Beeson, P., Hirsch, F., and Rewega, M. (2002). Successful single-word writing treatment: Experimental analyses of four cases. *Aphasiology*, **16**, 473–92.

Behrmann, M. (1987). The rites of righting writing. *Cognitive Neuropsychology*, **4**, 365–84.

Behrmann, M. and Bub, D. (1992). Surface dyslexia and dysgraphia – dual routes, single lexicon. *Cognitive Neuropsychology*, **9**, 209–51.

Belger, A., Puce, A., Krystal, J. H., Gore, J. C., Goldman-Rakic, P., and McCarthy, G. (1998). Dissociation of mnemonic and perceptual processes during spatial and nonspatial working memory using fMRI. *Human Brain Mapping*, **6**, 14–32.

Bell, M., Bryson, G., Greig, T., Corcoran, C., and Wexler, B. E. (2001). Neurocognitive enhancement therapy with work therapy: effects on neuropsychological test performance. *Archives of General Psychiatry*, **58**, 763–8.

Bell, B. D. and Roper, B. L. (1998). 'Myths of neuropsychology': Another view. *The Clinical Neuropsychologist*, **12**, 237–44.

Benedict, R. H. B., Brandt, J., and Bergey, G. (1993). An attempt at memory retraining in severe amnesia: An experimental single-case study. *Neuropsychological Rehabilitation*, **3**, 37–51.

Benedict, R. H. B., Schretlen, D., Groninger, L., and Brandt, J. (1998). Hopkins Verbal Learning Test – Revised: Normative data and analysis of inter-form and test-retest reliability. *The Clinical Neuropsychologist*, **12**, 43–55.

Benson, K. and Hartz, A. J. (2000). A comparison of observational studies and randomized controlled trials. *New England Journal of Medicine*, **342**, 1878–86.

Benton, A. L. and Hamsher, K. d. S. (1976). *Multilingual aphasia examination*. Iowa City: University of Iowa Press.

Ben-Yishay, Y. (1996). Reflections on the evolution of the therapeutic milieu concept. *Neuropsychological Rehabilitation*, **6**(4), 327–43.

Ben-Yishay, Y. and Daniels-Zide, E. (2000). Examined lives: Outcomes after holistic rehabilitation. *Rehabilitation Psychology*, **45**, 112–29.

Ben-Yishay, Y. and Diller, L. (1983). Cognitive remediation. In *Rehabilitation of the head injured adult* (ed. M Rosenthal). Philadelphia: F. A. Davis.

Ben-Yishay, Y. and Diller, L. (1993). Cognitive remediation in traumatic brain injury: update and issues. *Archives of Physical Medicine and Rehabilitation*, **74**, 204–13.

Berg, I. J., Koning-Haanstra, M., and Deelman, B. G. (1991). Long-term effects of memory rehabilitation. A controlled study. *Neuropsychological Rehabilitation*, **1**, 97–111.

Berndt, R. S., Wayland, S., Rochon, E., Saffran, E., and Schwartz, M. (2000). *Quantitative Production Analysis: A Training Manual for the Analysis of Aphasic Sentence Production.* Hove: Psychology Press.

Berthier, M. L., Hinajosa, J., del Carmen Martin, M., and Fernandez, I. (2003). Open-label study of donepezil in chronic poststroke aphasia. *Neurology, 60,* 1218–9.

Berti, A., Allport, D. A., Driver, J., Deines, Z., Oxbury, J., and Oxbury, S. (1992). Levels of processing of visual stimuli in the extinguished field. *Neuropsychologia, 30,* 403–15.

Bi, G.-q. and Poo, M.-m. (2001). Synaptic modification by correlated activity: Hebb's postulate revisited. *Annual Review of Neuroscience, 24,* 139–66.

Bird, M. J. (2000). Psychosocial rehabilitation for problems arising from cognitive deficits in dementia. In *Cognitive Rehabilitation in Old Age* (eds R. D. Hill, L. Backman and A. S. Neely). Oxford: Oxford University Press.

Bird, M. (2001). Behavioural difficulties and cued recall of adaptive behaviour in dementia: experimental and clinical evidence. *Neuropsychological Rehabilitation, 11,* 357–75.

Bird, M. and Luszcz, M. (1993). Enhancing memory performance in Alzheimer's disease: acquisition assistance and cue effectiveness. *Journal of Clinical and Experimental Neuropsychology, 15,* 921–32.

Birnboim, S. (1995). A metacognitive approach to cognitive rehabilitation. *British Journal of Occupational Therapy, 58,* 61–64.

Bisiach, E. and Luzzatti, C. (1978). Unilateral neglect of representational space. *Cortex, 14,* 128–33.

Blake, H., McKinney, M., Treece, K., Lee, E., and Lincoln, N. B. (2002). An evaluation of screening measures for cognitive impairment after stroke. *Age and Ageing, 31,* 451–6.

Blomert, L. (1995). Who's the 'expert'? Amateur and professional judgement of aphasic communication. *Topics in Stroke Rehabilitation, 2,* 64–71.

Blomert, L., Kean, M-L., Koster, C., and Schokker, J. (1994). Amsterdam-Nijmegen Everyday Language Test: Construction, reliability and validity. *Aphasiology, 8,* 381–407.

Boake, C. (1991). History of cognitive rehabilitation following head injury. In *Cognitive rehabilitation for persons with traumatic brain injury. A functional approach* (eds J. S. Kreutzer and P. H. Wehman), pp. 3–12. Baltimore, MD: Paul H. Brookes Publishing.

Bohnen, N. I. (1991). Mild head injury and post-concussive sequelae. Doctoral dissertation, Rijksuniversiteit Limburg, Maastricht, The Netherlands.

Boles, L. (1997). Conversation analysis as a dependent measure in communication therapy with four individuals with aphasia. *Asia Pacific Journal of Speech, Language and Hearing, 2,* 43–61.

Boles, L. (1998). Conducting conversation: A case study using the spouse in aphasia treatment. *Neurophysiology and Neurogenic Speech and Language Disorders (Newsletter),* September 24–30.

Boles, L. and Bombard, T. (1998). Conversational discourse analysis: Appropriate and useful sample sizes. *Aphasiology, 12,* 547–60.

Bollinger, R., Musson, N., and Holland, A. (1993). A study of group communication intervention with chronically aphasic persons. *Aphasiology, 7,* 301–13.

Bonhoeffer, K. (1901). *Die akuten Geisteskrankheiten der Gewohnheitstrinker.* Jena: Fischer.

Booth, S. and Perkins, L. (1999). The use of conversational analysis to guide individualized advice to carers and evaluate change in aphasia: a case study. *Aphasiology, 13,* 283–303.

Booth, S. and Swabey, D. (1999). Group training in communication skills for carers of adults with aphasia. *International Journal of Language and Communication Disorders, 34,* 291–310.

Borkowski, J. G., Benton, A. L., and Spreen, O. (1967). Word fluency and brain damage. *Neuropsychologia, 5,* 135–40.

Bourgeois, M. S. (1990). Enhancing conversation skills in patients with Alzheimer's disease using a prosthetic memory aid. *Journal of Applied Behavior Analysis, 23,* 29–42.

Bourgeois, M. S. (1991). Communication treatment for adults with dementia. *Journal of Speech and Hearing Research, 34,* 831–44.

Bourgeois, M. S. (1992). Evaluating memory wallets in conversations with persons with dementia. *Journal of Speech and Hearing Research, 35,* 1344–57.

Bowen, A., Lincoln, N. B., and Dewey, M. (2003). Cognitive rehabilitation for spatial neglect following stroke (Cochrane Review). In: *The Cochrane Library,* 2. Oxford: Update Software.

Bowen, A., McKenna, K., and Tallis, R. C. (1999). Reasons for variability in the reported rate of occurrence of unilateral spatial neglect after stroke. *Stroke, 30,* 1196–1202.

Bozeat, S., Lambon Ralph, M. A., Patterson, K., and Hodges, J. R. (2002). The influence of personal familiarity and context on object use in semantic dementia. *Neurocase*, **8**, 127–34.

Braga, L. W., A randomized controlled trial in the rehabilitation of the child with traumatic brain injury: conventional approach vs. family participation methodology. In press.

Brand, M. and Markowitsch, H. J. (2003). The bottleneck structures implicated in memory processing. In *Learning and memory* (eds R. H. Kluwe, G. Lüer and F. Rösler), pp. 171–84. Basel: Birkhäuser.

Brandt, J. (1991). The Hopkins Verbal Learning Test: Development of a new memory test with six equivalent forms. *The Clinical Neuropsychologist*, **5**, 125–42.

Brandt, J. and Rich, J. B. (1995). Memory disorders in the dementias. In *Handbook of Memory Disorders* (eds A. D. Baddeley, B. A. Wilson and F. N. Watts), pp. 243–270. Chichester: John Wiley and Sons Ltd.

Brazzelli, M., Colombo, N., Della Sala, and S., Spinnler, H. (1994). Spared and impaired cognitive abilities after bilateral frontal damage. *Cortex*, **30**, 27–51.

Brett, M., Johnsrude, I. S., and Owen, A. M. (2002). The problem of functional localization in the human brain. *Nature Neuroscience*, **3**, 243–50.

Breuil, V., Rotrou, J. d., Forette, F., Tortrat, D., Ganasia-Ganem, A., Frambourt, A., Moulin, F., and Boller, F. (1994). Cognitive stimulation of patients with dementia: preliminary results. *International Journal of Geriatric Psychiatry*, **9**, 211–17.

Bright, P., Jaldow, E., and Kopelman, M. D. (2002). The National Adult Reading Test as a measure of premorbid intelligence: A comparison with estimates derived from demographic variables. *Journal of the International Neuropsychological Society*, **8**, 847–54.

Brindley, P., Copeland, M., Demain, C., and Martyn, P. (1989). A comparison of the speech of ten chronic Broca's aphasics following intensive and non-intensive periods of therapy. *Aphasiology*, **3**, 695–707.

Broadbent, D. E. (1958). *Perception and communication*. London: Pergamon Press.

Broadbent, D. E., Cooper, P. F., FitzGerald, P., and Parkes, K. R. (1982). The Cognitive Failures Questionnaire (CFQ) and its correlates. *British Journal of Clinical Psychology*, **21**, 1–16.

Broca, P. (1865). Sur le siege de la faculté du langage articulé. *Bulletins de la Société d'Anthropologie* **6**, 337–93.

Brodmann, K. (1914). Physiologie des Gehirns. In *Neue deutsche Chirurgie, Bd.* **11**, Tl. **1**, (ed. P. von Bruns), pp. 85–426. Stuttgart: Enke.

Broida, H. (1977). Language therapy effects in long term aphasia. *Archives of Physical Medicine and Rehabilitation*, **58**, 248–53.

Brooks, D. N. (1987). Measuring neuropsychological and functional recovery. In *Neurobehavioral recovery from head injury* (eds H. S. Levin, J. Grafman and H. M. Eisenberg), pp. 57–72. Oxford: Oxford University Press.

Brooks, D. N. and McKinlay, W. (1987). Return to work within the first seven years of severe head injury. *Brain Injury*, **1**, 5–15.

Brooks, N., McKinlay, W., Symington, C., Beattie, A., and Campsie, L. (1987). Return to work within the first seven years of severe head injury. *Brain Injury*, **1**(1), 5–19.

Brookshire, R. H. and Nicholas, M. E. (1993). Word choice in the connected speech of aphasic and non-brain damaged speakers. In *Clinical Aphasiology* (ed. M. L. Lemme). Vol. 21. Austin, TX:Pro Ed.

Brouwer, W. H. (2002). Attention et aptitude a la conduite: approche neuropsychologique. In *La Neuropsychologie de l'Attention* (eds J. Couillet, M. Leclercq and C. Mouroni et Ph. Azouvi). Marseille: Solal.

Brouwer, W. H., Rothengatter, J. A., and Van Wolffelaar, P. C. (1988). Compensatory potential in elderly drivers. In *Road user behaviour: Theory and research* (eds J. A. Rothengatter and R. A. de Bruin), pp. 296–301. Assen: van Gorcum.

Brumfitt, S. M. and Sheeran, P. (1999). *VASES: Visual Analogue Self-Esteem Scale*. Bicester, Oxon: Winslow Press.

Brunsdon, R., Coltheart, M., and Nickels, L. (in press). Treatment of irregular word spelling in a case of developmental surface dysgraphia. *Cognitive Neuropsychology*.

Bub, D. N., Arguin, M., and Lecours, A. R. (1993). Dejerine, Jules and his interpretation of pure alexia. *Brain and Language*, **45**, 531–59.

Büchel, C. and Friston, K. J. (1997). Modulation of connectivity in visual pathways by attention: Cortical interactions evaluated with structural equation modelling and fMRI. *Cerebral Cortex,* **7,** 768–78.

Buchman, A., Garron, D., Trost-Cardamone, J., Wichter, M., and Schwartz, D. (1986). Word deafness: one hundred years later. *Journal of Neurology, Neurosurgery and Psychiatry,* **49,** 489–99.

Buchtel, H. A. (1987). Attention and vigilance after head trauma. In *Neurobehavioral recovery from head injury* (eds H. S. Levin, J. Grafman and H. M. Eisenberg), pp. 372–8. New York: Oxford University Press.

Bullinger, M. and TBI Consensus Group (2002). Quality of life in participants with traumatic brain injury-basic issues, assessment and recommendations. *Restorative Neurology and Neuroscience* **20,** 111–24.

Burgess, P. W. (1997). Theory and methodology in executive function research. In *Methodology of Frontal and Executive Function* (ed. P. Rabbitt), pp. 81–111. Hove: Psychology Press.

Burgess, P. W. (2000a). Real-world multitasking from a cognitive neuroscience perspective. In *Control of Cognitive Processes: Attention and Performance XVIII* (eds S. Monsell and J. Driver), pp. 465–72. Cambridge, MA: MIT Press.

Burgess, P. W. (2000b). Strategy application disorder: The role of the frontal lobes in human multitasking. *Psychological Research,* **63,** 279–88.

Burgess, P. W. and Alderman, N. (1990). Rehabilitation of dyscontrol syndromes following frontal lobe damage: A cognitive neuropsychological approach. In *Cognitive rehabilitation in perspective* (eds R. L. l. Wood and I. Fussey), pp. 183–203. London: Taylor and Francis.

Burgess, P. W. and Alderman, N. (2004). Executive dysfunction. In *Clinical Neuropsychology: A Practical Guide to Assessment and Management for Clinicians* (eds L. H. Goldstein and J. E. McNeil), pp. 185–210. Chichester: John Wiley.

Burgess, P. W. and McNeil, J. E. (1999). Content-specific confabulation. *Cortex,* **35,** 163–82.

Burgess, P. W. and Robertson, I. H. (2002). Principles of the rehabilitation of frontal lobe function. In *Principles of Frontal Lobe Function* (eds D. T. Stuss and R. T. Knight), pp. 557–72. New York: Oxford University Press.

Burgess, P. W. and Shallice, T. (1994). Fractionnement du syndrome frontal. *Revue de Neuropsychologie,* **4,** 345–70.

Burgess, P. W. and Shallice, T. (1996a). Bizarre responses, rule detection and frontal lobe lesions. *Cortex,* **32,** 241–60.

Burgess, P. W. and Shallice, T. (1996b). Confabulation and the control of recollection. *Memory,* **4,** 359–411.

Burgess, P. W. and Shallice, T. (1996c). Response suppression, initiation and strategy use following frontal lobe lesion. *Neuropsychologia,* **34,** 263–76.

Burgess, P. W. and Shallice, T. (1997). *The Hayling and Brixton Tests. Test Manual.* Bury St Edmunds: Thames Valley Test Company.

Burgess, P. W. and Shallice, T. (1997). The relationship between prospective and retrospective memory: Neuropsychological evidence. In *Cognitive Models of Memory* (eds M. A. Conway), pp. 74–90. Hove: Psychology Press.

Burgess, P. W., Alderman, N., Emslie, H., Evans, J. J., and Wilson, B. A. (1996a). The dysexecutive questionnaire. In *Behavioural Assessment of the Dysexecutive Syndrome* (eds B. A. Wilson, N. Alderman, P. W. Burgess, H. Emslie and J. J. Evans) . Bury St Edmunds: Thames Valley Test Company.

Burgess, P. W., Alderman, N., Emslie, H., Evans, J. J., Wilson, B. A., and Shallice, T. (1996b). The simplified six element test. In *Behavioural Assessment of the Dysexecutive Syndrome* (eds B. A. Wilson, N. Alderman, P. W. Burgess, H. Emslie and J. J. Evans). Bury St. Edmunds: Thames Valley Test Company.

Burgess, P. W., Alderman, N., Evans, J., Emslie, H., and Wilson, B. A. (1998). The ecological validity of tests of executive function. *Journal of the International Neuropsychological Society,* **4,** 547–58.

Burgess, P. W., Baxter, D., Rose, M., and Alderman, N. (1996c). Delusional paramnesic misidentification In *Method in Madness: Case Studies in Neuropsychiatry* (eds P. W. Halligan and J. C. Marshall), pp. 51–78. Hove: Psychology Press.

Burgess, P. W., Simons, J. S., Coates, L. M., and Channon, S. (2005) The search for specific planning processes. In *The Cognitive Psychology of Planning* (ed. R. G. Morris), pp. 199–227. Oxford: Oxford University Press.

Burgess, P. W., Veitch, E., Costello, A., and Shallice, T. (2000). The cognitive and neuroanatomical correlates of multitasking. *Neuropsychologia,* **38,** 848–63.

Burgess, I. S., Wearden, J. H., Cox, T., and Rae, M. (1992). Operant conditioning with subjects suffering from dementia. *Behavioural Psychotherapy*, **20**, 219–37.

Burke, W. H., Zenicus, A. H., Wesolowski, M. D., and Doubleday, F. (1991). Improving executive function disorders in brain-injured patients. *Brain Injury*, **5**, 241–52.

Burleigh, S. A., Farber, R. S., and Gillard, M. (1998). Community integration and life satisfaction after traumatic brain injury: Long-term findings. *American Journal of Occupational Therapy*, **52**, 45–52.

Buschke, H. (1973). Selective reminding for analysis of memory and learning. *Journal of Verbal Learning and Verbal Behaviour*, **12**, 543–50.

Buschke, H. and Fuld, P. A. (1974). Evaluating storage, retention, and retrieval in disordered memory and learning. *Neurology*, **24**, 1019–25.

Butfield, E. and Zangwill, O. L. (1946). Re-education in aphasia: a review of 70 cases. *Journal of Neurology, Neurosurgery and Psychiatry*, **9**, 75–9.

Butler, R. W. and Copeland, D. R. (2002). Attentional processes and their remediation in children treated for cancer: A literature review and the devleopment of a therapeutic approach. *Journal of International Neuropsychological Society*, **8**, 115–24.

Butler, R. W., Rorsman, I., Hill, J. M., and Tuma, R. (1993). The effects of frontal brain impairment on fluency: Simple and complex paradigms. *Neuropsychology*, **4**, 519–29.

Butters, M. A., Soety, E. M., and Glisky, E. L. (1998). Memory rehabilitation. In *Clinical neuropsychology* (eds P. J. Snyder and P. D. Nussbaum), pp. 450–66. Washington, DC: American Psychological Association.

Butterworth, B. L. (1979). Hesitation and the production of verbal paraphasias and neologisms in jargon aphasia. *Brain and Language*, **8**, 133–61.

Buxbaum, L. J., Schwartz, M. F. and Montgomery, M. W. (1998). Ideational apraxia and naturalistic action. *Cognitive Neuropsychology*, **15**, 617–43.

Byng, S. (1988). Sentence processing deficits: Theory and therapy. *Cognitive Neuropsychology*, **5**, 629–76.

Byng, S. (1993). Hypothesis testing and aphasia therapy. In *Aphasia treatment: World perspectives* (eds A. Holland and M. Forbes). San Diego, CA: Singular Publishing group.

Byng, S., Kay, J., Edmundson, A., and Scott, C. (1990). Aphasia tests reconsidered. *Aphasiology*, **4**, 67–91.

Byng S., Pound, C., and Parr, S. (2000). Living with aphasia: a framework for therapy interventions. In *Acquired neurogenic communication disorders: A clinical perspective* (ed. I. Papathanasiou). London: Whurr Publishers.

Byng, S. Van Der Gaag, A., Parr, S., Swain, J., Finkelstein, V., French, S., and Oliver, M. (1998). International Initiatives in outcome measurements: a perspective from the UK. In *Measuring outcomes in speech language pathology* (ed. C. Frattali). New York: Thieme Medical Publishers.

Cabana, M. D., Rand, C. S., Powe, N. R. *et al.* (1999). Why don't physicians follow clinical practice guidelines? *Journal of the American Medical Association*, **282**, 1458–65.

Cabeza, R., Locantore, J. K., and Anderson, N. D. (2003). Lateralization of prefrontal activity during episodic memory retrieval: evidence for the production-monitoring hypothesis. *Journal of Cognitive Neuroscience*, **15**, 249–59.

Cahill, L., Babinsky, R., Markowitsch, H. J., and McGaugh, J. L. (1995). Involvement of the amygdaloid complex in emotional memory. *Nature*, **377**, 295–6.

Calabrese, P., Markowitsch, H. J., Harders, A. G., Scholz, A., and Gehlen, W. (1995). Fornix damage and memory: a case report. *Cortex*, **31**, 555–64.

Callahan, C. D. (2001). The assessment and rehabilitation of executive function disorders. In *Rehabilitation of neuropsychological disorders* (eds B. Johnstone and H. H. Stonnington), pp. 87–124. Philadelphia, PA: Psychology Press.

Camp, C. J. (1989). Facilitation of new learning in Alzheimer's disease. In *Memory and Aging: Theory, Research and Practice* (eds G. Gilmore, P. Whitehouse and M. Wykle), pp. 212–25. New York: Springer.

Camp, C. J., Bird, M. J., and Cherry, K. E. (2000). Retrieval strategies as a rehabilitation aid for cognitive loss in pathological aging. In *Rehabilitation in Old Age Cognitive* (eds R. D. Hill, L. Backman and A. S. Neely), pp. 224–248. Oxford: Oxford University Press.

Camp, C. J., Foss, J. W., Stevens, A. B., Reichard, C. C., McKitrick, L. A., and O'Hanlon, A. M. (1993). Memory training in normal and demented elderly populations: the E-I-E-I-O model. *Experimental Aging Research,* **19**, 277–90.

Caplan, D. (1987). *Neurolinguistics and linguistic aphasiology: an introduction.* Cambridge: Cambridge University Press.

Caplan, L. R. (2001). Evidence based medicine: concerns of a clinical neurologist. *Journal of Neurology Neurosurgery and Psychiatry,* **71**, 569–76.

Caplan, D., Alpert, N., and Waters, G. (1999). PET studies of syntactic processing with auditory sentence presentation. *Neuroimage,* **9**, 343–51.

Caplan, D., Vanier, M., and Baker, C. (1986). A case study of reproduction conduction aphasia. I: Word production. *Cognitive Neuropsychology,* **3**, 99–128.

Caporali, A. and Basso, A. (2003). A survey of long-term outcome of aphasia and of chances of gainful employment. *Aphasiology,* **17**, 815–34.

Cappa, S. (1998). Spontaneous recovery from aphasia. In *Handbook of neurolinguistics* (eds B. Stemmer, and H. A. Whitaker), pp. 535–45. San Diego: Academic Press.

Cappa, S. F., Perani, D., Grassi, F. *et al.* (1997). A PET follow-up study of recovery after stroke in acute aphasics. *Brain and Language,* **56**, 55–67.

Cappa, S. F., Sterzi, R., Vallar, G., and Bisiach, E. (1987). Remission of hemineglect and anosognosia during vestibular stimulation. *Neuropsychologia,* **25**, 775–82.

Caramazza, A. (1989). Cognitive Neuropsychology and rehabilitation: an unfulfilled promise? In *Cognitive approaches in neuropsychological rehabilitation* (eds X. Seron and G. Deloche). Hillsdale, NJ: Lawrence Erlbaum Associates.

Caramazza, A. and Hillis, A. E. (1990). Where do semantic errors come from? *Cortex,* 26, 95–122.

Caramazza, A., Hillis, A. E. (1993). For a theory of remediation of cognitive deficits. *Neuropsychological Rehabilitation,* **3**, 217–34.

Carney, N., Chesnut, R. M., Maynard, H., Mann, N. C., Patterson, P., and Helfand, M. (1999). Effect of cognitive rehabilitation on outcomes for persons with traumatic brain injury: A systematic review. *Journal of Head Trauma Rehabilitation,* **14**(3), 277–307.

Carter, L. T., Oliveira, D. O., Duponte, J., and Lynch, S. V. (1988). The relationship of cognitive skills performance to activities of daily living in stroke patients. *The American Journal of Occupational Therapy,* **42**, 449–55.

Cartoni, A., Lincoln, N. B. (in press). The sensitivity and specificity of the Middlesex Elderly Assessment of Mental State (MEAMS) for detecting cognitive impairment after stroke. Neuropsychological Rehabilitation.

Chambless, D. L., Baker, M. J., Baucom, D. H., Beutler, L. E., Calhoun, K. S., CritsChristoph, P., Daiuto, A., DeRubeis, R., Detweiler, J., Haaga, D. A. F., Johnson, S. B., McCurry, S., Mueser, K. T., Pope, K. S., Sanderson, W. C., Shoham, V., Stickle, T., Williams, S. A., and Woody, S. R. (1998). Update on empirically validated therapies II. *The Clinical Psychologist,* **51**, 3–16.

Chan, R. C. K. (2001). Dysexecutive symptoms among a non-clinical sample: A study with the use of the Dysexecutive Questionnaire. *British Journal of Psychology,* **92**, 551–65.

Chapey, R. (2001). *Language intervention strategies in adult aphasia,* 4th edn. Baltimore, MD: Williams and Wilkins.

Chapey, R., Duchan, J. F., Elman, R. J., Garcia, L. J., Kagan, A., Lyon, J. G., and Simmons-Mackie, N. (2001). Life participation approach to aphasia: A statement of values for the future. In *Language intervention strategies in aphasia and related neurogenic communication disorders* (ed. R. Chapey), 4th edn, pp. 55–126). Philadelphia: Lippincott, Williams and Wilkins.

Chesnut, R. M., Carney, N., Maynard, H., Mann, N. C., Patterson, P., and Helfand, M. (1999). Summary report: Evidence for the effectiveness of rehabilitation for persons with traumatic brain injury. *Journal of Head Trauma Rehabilitation,* **14**, 176–88.

Chesnut, R. M., Carney, N., Maynard, H., Patterson, P., Mann, N. C., and Helfand, M.(1999). Rehabilitation for traumatic brain injury. AHRQ Publ. No. 99-#006.

Chow, K. L. (1967). Effects of ablation. In *The Neurosciences* (eds G. C. Quarton, T. Melnechuk and F. O. Schmitt), pp. 705–13. New York: Rockefeller University Press.

Christensen, A.-L. and Caetano, C. (1996). Alexandr Romanovich Luria (1902–1977): Contributions to neuropsychological rehabilitation. *Neuropsychological Rehabilitation,* **6**(4), 279–303.

Christensen, H., Kopelman, M. D., Stanhope, N., Lorentz, L., and Owen, P. (1998). Rates of forgetting in Alzheimer dementia. *Neuropsychologia, 36*, 547–57.

Cicerone, K. D. (2002). Remediation of 'working attention' in mild traumatic brain injury. *Brain Injury, 16*(3), 185–95.

Cicerone, K. D. and Giacino, J. T. (1992). Remediation of executive function deficits after traumatic brain injury. *NeuroRehabilitation, 2*(3), 12–22.

Cicerone, K. D. and Tupper, D. E. (1991). Neuropsychological rehabilitation: treatment of errors in everyday functioning. In *The neuropsychology of everyday life: issues in development and rehabilitation* (eds D. E. Tupper and K. D. Cicerone), pp. 271–92. Boston: Kluwer Academic.

Cicerone, K. D. and Wood, J. C. (1987). Planning disorder after closed head injury: a case study. *Archives of Physical Medicine and Rehabilitation, 68*, 111–15.

Cicerone, K. D., Mott, T., and Azulay, J. (2002). Community integration and satisfaction with functioning after intensive cognitive rehabilitation for acquired brain injury. *Archives of Physical Medicine & Rehabilitation, 83*, 1480.

Cicerone, K. D., Smith, L. C., Ellmo, W. *et al.* (1996). Neuropsychological rehabilitation of mild traumatic brain injury. *Brain Injury, 10*(4), 277–86.

Cicerone, K. D., Dahlberg, C., Kalmar, K., Langenbahn, D. M., Malec, J. F., Bergquist, T. F. *et al.* (2000). Evidence-based cognitive rehabilitation: Recommendations for clinical practice. *Archives of Physical Medicine and Rehabilitation, 81*, 1596–615.

Clare, L. (2003). Cognitive training and cognitive rehabilitation for people with early-stage dementia. *Reviews in Clinical Gerontology, 13*, 75–83.

Clare, L. and Woods, R. T. (eds.) (2001). *Cognitive Rehabilitation in Dementia.* Hove: Psychology Press.

Clare, L. and Woods, R. T. (2004). Cognitive training and cognitive rehabilitation for people with early-stage Alzheimer's disease: a review. *Neuropsychological Rehabilitation, 14*, 385–401.

Clare, L., Wilson, B. A., Breen, K., and Hodges, J. R. (1999). Errorless learning of face-name associations in early Alzheimer's disease. *Neurocase, 5*, 37–46.

Clare, L., Wilson, B. A., Carter, G., Breen, E. K., Gosses, A., and Hodges, J. R. (2000). Intervening with everyday memory problems in dementia of Alzheimer type: An errorless learning approach. *Journal of Clinical and Experimental Neuropsychology, 22*, 132–46.

Clare, L., Wilson, B. A., Carter, G., Hodges, J. R., and Adams, M. (2001). Long-term maintenance of treatment gains following a cognitive rehabilitation intervention in early dementia of Alzheimer type: a single case study. *Neuropsychological Rehabilitation, 11*, 477–94.

Clare, L., Wilson, B. A., Carter, G., Roth, I., and Hodges, J. R. (2002). Relearning of face-name associations in early-stage Alzheimer's disease. *Neuropsychology, 16*, 538–47.

Clare, L., Wilson, B. A., Carter, G., Roth, I., and Hodges, J. R. (2004). Awareness in early-stage Alzheimer's disease: relationship to outcome of cognitive rehabilitation. *Journal of Clinical and Experimental Neuropsychology, 26*, 215–26.

Clare, L., Wilson, B. A., Carter,G., and Hodges, J. R. (2003b). Cognitive rehabilitation as a component of early intervention in dementia: a single case study. *Aging and Mental Health, 7*, 15–21.

Clare, L., Woods, R. T., Moniz-Cook, E. D., Orrell, M., and Spector, A. (2003a). Cognitive rehabilitation and cognitive training for early-stage Alzheimer's disease and vascular dementia (Cochrane Review). In *The Cochrane Library*, Issue **4**, 2003. Chichester: John Wiley and Sons Ltd.

Clayton, N. S. and Dickinson, A. (1998). Episodic-like memory during cache recovery by scrub jays. *Nature, 395*, 272–4.

Cluzeau, F., Littlejohns, P., Grimshaw, J., Feder, G., and Moran, S. Development and application of a generic methodology to assess the quality of clinical guidelines. *International Journal for Quality in Health Care, 11*, 21–8.

Code, C. and Müller, D. (1992). *The Code-Müller Protocols: Assessing perceptions of psychosocial adjustment to aphasia and related disorders.* London: Whurr.

Code, C., Müller, D., Hogan, A., and Hermann, M. (1999). Perceptions of psychosocial adjustment to acquired communication disorders: applications of the Code-Müller Protocols. *International Journal of Language and Communication Disorders, 34*, 193–207.

Cohelho, C. A., DeRuyter, F., and Stein, M. (1996). Treatment efficacy: Cognitive-communicative disorders resulting from traumatic brain injury in adults. *Journal of Speech and Hearing Research, 39*, S5–17.

Cohen, J. (1977). *Statistical power analysis for the behavioral sciences*, 2nd edn. Hillsdale, NJ: Lawrence Erlbaum Associates.

Cohen, J. and Cohen, P. (1983). *Applied multiple regression/correlation analysis for the behavioral sciences*, 2nd edn. London: Lawrence Erlbaum Associates.

Cohen, D. and Eisdorfer, C. (1986). *The Loss of Self: a Family Resource for the Care of Alzheimer's Disease and Related Disorders*. New York: W W Norton and Company.

Cohen, J. D. and Servan-Schreiber, D. (1992). Context, cortex and doapmine: a connectionist approach to behaviour and biology in schizophrenia. *Psychological Review*, **99**, 45–77.

Cohen, J. D., Braver, T. S., and O'Reilly, R. C. (1998). A computational approach to prefrontal cortex, cognitive control, and schizophrenia: recent developments and current challenges. In *The Prefrontal Cortex: Executive and Cognitive Functions* (eds A. C. Roberts, T. W. Robbins and L. Weiskrantz). Oxford: Oxford University Press.

Cohen, J. D., Dunbar, K., and McClelland, J. L. (1990). On the control of automatic processes: a parallel distributed processing account of the Stroop effect. *Psychological Review*, **97**, 332–61.

Cohen, L., Dehaene, S., Naccache, L., Lehericy, S., Dehaene-Lambertz, G., Henaff, M. A., and Michel, F. (2000). The visual word form area – Spatial and temporal characterization of an initial stage of reading in normal subjects and posterior split-brain patients. *Brain*, **123**, 291–307.

Cohen, L., Lehericy, S., Chochon, F., Lemer, C., Rivaud, S., and Dehaene, S. (2002). Language-specific tuning of visual cortex functional properties of the Visual Word Form Area. *Brain*, **125**, 1054–69.

Cole, J. C. (1993). Remediation of an acquired dyslexic: a case study. Paper presented at the first National Aphasiology Symposium of Australia, Sydney.

Colotla V. A. and Bach-y-Rita, P. (2002). Shepherd Ivory Franz: His contributions to neuropsychology and rehabilitation. *Cognitive, Affective, and Behavioral Neuroscience*, 2(**2**), 141–8.

Coltheart, M. (1983). Aphasia therapy research: a single case study approach. In *Aphasia therapy* (eds C. Code and D. C. Muller). London: Edward Arnold.

Coltheart, M. (1991). Cognitive psychology applied to the treatment of acquired language disorders. In *Handbook of behavior therapy and psychological science: An integrative approach* (ed. P. Martin), pp. 216–26. New York: Pergamon Press.

Coltheart, M. and Byng, S. (1989). A treatment for surface dyslexia. In X. Seron (ed.) *Cognitive approaches in neuropsychological rehabilitation*. London: Lawrence Erlbaum Associates.

Coltheart, M. and Byng, S. (1989). A treatment for surface dyslexia. In *Cognitive approaches in neuropsychological rehabilitation* (eds S. Seron and G. Deloche), pp. 159–74. Hillsdale, NJ: Lawrence Erlbaum Associates.

Coltheart, M. and Leahy, J. (1996). Assessment of lexical and nonlexical reading abilities in children: Some normative data. *Australian Journal of Psychology*, **48**, 136–40.

Coltheart, M., Bates, A., and Castles, A. (1994). Cognitive neuropsychology and rehabilitation. In *Cognitive neuropsychology and cognitive rehabilitation* (eds G. W. Humphreys and M. J. Riddoch). London: Lawrence Erlbaum Associates.

Coltheart, M., Rastle, K., Perry, C., Langdon, R., and Ziegler, J. (2001). DRC: A dual route cascaded model of visual word recognition and reading aloud. *Psychological Review*, **108**, 204–56.

Concato, J., Shah, N., and Horwitz, R. I. (2000). Randomized, controlled trials, observational studies, and the hierarchy of research designs. *New England Journal of Medicine*, **342**, 1887–92.

Condeluci, A. (1992). Brain injury rehabilitation: the need to bridge paradigms. *Brain Injury*, **6**, 543–51.

Cooper, R. and Shallice, T. (2000). Contention scheduling and the control of routine activities. *Cognitive Neuropsychology*, **17**, 297–338.

Cope, D. N. (1995). The effectiveness of traumatic brain injury rehabilitation: a review. *Brain Injury*, **9**, 649–70.

Corkin, S. (2002). What's new with the amnesic patient H. M.? *Neuroscience*, **3**, 153–60.

Corrigan, J. D., Bogner, J. A., Mysiw, W. J., Clinchot, D., and Fugate, L. (2001). Life satisfaction after traumatic brain injury. *Journal of Head Trauma Rehabilitation*, **16**, 543–55.

Corwin, J. and Bylsma, F. W. (1993). Translations of excerpts from Andre Rey's Psychological Examination of Traumatic Encephalopathy and P. A. Osterreith's The Complex Figure Copy Test. *The Clinical Neuropsychologist*, **7**, 3–15.

Coughlan, A. K. and Hollows, S. E. (1985). *The Adult Memory and Information Processing Battery.* Leeds: A. K. Coughlan, Psychology Department, St James's University Hospital.

Coull, J. T., Sahakian, B. J., and Hodges, J. R. (1996). The alpha-2 antagonist idazoxan remediates certain attentional and executive dysfunction in patients with dementia of the frontal type. *Psychopharmacology,* **123**, 239–49.

Courtney, S. M., Ungerleider, L. G., Keil, K., and Haxby, J. V. (1996). Object and spatial visual working memory activate separate neural systems in human cortex. *Cerebral Cortex,* **6**, 39–49.

Cowan, N. (2000). The magical number 4 in short-term memory: a reconsideration of mental storage capacity. *Behavioral and Brain Sciences,* **24**, 87–185.

Cramon, D. Y. von and Markowitsch, H. J. (2000). The septum and human memory. In *The behavioral neuroscience of the septal region* (ed. R Numan), pp. 380–413. Berlin: Springer.

Cramon, D. Y. von, Markowitsch, H. J., and Schuri, U. (1993). The possible contribution of the septal region to memory. *Neuropsychologia,* **31**, 1159–80.

Cramon, D. Y. von and G. Matthes-von Cramon (1994). Back to work with a chronic dysexecutive syndrome? A case report. *Neuropsychological Rehabilitation,* **4**, 399–417.

Crawford, J. R. (1996). Assessment. In *The Blackwell dictionary of neuropsychology* (eds J. G. Beaumont, P. M. Kenealy, and M. J. Rogers), pp. 108–16, Oxford: Blackwell Publishing.

Crawford, J. R. (2004). Psychometric foundations of neuropsychological assessment. In *Clinical neuropsychology: A practical guide to assessment and management for clinicians* (eds L. H. Goldstein and J. E. McNeil), pp. 121–40, Chichester: Wiley.

Crawford, J. R. and Warrington, E. K. (2002). The Homophone Meaning Generation Test: Psychometric properties and a method for estimating premorbid performance. *Journal of the International Neuropsychological Society,* **8**, 547–54.

Crawford, J. R., Blackmore, L. M., Lamb, A. E., and Simpson, S. A. (2000b). Is there a differential deficit in fronto-executive functioning in Huntington's disease? *Clinical Neuropsychological Assessment,* **1**, 3–19.

Crawford, J. R., Burgess, P. W., and Downey, B. (in preparation). The Brixton Test: psychometric properties, an equation for inferring change, and *T* score norms based on an enlarged normative sample.

Crawford, J. R., Deary, I. J., Starr, J. M., and Whalley, L. J. (2001). The NART as an index of prior intellectual functioning: A retrospective validity study covering a 66 year interval. *Psychological Medicine,* **31**, 451–8.

Crawford, J. R., Moore, J. W., and Cameron, I. M. (1992). Verbal fluency: A NART-based equation for the estimation of premorbid performance. *British Journal of Clinical Psychology,* **31**, 327–9.

Crawford, J. R., Obonsawin, M. C., and Bremner, M. (1993). Frontal lobe impairment in schizophrenia: Relationship to intellectual functioning. *Psychological Medicine,* **23**, 787–90.

Crawford, J. R., Smith, G. V., Maylor, E. A. M., Della Sala, S., and Logie, R. H. (2003). The Prospective and Retrospective Memory Questionnaire (PRMQ): Normative data and latent structure in a large non-clinical sample. *Memory,* **11**, 261–75.

Crawford, J. R., Venneri, A., and O'Carroll, R. E. (1998). Neuropsychological assessment of the elderly. In *Comprehensive clinical psychology, vol. 7: Clinical geropsychology* (eds A. S. Bellack and M. Hersen), pp. 133–69, Oxford: Pergamon.

Crawford, J. R., Wright, R., and Bate, A. (1995). Verbal, figural and ideational fluency in CHI. *Journal of the International Neuropsychological Society,* **1**, 321.

Crawford, J., Bryan, J., Luszcz, M., Obonsawin, M., and Stewart, L. (2000a). The executive decline hypothesis of cognitive ageing: Do executive deficits qualify as differential deficits and do they mediate age-related memory decline? *Aging, Neuropsychology and Cognition,* **7**, 9–31.

Crepeau, F., Scherzer, B. P., Belleville, S., Desmarais, G. (1997). A qualitative analysis of central executive disorders in a real-life work situation. *Neuropsychological Rehabilitation,* **7**, 147–65.

Crick, F. and Koch, C. (1990). Towards a neurobiological theory of consciousness. *Seminars in the Neurosciences,* **2**, 263–75.

Crovitz, H. F. and Schiffman, H. (1974). Frequency of episodic memories as a function of their age. *Bulletin of the Psychonomic Society,* **4**, 517–8.

Cruice, M., Worrall, L., Hickson, L., and Murison, R. (2003). Finding a focus for quality of life with aphasia: Social and emotional health and psychological well-being. *Aphasiology,* **17**, 333–53.

Curran, M. C. (2002). Scaffolded training facilitates learning of naturalistic actions after stroke. Unpublished Ph.D., York University, Toronto.

Curran, C., Hussain, Z., and Park, N. W. (2001). *Scaffolded training facilitates learning of naturalistic actions after stroke.* Paper presented at the 109th Annual Convention of the American Psychological Association, San Francisco, CA.

D'Esposito, M., Detre, J. A., Aguirre, G. K., Stallcup, M., Alsop, D. C., Tippet, L. J., and Farah, M. J. (1997). A functional MRI study of mental image generation. *Neuropsychologia, 35,* 725–30.

D'Esposito, M. and Postle, B. R. (2002). The organization of working memory function in lateral prefrontal cortex: Evidence from event-related functional MRI. In *Principles of Frontal Lobe Function* (eds D. T. Stuss and R. K. Knight), pp. 168–187. New York: Oxford University Press.

D'Zurilla, T. J. and Goldfried, M. R. (1971). Problem-solving and behaviour modification. *Journal of Abnormal Psychology, 78,* 107–26.

Dab, S., Claes, T., Morais, J., and Shallice, T. (1999). Confabulation with a selective descriptor process impairment. *Cognitive Neuropsychology, 16,* 215–42.

Dalla Barba, G., Capaletti, Y. J., Signorini, M., and Denes, G. (1997). Confabulation: Remembering 'another' past, planning 'another' future. *Neurocase 3,* 425–36.

Damasio, A. R., Graf-Radford, N. R., Eslinger, P. J., Damasio, H., and Kassell, N. (1985). Amnesia following basal forebrain lesions. *Archives of Neurology, 42,* 263–71.

Darley, F. L. (1972). The efficacy of language rehabilitation in aphasia. *Journal of Speech and Hearing Disorders, 37,* 3–21.

David, R. M. (1990). Aphasia assessment: The acid test. *Aphasiology, 4,* 103–7.

David, R. M., Enderby, P., and Bainton, D. (1982). Treatment of acquired aphasia: speech therapists and volunteers compared. *Journal of Neurology, Neurosurgery and Psychiatry, 45,* 957–61.

David, R. M., Enderby, P., and Bainton, D. (1983). Speech-therapists and volunteers – some comments on recent investigations of their effectiveness in the treatment of aphasia. Response to T. R. Pring. *British Journal of Disorders of Communication, 18,* 73–7.

Davidson, B. and Worrall, L. (2000). The assessment of activity limitation in functional communication: Challenges and choices. In *Neurogenic commmunication disorders: a functional approach* (eds L. E. Worrall and C. M. Frattali). New York: Thieme Medical Publishers.

Davis, R. N., Massman, P. J., and Doody, R. S. (2001). Cognitive intervention in Alzheimer Disease: a randomized placebo-controlled study. *Alzheimer Disease and Associated Disorders, 15,* 1–9.

Dayns, B., and Van den Broek, M. D. (2000). Treatment of stable delusional confabulations using self-monitoring training. *Neuropsychological Rehabilitation, 10,* 415–27.

De Haan, E., Young, A., and Newcombe, F. (1991). Covert and overt recognition in prosopagnosia, *Brain 114,* 2575–91.

De Vreese, L. P., Neri, M., Fioravanti, M., Belloi, L., and Zanetti, O. (2001). Memory rehabilitation in Alzheimer's disease: a review of progress. *International Journal of Geriatric Psychiatry, 16,* 794–809.

De Vreese, L. P., Verlato, C., Emiliani, S., Schioppa, S., Belloi, L., Salvioli, G., and Neri, M. (1998). Effect size of a three-month drug treatment in AD when combined with individual cognitive retraining: preliminary results of a pilot study. Abstract. *Neurobiology of Aging, 19*(4S), S213.

De Weerdt, W., Selz, B., Nuyens, G. *et al.* (2000). Time use of stroke patients in an intensive rehabilitation unit: a comparison between a Belgian and Swiss setting. *Disability and Rehabilitation, 22,* 181–6.

Deacon, D. and Campbell, K. (1991). Decision making following closed head injury: Can response speed be trained? *Journal of Clinical Neuropsychology, 13,* 639–51.

Dean, C. M. and Shepherd, R. B. (1997). Task-related training improves performance of seated reaching tasks after stroke. A randomised controlled trial. *Stroke, 28,* 722–8.

Dean, C. M., Richards, C. L., and Malouin, F. (2000). Task-related circuit training improves performance of locomotor tasks in chronic stroke: a randomised controlled pilot trial. *Archives of Physical Medicine and Rehabilitation, 81,* 409–17.

DeFocket, J. W., Rees, G., Frith, C., and Lavie, N. (2001). The role of working memory in visual selective attention. *Science, 2,* 291(5509), 1684–5.

Dehaene, S., Le Clec'H, G., Poline, J.-B., Le Bihan, D., and Cohen, L. (2002). The visual word form area: a prelexical representation of visual words in the fusiform gyrus. *Neuroreport, 13,* 321–5.

Dejerine, J. (1891). Sur un cas de cécité verbale avec agraphie, suivi d'autopsie. *Mémoires de la Société de Biologie*, **3**, 197–201.

Delahunty, A. and Morice, R. (1993). *A Training Programme for the Remediation of Cognitive Deficits in Schizophrenia*. Albury, New South Wales: Department of Health.

Delis, D. C., Kaplan, E., Kramer, J. H., and Ober, B. A. (2001). *California Verbal Learning Test*, 2nd UK edn. San Antonio, TX: The Psychological Corporation.

Delis, D. C., Kramer, J. H., Kaplan, E., and Ober, B. A. (1987). *The California Verbal Learning Test*. New York: The Psychological Corporation.

Delis, D. C., McKee, R., Massman, P. J. *et al.* (1991). Alternate form of the California Verbal Learning Test: Development and reliability. *The Clinical Neuropsychologist*, **5**, 154–62.

Dell, G. S. (1986). A spreading activation theory of retrieval in sentence production. *Psychological Review*, **93**, 283–321.

Dell, G. S., Schwartz, M. F., Martin, N., Saffran, E. M., and Gagnon, D. A. (1997). Lexical access in aphasic and nonaphasic speakers. *Psychological Review*, **104**, 801–38.

Denes, G., Perazzolo, C., Piani, A., and Piccione, F. (1996). Intensive versus regular speech therapy in global aphasia: a controlled study. *Aphasiology* **10**, 385–94.

Desimone, R. and Duncan, J. (1995). Neural mechanisms of selective visual attention. *Annual Review of Neuroscience*, **18**, 193–221.

Desmond, D. W., Moroney, J. T., Sano, M., and Stern, Y. (1996). Recovery of cognitive function after stroke. *Stroke*, **27**, 1798–803.

Devlin, J. T., Moore, C. J., Mummery, C. J., Gorno-Tempini, M. L., Phillips, J. A., Noppeney, U., Frackowiak, R. S. J., Friston, K. J., and Price, C. J. (2002). Anatomic constraints on cognitive theories of category specificity. *Neuroimage*, **15**, 675–85.

Dewart, H. and Summers, S. (1996). *Pragmatics profile of everyday communication skills in adults*. Windsor: NFER Nelson.

Diamond, A. (1998). Evidence for the importance of dopamine for prefrontal cortex functions early in life. In *The Prefrontal Cortex: Executive and Cognitive Functions* (eds A. C. Roberts, T. W. Robbins and L. Weiskrantz), pp. 117–130. Oxford: Oxford University Press.

Diller, L. and Ben-Yishay, Y. (2003). The clinical utility and cost-effectiveness of comprehensive (holistic) brain injury day-treatment programs. In *Clinical neuropsychology and cost outcome research* (eds G Prigatano and N H Pliskin), pp. 293–312. New York: Psychology Press.

Diller, L. and Gordon, W. A. (1981). Interventions for cognitive deficits in brain-injured adults. *Journal of Consulting and Clinical Psychology*, **49**, 822–34.

Dimitrov, M., Grafman, J., and Hollnagel, C. (1996). The effects of frontal lobe damage on everyday problem solving. *Cortex*, **32**, 357–66.

Dirette, D. and Hinojosa, J. (1999). The effects of a compensatory intervention on processing deficits of adults with acquired brain injuries. *The Occupational Therapy Journal of Research*, **19**(4), 223–40.

Dirette, D. K., Hinojosa, J. and Carnevale, G. J. (1999). Comparison of remedial and compensatory interventions for adults with acquired brain injuries. *Journal of Head Trauma Rehabilitation* **14**, 595–601.

Dixon, R. A. and Bäckman, L. (1999). Principles of compensation in cognitive neurorehabilitation. In *Cognitive Neurorehabilitation* (eds D. T. Stuss, G. Winocur and I. H. Robertson), pp. 59–72. Cambridge: Cambridge University Press.

Dixon, R. A. and Bäckman, L. (1995). *Compensating for psychological deficits and declines*. Manwah, NJ: Lawrence Erlbaum.

Dixon, R. A., de Frias C. M., and Bäckman, L. (2001). Characteristics of self-reported memory compensation in older adults. *Journal of Clinical and Experimental Neuropsychology*, **23**, 650–61.

Dobrossy, M. D., LeMoal, M., Montaron, M. F., and Abrous, N. (2000). Influence of environment on the efficacy of intrastriatal dopaminergic grafts. *Experimental Neurology*, **165**, 172–83.

Dodrill, C. B. (1997). Myths of neuropsychology. *The Clinical Neuropsychologist*, **11**, 1–17.

Dodrill, C. B. (1999). Myths of neuropsychology: Further considerations. *The Clinical Neuropsychologist*, **13**, 562–72.

Doesborgh, S. J. C., van de Sandt-Koenderman, W. M. E., Dippel, D. W. J., van Harskamp, F., Koudstaal, P. J., and Visch-Brink, E. G. (2002). The impact of linguistic deficits on verbal communication. *Aphasiology*, **16**, 413–23.

Donaghy, S. and Williams, W. (1998). A new protocol for training severely impaired patients in the usage of memory journals. *Brain Injury*, **12**(12), 1061–70.

Doody, R. S., Stevens, J. C., Beck, C., Dubinsky, R. M., Kaye, J. A., Gwyther, L., Mohs, R. C., Thal, L. J., Whitehouse, P. J., DeKosky, S. T., and Cummings, J. L. (2001). Practice parameter: management of dementia (an evidence-based review). *Neurology*, **56**, 1154–66.

Douglas, J. M., O'Flaherty, C. A., and Snow, P. C. (2000). Measuring perception of communicative ability: the development and evaluation of the La Trobe communication questionnaire. *Aphasiology*, **14**, 251–68.

Downes, J. J., Sharp, H. M., Costall, B. M., Sagar, H. J., and Howe, J. (1993). Alternating fluency in Parkinson's disease. *Brain*, **116**, 887–902.

Dritschel, B. H. Kogan L., Burton A., Burton E., and Goddard, L. (1998). Everyday planning difficulites following brain injury: a role for autobiographical memory. *Brain Injury*, **12**, 875–86.

Driver, J. (1996). Enhancement of selective listening by illusory mislocation of speech sounds due to lip-reading. *Nature*, **381**, 66–8.

Driver, J. and Halligan, P. W. (1991). Can visual neglect operate in object centred co-ordinates? An affirmative case study. *Cognitive Neuropsychology*, **8**, 475–96.

Driver, J. and Spence, C. J. (1999). Cross-modal links in spatial attention. In *Attention, space and action* (eds G. W. Humphreys, J. Duncan and A. Treisman), pp. 130–49. Oxford: Oxford University Press.

Dromerick, A. W., Edwards, D. F., and Hahn, M. (2000). Does the application of constraint-induced movement therapy during acute rehabilitation reduce arm impairment after ischemic stroke? *Stroke*, **31**, 2984–8.

Dronkers, N. F. (1996). A new brain region for coordinating speech articulation. *Nature*, **384**, 159–61.

Duchan, J. and Black, M. (2001). Progressing towards life goals: A person centred approach to therapy. *Topics in Language Disorders*, **21**, 37–49.

Ducharme, J. M. (1999). A conceptual model for treatment of externalizing behavior in acquired brain injury. *Brain Injury*, **13**, 645–68.

Duncan, J. (1986). Disorganisation of behaviour after frontal lobe damage. *Cognitive Neuropsychology*, **3**, 271–90.

Duncan, J. (1995). Attention, intelligence and the frontal lobes. In *The Cognitive Neurosciences* (ed. M. S. Gazzaniga), pp. 721–733. Cambridge, MA: MIT Press.

Duncan, J. (1999). Converging levels of analysis in the cognitive neurosciences. In *Attention, space and action* (eds G. W. Humphreys, J. Duncan and A. Treisman). Oxford: Oxford University Press.

Duncan, J. and Humphreys, G. W. (1989). Visual search and visual similarity. *Psychological Review*, **96**, 433–58.

Duncan, J. and Humphreys, G. W. (1992). Beyond the search surface: Visual search and attentional engagement theory. *Journal of Experimental Psychology: Human Perception and Performance*, **18**, 578–88.

Duncan, J. and Miller, E. K. (2002). Cognitive focus through adaptive neural coding in the primate prefrontal cortex. In *Principles of Frontal Lobe Function* (eds D. T. Stuss and R. K. Knight), pp. 278–291. New York: Oxford University Press.

Duncan, J., Burgess, P. W., and Emslie, H. (1995). Fluid intelligence after frontal lobe lesions. *Neuropsychologia*, **33**, 261–68.

Duncan, J., Emslie, H., Williams, P., Johnson, R., and Freer, C. (1996). Intelligence and the frontal lobe: The organisation of goal-directed behaviour. *Cognitive Psychology*, **30**, 257–303.

Duncan, J., Johnson, R., Swales, M., and Freer, C. (1997). Frontal lobe deficits after head injury: Unity and diversity of function. *Cognitive Neuropsychology*, **14**, 713–41.

Duncan, J., Seitz, R. J., Kolodny, J., Bor, D., Herzog, H., Ahmed, A., Newell, F. N., and Emslie, H. (2000). A neural basis for intelligence. *Science*, **289**(5478), 457–60.

Dusoir, H., Kapur, N., Byrnes, D. P., McKinstry, S., and Hoare, R. D. (1990). The role of diencephalic pathology in human memory disorder. *Brain*, **113**, 1695–706.

Eakman, A. and Nelson, D. (2001). The effect of hands-on occupation on recall memory in men with traumatic brain injury. *The Occupational Therapy Journal of Research*, **21**(2), 109–114.

Eames, P., Cotterill, G., Kneale, T. A., Storrar, A. L., and Yeomans, P. (1996). Outcome of intensive rehabilitation after severe brain injury: a long-term follow-up study. *Brain Injury*, **10**, 631–50.

Ebbinghaus, H. (1885). *Über das Gedächtnis*. Leipzig: Duncker and Humblot.

Edmans, J., Champion, A., Hill, L., Ridley, M., Skelly F., Jackson, T., and Neale, M. (2000). *Occupational Therapy and Stroke*. London: Whurr Publishers.

Eichenbaum, H. and Cohen, N. J. (2001). Habits, skills, and procedural memory. In *From coditioning to conscious recollection* (eds H. Eichenbaum and N. J. Cohen), pp. 435–70. Oxford: Oxford University Press.

Ellis, A. W. and Young, A. W. (1988). *Human cognitive neuropsychology*. London: Lawrence Erlbaum Associates.

Ellis, H. and Young, A. (1988). Training in face-processing skills for a child with acquired prosopagnosia. *Developmental Neuropsychology*, **4**, 283–94.

Elman, R. (1999). *Group treatment of neurogenic communication disorders: The expert clinician's approach*. Woburn: Butterworth-Heinemann.

Elman R. and Bernstein-Ellis E. (1999). The efficacy of group communication treatment in adults with chronic aphasia. *Journal of Speech, Language and Hearing Research*, **42**, 411–19.

Enderby, P. and Crow, E. (1996). Frenchay aphasia screening test: Validity and comparability. *Disability and Rehabilitation*, **18**, 238–40.

Enderby, P. and John, A. (1997). *Therapy outcome measures for speech and language pathology*. SanDiego, CA: Singular Publishing Group.

Enderby, P., Wood, V., Wade, D., and Langton Hewer, R. (1987). The Frenchay Aphasia Screening Test: A short simple test appropriate for nonspecialists. *Int. J. Rehab med*, **8**, 166–70.

Engel, G. L. (1977). The need for a new medical model: a challenge for biomedicine. *Science* **196**, 129–36.

Engelberts, N. H., Klein, M., Ader, H. J., Heimans, J. J., Trenite, D. G., and van der Ploeg, H. M. (2002). The effectiveness of cognitive rehabilitation for attention deficits in focal seizures: a randomized controlled study. *Epilepsia*, **43**, 587–95.

Eriksson, P. S., Perfilieva, E., Bjork-Eriksson, T., Alborn, A. M., Nordborg, C., Peterson, D. A., and Gage, F. H. (1998). Neurogenesis in the adult human hippocampus. *Nature Medicine*, **4**(11), 1313–17.

Eslinger, P. J. and Damasio, A. R. (1985). Severe disturbance of higher cognition after bilateral frontal lobe ablation: patient EVR. *Neurology*, **35**, 1731–41.

Eslinger, P. J. and Grattan, L. M. (1993). Frontal lobe and frontal-striatal substrates for different forms of human cognitive flexibility. *Neuropsychologia*, **31**, 17–28.

Evans, J. J. (2001). Rehabilitation of the Dysexecutive Syndrome. In *Neurobehavioural disability and social handicap following traumatic brain injury* (eds R. Ll. Wood and T. M. McMillan), pp. 209–27. Hove: Psychology Press.

Evans, J. J. (2003). Rehabilitation of executive deficits. In *Neuropsychological Rehabilitation: Theory and Practice* (ed. B. A. Wilson). Lisse: Swets and Zeitlinger.

Evans, J. J., Emslie, H., and Wilson, B. A. (1998). External cueing systems in the rehabilitation of executive impairments of action. *Journal of the International Neuropsychological Society*, **4**, 399–408.

Evans, J., Wilson, B. A., Needham, P., and Brentnall, S. (2003). Who makes good use of memory aids? Results of a survey of people with acquired brain injury. *Journal of the International Neuropsychological Society*, **9**, 925–35.

Evans, J. J., Wilson, B. A., Schuri, U., rade, J., Baddeley, A., Bruna, O., Canavan, T., Della Sala, S., Green, R., Laaksonen, R., Lorenzi, L., and Taussik, I. (2000). A comparison of "errorless" and "trial-and-error" learning methods for teaching individuals with acquired memory deficits. *Neuropsychological Rehabilitation*, **10**, 67–101.

Everitt, B. (1995). *Cambridge dictionary of statistics in the medical sciences*. Cambridge: Cambridge University Press.

Eysenck, M. (1982). *Attention and arousal: Cognition and performance*. New York: Springer.

Ezrachi, O., Ben-Yishay, Y., Kay T., Diller L. and Rattok, J. (1991). Predicting employment in traumatic brain injury following neuropsychological rehabilitation. *Journal of Head Trauma Rehabilitation*, **6**(3), 71–84.

Fabiano, R. J. and Crewe, N. (1995). Variables associated with employment following severe traumatic brain injury. *Rehabilitation Psychology*, **40**(3), 223–31.

Farah, M. J., Wong, A. B., Monheit, M. A., and Morrow, L. A. (1989). Parietal lobe mechanisms of spatial attention: modality specific or supra-modal? *Neuropsychologia*, **27**, 461–70.

Fasotti, L., Kovacs, F., Eling, P. A. T. M., and Brouwer, W. H. (2000). Time pressure management as a compensatory strategy training after closed head injury. *Neuropsychological Rehabilitation*, **10**, 47–65.

Ferguson, A. (1994). The influence of aphasia, familiarity and activity on conversational repair. *Aphasiology*, **8**, 143–57.

Ferguson, A. (2002). Information exchange in conversational interaction: the development of replicable sampling and measurement methods. Paper presented at the 10th International Aphasia Rehabilitation Conference, Brisbane, Australia.

Fillingham, J. K., Hodgson, C., Sage, K., and Lambon Ralph, M. A. (2003). The application of errorless learning to aphasic disorders: A review of theory and practice. *Neuropsychological Rehabilitation*, **13**(3), 337–63.

Finger, S. (1994). *Origins of neuroscience: A history of exploration into brain function*. New York: Oxford University Press.

Fink, G. R., Markowitsch, H. J., Reinkemeier, M., Bruckbauer, T., Kessler, J., and Heiss, W.-D. (1996). A PET-study of autobiographical memory recognition. *Journal of Neuroscience*, **16**, 4275–82.

Finlayson, M. A. and Garner, S. G. (1994). *Brain injury rehabilitation: Clinical considerations*. Baltimore: Williams and Wilkins.

Fischer, J. S., Priore, R. L., Jacobs, L. D., Cookfair, D. L., Rudik, R. A., Herndon, R. M., Richert J. R. *et al*. (2000). Neuropsychological effects of interferon beta-1a in relapsing multiple sclerosis. *Annals of Neurology*, **48**, 885–92.

Fletcher, P. C., Shallice, T., and Dolan, R. J. (1998). The functional roles of prefrontal cortex in episodic memory. I. Encoding. *Brain*, **121**, 1239–48.

Fluharty, G. and Glassman, N. (2001). Use of antecedent control to improve the outcome of rehabilitation for a client with frontal lobe injury and intolerance for auditory and tactile stimuli. *Brain Injury*, **15**, 995–1002.

Fodor, J. (1983). *Modularity of mind*. Cambridge, MA: MIT Press.

Forde, E. M. E. and Humphreys, G. W. (2002). The cognitive neuropsychology of everyday actions. *Neurocase*, **8**, 59–60.

Forer, S. (1990). *Functional Assessment measures – revised*. Santa Clara, CA: Santa Clara Medical Center.

Foundas, A. L., Macauley, B. L., Raymer, A. M., Maher, L. M., Heilman, K. M., and Gonzalez Rothi, L. J. (1995). Ecological implications of limb apraxia: Evidence from mealtime behavior. *Journal of the International Neuropsychological Society*, **1**, 62–6.

Franklin, S. (1989). Dissociations in auditory word comprehension: evidence from nine 'fluent' aphasic patients. *Aphasiology*, **3**, 189–207.

Franklin, S., Howard, D., and Patterson, K. (1994). Abstract word meaning deafness. *Cognitive Neuropsychology*, **11**, 1–34.

Franz, S. I. (1924). Studies in re-education. The aphasias. *Comparative Psychology*, 4 (4), 349–429.

Franz, S. I. and Lashley, K. S. (1917). The retention of habits by the rat after destruction of the frontal portion of the cerebrum. *Psychobiology*, **1**, 3–18.

Fraser, R., Dikmen, S., McLean, A., Miller, B. and Temkin, N. (1988). Employability of head injury survivors: First year post-injury. *Rehabilitation Counseling Bulletin*, **31**, 276–88.

Frassinetti, F., Angeli, V., Meneghello, F., Avanzi, S., and Ladavas, E. (2002). Long-lasting amelioration of visuospatial neglect by prism adaptation. *Brain*, **125**, 608–23.

Frattali, C. (1992). Functional assessment of communication: merging public policy with clinical views. *Aphasiology*, **6**, 63–83.

Frattali, C., Thompson, C. K., Holland, A. L., Wohl, C. B., and Ferketic, M. K. (1995). *American Speech-Language Hearing Association functional assessment of communication skills for adults*. (ASHA FACS) Rockville, MD: American Speech-Language-Hearing Association.

Freud, S. (1891). *Zur Auffassung der Aphasien*. Vienna; Deuticke. Translated by E. Stengel (1953). *On aphasia*. New York: International Universities Press.

Fujii, T., Okuda, J., Tsukiura, T. *et al*. (2002). The role of basal forebrain in episodic memory retrieval: a positron emission tomography study. *NeuroImage*, **15**, 501–8.

Fuster, J. M. (1997). *The Prefrontal Cortex: Anatomy, Physiology and Neuropsychology of the Frontal Lobe*. Philadelphia, PA: Lippincott-Raven.

Fuster, J. M. (2002). Physiology of executive functions: The perception-action cycle. In *Principles of Frontal Lobe Function* (eds D. T. Stuss and R. K. Knight), pp. 96–108. New York: Oxford University Press.

Gade, A. (1994). Imagery as a mnemonic aid in amnesia patients: Effects of amnesia subtype and severity. In *Cognitive neuropsychology and cognitive rehabilitation* (eds M. J. Riddoch and G. W. Humphreys), pp. 571–89. Hillsdale, NJ: Lawrence Erlbaum Associates.

Gagné, R. M. (1965). *The conditions of learning*. New York: Holt, Rinehart and Winston.

Gainotti, G. (1993). Emotional and psychosocial problems after brain injury. *Neuropsychological Rehabilitation*, **3**, 259–77.

Galaburda, A. M. (1985): Norman Geschwind: 1926–1984. *Neuropsychologia*, **23**, 297–304.

Gamper, E. (1929). Schlaf – Delirium tremens – Korsakowsches Syndrom. *Zentralbaltt für Neurologie*, **51**, 236–9.

Garrard, P., and Hodges, J. R. (2000). Semantic dementia: clinical, radiological and pathological perspectives. *Journal of Neurology*, **247**, 409–22.

Garrett, K. and Huth, C. (2002). The impact of graphic contextual information and instruction on the conversational behaviours of a person with severe aphasia. *Aphasiology*, **16**, 523–36.

Gatz, M., Fiske, A., Fox, L., Kaskie, B., Kasl-Godley, J. E., McCallum, T. J., and Wetherell, J. L. (1998). Empirically validated psychological treatments for older adults. *Journal of Mental Health and Aging*, **4**, 9–45.

Gazzaniga, M. S. (ed.) (2000). *The new cognitive neurosciences*. Cambridge, MA: MIT Press.

Geschwind, N. (1979). Specializations of the human brain, *The Brain*. San Francisco: W.H. Freeman.

Geshwind, N. (1985). Mechanisms of change after brain lesions. In *Hope for a new neurology* (ed. F. Nottebohm). New York: New York Academy of Sciences, 4–11.

Getzels, J. W. and Jackson, P. W. (1961). *Creativity and intelligence*. New York: Wiley.

Gianutsos, R. (1989). Foreword to *Introduction to cognitive rehabilitation*. In *Introduction to cognitive rehabilitation: Theory and practice* (eds M. Sohlberg and C. Mateer), pp. vii–viii. New York: Guilford Press.

Gianutsos, R. and Gianutsos, J. (1979). Rehabilitating the verbal recall of brain injured patients by mnemonic training: An experimental demonstration using single case methodology. *Journal of Clinical Neuropsychology*, **1**, 117–35.

Giles, G. M. and Clark-Wilson, J. (1999). Functional skills training following severe brain injury. In *Rehabilitation of the severely injured adult: a practical approach* (eds G. M. Giles and J. Clark-Wilson), 2nd edn, pp. 97–134. Cheltenham: Stanley Thornes.

Gillen, R., Tennen, H., McKee, T. E., Gernert-Dott, P., and Affleck, G. (2001). Depressive symptoms and history of depression predict rehabiliation efficiency in stroke patients. *Archives of Physical Medicine and Rehabilitation*, **82**, 1645–49.

Girard, D., Brown, J., Burnett-Stolnack, M., *et al.* (1996). The relationship of neuropsychological status and productive outcomes following traumatic brain injury. *Brain Injury*, **10**(9), 663–76.

Giraud, A. L. and Price, C. J. (2001). The constraints functional neuroimaging places on classical models of auditory word processing. *Journal of Cognitive Neuroscience*, **13**, 754–65.

Glang, A., Singer, G., Cooley, E., and Tish, N. (1992). Tailoring direct instruction techniques for use with elementary students with brain injury. *Journal of Head Trauma Rehabilitation*, **7**(4), 93–108.

Glasgow, R. E., Zeiss, R. A., Barrera, M., and Lewinsohn, P. M. (1977). Case studies on remediating memory deficits in brain damaged individuals. *Journal of Clinical Psychology*, **33**,1049–54.

Glenn, M. B., Yablon, S. A., Whyte, J., and Zafonte, R. (2001). Letter to the editor. *Journal of Head Trauma Rehabilitation*, **16**, vii–viii.

Glisky, E. L. (1998). Differential contribution of frontal and medial temporal lobes to memory: evidence from focal lesions and normal aging. In *The Other Side of the Error Term* (ed. N. Raz). Amsterdam: Elsevier.

Glisky, E. L. and Glisky, M. L. (2002). Learning and memory impairments. In *Neuropsychological Interventions* (ed. P. J. Eslinger), pp. 137–62. New York: Guildford Press.

Glisky, E. L. and Schacter, D. L. (1986). Long-term retention of computer learning by patients with memory disorders. *Neuropsychologia*, **26**, 173–8.

Glisky, E. L. and Schacter, D. L. (1989). Models and methods of memory rehabilitation. In *Handbook of neuropsychology* (eds F. Boller and J. Grafman), Vol. 3. Amsterdam: Elsevier Publications.

Glisky, E. L., Schacter, D. L., and Tulving, E. (1986). Learning and retention of computer-related vocabulary in memory impaired patients: method of vanishing cues. *Journal of Clinical and Experimental Neuropsychology,* **8***,* 292–312.

Glisky, E. L., Schacater, D. L., and Tulving, E. (1986). Computer learning by momory-impaired patients: Acquisition and retention of complex knowledge. *Neuropsychologia,* **24***,* 313–28.

Gloning, K., Trappl, R., Heiss, W. D., and Quatember, R. (1976). Prognosis and speech therapy in aphasia. In *Recovery in aphasics* (eds Y. Lebrun and R. Hoops), pp. 57–62. Atlantic Highlands NJ: Humanities Press.

Godfrey, H. P. D. and Knight, R. G. (1985). Cognitive rehabilitation of memory functioning in amnesiac alcoholics. *Journal of Consulting and Clinical Psychology,* **53***,* 555–7.

Goel, V. and Grafman, J. (1995). Are the frontal lobes implicated in 'planning' functions? Interpreting data from the Tower of Hanoi. *Neuropsychologia,* **33***,* 623–42.

Goel, V. and Grafman, J. (2000). Role of the right prefrontal cortex in ill-structured planning. *Cognitive Neuropsychology,* **17***,* 415–36.

Goel, V., Grafman, J., Tajik, J., Gana, S., and Danto, D. (1997). A study of the performance of patients with frontal lobe lesions in a financial planning task. *Brain,* **120***,* 1805–22.

Goldberg, E. (2001). *The executive brain. Frontal lobes and the civilized mind.* New York: Oxford University Press.

Golding, E. (1989). *The Middlesex Elderly Assessment of Mental State.* Bury St Edmunds: Thames Valley Test Company.

Goldman-Rakic, P. S. (1995). Architecture of the prefrontal cortex and the central executive. *Annals of the New York Academy of Science,* **769***,* 212–20.

Goldman-Rakic, P. S. (1998). The prefrontal landscape: implications of functional architecture for understanding human mentation and the central executive. In *The Prefrontal Cortex: Executive and Cognitive Functions* (eds A. C. Roberts, T. W. Robbins and L. Weiskrantz), pp. 87–102. Oxford: Oxford University Press.

Goldman-Rakic, P. (2000). Localization of function all over again. *NeuroImage,* **11***,* 451–7.

Goldman-Rakic, P. S., Scalaidhe S. P. O., and Chafee, M. V. (2000). Domain specificity in cognitive systems. In *The new cognitive neurosciences* (ed. M. S. Gazzaniga), 2nd edn, pp. 733–42. Cambridge, MA: MIT Press.

Goldstein, K. (1942). *Aftereffects of brain injuries in war.* New York: Grune and Stratton.

Goldstein, L. B. (1998). Potential effects of common drugs on stroke recovery. *Archives of Neurology* **55***,* 454–6.

Goldstein, L. B., Matchar, D. B., Morgandlander, J. C., and Davis, J. C. (1990). The influence of drugs on the recovery of sensorimotor function after stroke. *Journal of Neurological Rehabilitation,* **4***,* 137–44.

Goldstein, G., McCue, M., Turner, S., Spainer, C., Malec, E., and Shelly, C. (1988). An efficacy study of memory training for persons with closed-head injury. *Clinical Neuropsychology,* **2***,* 251–59.

Goodglass, H. (1990). Cognitive psychology and clinical aphasiology: Commentary. *Aphasiology,* **4***,* 93–5.

Goodglass, H., and Kaplan, E. (1983). *The assessment of aphasia and related disorders.* Philadelphia, PA: Lea and Febiger.

Goodglass, H., and Kaplan, E. (1983). *Boston diagnostic aphasia examination,* 2nd edn. Philadelphia: Lea and Febiger.

Goodglass, H., and Kaplan, E. (1983). *Boston Naming Test.* Philadelphia, PA: Lea and Febiger.

Goodglass, H., Kaplan, E., and Barresi, B. (2001). The Boston Diagnostic Aphasia Examination. 3rd edn. Philadelphia: Lippincott Williams and Wilkins.

Gordon, W. A. (1990). Cognitive remediation: an approach to the amelioration of behavioral disorders. In *Neurobehavioural sequelae of traumatic brain injury* (ed. R. Ll. Wood), pp. 175–93. London: Taylor and Francis.

Gould, E., Beylin, A., Tanapat, P., Reeves, A., and Shors, T. J. (1999). Learning enhances adult neurogenesis in the hippocampal formation. *Nature Neuroscience,* **2***,* 260–5.

Grace, J. and Malloy, P. F. (2001). *Frontal Systems Behavior Scale. Professional manual.* Lutz, FL: Psychological Assessment Resources, Inc.

Grace, J., Nadler, J. D., White, D. A., Guilmette A. J., Monsch A. U., and Snow, M. G. (1995). Folstein vs. modified mini-mental state examination in geriatric stroke: stability, validity and screening utility. *Archives of Neurology,* **52***,* 477–84.

Grace, J., Stout, J. C., and Malloy, P. F. (1999). Assessing frontal lobe behavioral syndromes with the Frontal Lobe Personality Scale. *Assessment,* **6,** 269–84.

Grafman, J. (2002). The structured event complex and the human prefrontal cortex. In *Principles of Frontal Lobe Function* (eds D. T. Stuss and R. K. Knight), pp. 292–310. New York: Oxford University Press.

Graham, I. D., Calder, L. A., Hebert, P. C., Carter, A. P., and Tetro, J. M. (2000). A comparison of clinical practice guideline appraisal instruments. *International Journal of Assessment of Health Care* **16,** 1024–38.

Granger, C. V. and Hamilton, B. B. (1987). *Uniform data set or medical rehabiltation.* Buffalo: Research Foundation, State University of New York.

Grant, D. A. and Berg, E. A. (1948). A behavioural analysis of degree of reinforcement and ease of shifting to new responses in a Weigl-type card-sorting problem. *Journal of Experimental Psychology,* **38,** 404–11.

Gray, D. B. and Hendershot, G. E. (2000). The ICIDH-2: developments for a new era of outcomes research. *Archives of Physical Medicine and Rehabilitation,* **81,** (Suppl. 2) S10–14.

Gray, J. M., Robertson, I., Pentland, B., Anderson, S. (1992). Microcomputer-based attentional retraining after brain damage: A randomized group controlled trial. *Neuropsychological Rehabilitation,* **2,** 97–115.

Grealy, M., Johnson D., and Rushton, S. (1999). Improving cognitive function after brain injury: the use of exercise and virtual reality. *Archives of Physical Medicine and Rehabilitation,* **80,** 661–67.

Green, P. and Astner, K. (1995). *The Word memory Test.* Edmonton: Neurobehavioural Associates.

Green, P., Allen, L., and Astner, K. (1996). *Manual for Computerized Word memory Test.* Durham, NC: Cognisyst.

Green, S. M., Rich, J. B., and Park, N. W. (2003). *Moderators of verbal cueing effects on novel naturalistic actions in stroke.* Paper presented at the Thirty-first Annual Meeting of the International Neuropsychological Society, Honolulu, Hawaii.

Greene, J. D. W., Hodges, J. R., and Baddeley, A. D. (1995). Autobiographical memory and executive function in early dementia of Alzheimer type. *Neuropsychologia,* **33,** 1647–70.

Greener, J., Enderby, P., and Whurr, R. (1999). Speech and language therapy for aphasia following stroke (Cochrane review). In *The Cochrane Library,* Issue 4. Oxford: Update software.

Greener, J., Enderby, P., Whurr, R., and Grant, A. (1998). Treatment for aphasia following stroke: evidence for effectiveness. *International Journal of Language and Communication Disorders,* **33,** 158–161.

Grodzinsky, Y. (2000). The neurology of syntax: Language use without Broca's area. *Behavioral and Brain Sciences,* **23,** 1–21.

Gronwall, D. and Sampson, H. (1974). *The psychological effects of concussion.* Auckland: Auckland University Press.

Guariglia, C. and Antonucci, G. (1992). Personal and extrapersonal space: a case of neglect dissociation. *Neuropsychologia,* **30,** 1001–9.

Gudden, B. von (1886). Ueber die Frage der Localisation der Functionen der Grosshirnrinde [On the question of localization of functions in the brain]. *Allgemeine Zeitschrift für Psychiatrie und ihre Grenzgebiete,* **42,** 478–99.

Hagen, C. (1973). Communication abilities in hemiplegia: effect of speech therapy. *Archives of Physical Medicine and Rehabilitation,* **54,** 454–63.

Haggard, P., Cockburn, J., Cock, J., Fordham, C., and Wade, D. (2000). Interference between gait and cognitive tasks in a rehabilitating neurological population. *Journal of Neurology, Neurosurgery and Psychiatry,* **69,** 479–86.

Hall, K. M. and Cope, D. N. (1995). The benefit of rehabilitation in traumatic brain injury: A literature review. *Journal of Head Trauma Rehabilitation,* **10,** 1–13.

Hall, C. S. and Lindzey, C. (1978). *Theories of personality,* 3rd edn. New York: John Wiley and Sons.

Halliday, M. A. K. (1994). *Introduction to functional grammar.* London: Edward Arnold.

Hameroff, S. R. (1998). 'Funda-mentality': is the conscious mind subtly linked to a basic level of the universe? *Trends in Cognitive Sciences,* **2,** 119–27.

Hamm, R. J., Temple, M. D., Buck, D. L., Deford, S. M., and Floyd, C. L. (2000). Cognitive recovery from traumatic brain injury: Results of post traumatic experimental interventions. In *Cerebral reorganization of function after brain damage* (eds H. S. Levin and J. Grafman), pp. 49–67. Oxford: Oxford University Press.

Hanks, R. A., Rapport, L. J., Millis, S. R., and Deshpande, S. A. (1999). Measures of executive functioning as predictors of functional ability and social integration in a rehabilitation sample. *Archives of Physical Medicine and Rehabilitation*, **80**, 1030–7.

Hanson, W. R., Metter, J. F., and Riege, W. H. (1989). The course of chronic aphasia. *Aphasiology* **3**, 19–29.

Hart, J. Berndt, R., and Caramazza, A. (1985). Category-specific naming deficit following cerebral infarction. *Nature*, **316**, 338.

Hartman, J. and Landau, W. M. (1987). Comparison of formal language therapy with supportive counseling for aphasia due to acute vascular accident. *Archives of Neurology*, **24**, 646–9.

Haut, M. W., Franzen, M. D., and Rogers, M. J. C. (1992). Assessment of Memory. *Physical Medicine and Rehabilitation*, **6**, 451–66.

Hayden, M. E., Moreault, A., LeBlanc, J., and Plenger, P. M. (2000). Reducing level of handicap in traumatic brain injury: an environmentally based model of treatment. *Journal of Head Trauma and Rehabilitation*, **15**, 1000–21.

Head, H. (1926). *Aphasia and kindred disorders of speech.* Cambridge: Cambridge University Press.

Heald, A., Bates, D., Cartlidge, N. E. F., French, J. M., and Miller, S. (1993). Longitudinal study of central motor conduction time following stroke: 2 – Central motor conduction measured within 72 h after stroke as a predictor of functional outcome at 12 months. *Brain*, **116**, 1371–85.

Heaton, R. K. (1981). *Wisconsin Card Sorting Test manual.* Odessa, FL: Psychological Assessment Resources, Inc.

Hebb, D. O. (1949). *The organization of behavior: A neuropsychological theory.* New York: Wiley.

Hedges, L. V. (1982). Estimate of effect size from a series of independent experiments. *Psychological Bulletin*, **92**, 490–9.

Hedges, L. V. (1994). Fixed effects models. In *The handbook of research synthesis* (eds H. Cooper and L. V. Hedges), pp. 285–99. New York: Russell Sage Foundation.

Hedges, L. V. and Olkin, I. (1985). *Statistical methods for meta-analysis.* New York: Academic Press.

Heilman, K. M., Rothi, L. J., and Valenstein, E. (1982). Two forms of ideomotor apraxia. *Neurology*, **32**, 342–6.

Heilman, K. M., Watson, R. T., and Valenstein, E. (1985). Neglect and related disorders. In *Clinical neuropsychology.* New York: Oxford University Press.

Heilman, K. M., Watson, R. T., Valenstein, E., and Goldberg, M. E. (1987). Attention: Behavioral and neural mechanisms. In *Handbook of physiology, Section 1: The nervous system* (ed. F. Plum), Vol. 5, pp. 461–481. Bethesda, MD: American Physiological Society.

Heindel, W. C., Salmon, D. P., Shults, C. W., Walicke, P. A., and Butters, N. (1989). Neuropsychological evidence for multiple implicit memory systems: a comparison of Alzheimer's, Huntington's, and Parkinson's disease patients. *Journal of Neuroscience*, **9**, 582–7.

Heinemann, A. W. (1989). *Rehabilitation Institute of Chicago Functional Assessment Scale – Revised.* Chicago, IL: Rehabilitation Institute of Chicago.

Heinrichs, R. W., Levitt, H., Arthurs, A., Gallardo, C., Hirscheimer, K., MacNeil, M., Olshansky, E., and Richards, K. (1992). Learning and retention of a daily activity schedule in a patient with alcoholic Korsakoff's syndrome. *Neuropsychological Rehabilitation*, **2**, 43–58.

Heiss, W. D., Karbe, H., Weber-Luxenburger, G. *et al.* (1997). Speech-induced cerebral metabolic activation reflects recovery from aphasia. *Journal of Neuroscience*, **145**, 213–17.

Heiss, W. D., Kessler, J., Thiel, A. *et al.* (1999). Differential capacity of left and right hemispheric areas for compensation of poststroke aphasia. *Annals of Neurology*, **45**, 430–38.

Heiss, W.-D., Kessler, J., Mielke, R., Szelies, B., and Herholz, K. (1994). Long-term effects of phosphatidylserine, pyritinol and cognitive training in Alzheimer's disease. *Dementia*, **5**, 88–98.

Helfenstein, D. and Wechsier, R. (1982). The use of interpersonal process recall (IPR) in the remediation of interpersonal and communication skill deficits in the newly brain injured. *Clinical Neuropsychologist*, **4**, 139–43.

Henry, J. D. and Crawford, J. R. (2004a). A meta-analytic review of verbal fluency performance following focal cortical lesions. *Neuropsychology*, **18**, 284–95.

Henry, J. D. and Crawford, J. R. (2004b). A meta-analytic review of verbal fluency performance following traumatic brain injury. *Neuropsychology*, **18**, 621–8.

Henry, J. D. and Crawford, J. R. (2004c). Verbal fluency deficits in Parkinson's disease: A meta-analysis. *Journal of the International Neuropsychological Society,* **10**, 608–23.

Henry, J. D. and Crawford, J. R. (2005a). A meta-analytic review of verbal fluency deficits in depression. *Journal of Clinical and Experimental Neuropsychology,* **27**, 1–24.

Henry, J. D. and Crawford, J. R. (2005b). A meta-analytic review of verbal fluency deficits in schizophrenia relative to other neurocognitive deficits. *Cognitive Neuropsychiatry,* **10**, 1–33.

Henry, J. D., Crawford, J. R., and Phillips, L. H. (2004). Verbal fluency performance in dementia of the Alzheimer's type: A meta-analysis. *Neuropsychologia,* **42**, 1212–22.

Henry, J. D., Crawford, J. R., and Phillips, L. H. (in press). A meta-analytic review of verbal fluency deficits in Huntington's disease. *Neuropsychology.*

Herbert, R., Best, W., Hickin, J., Howard, D., and Osborne, F. (2004). Measuring lexical retrieval in aphasic conversation: Reliability of a quantitative approach. *Manuscript in preparation.*

Hering, E. (1870). *Ueber das Gedächtnis als eine allgemeine Funktion der organisierten Materie. Vortrag gehalten in der feierlichen Sitzung der Kaiserlichen Akademie der Wissenschaften in Wien am XXX. Mai MDCCCLXX.* Leipzig: Akademische Verlagsgesellschaft.

Herlitz, A. and Viitanen, M. (1991). Semantic organisation and verbal episodic memory in patients with mild and moderate Alzheimer's disease. *Journal of Clinical and Experimental Neuropsychology,* **13**, 559–74.

Hersch, N. and Treadgold, L. (1994). NeuroPage: The rehabilitation of memory dysfunction by prosthetic memory and cueing. *NeuroRehabilitation,* **4**, 187–97.

Heruti, R. J., Lusky, A., Dankner, R. *et al.* (2002). Rehabilitation outcome of elderly patients after a first stroke: effect of cognitive status at admission on the functional outcome *Arch Phys Med Rehabil,* **83**, 742–49.

Hesse, S., Bertelt, C., Jahnke, M. T., Schaffrin, A., Baake, P., Malezie, M., and Mauritz, K. H. (1995). Treadmill training with partial body weight support compared with physiotherapy in nonambulatory hemiparetic patients. *Stroke,* **26**, 976–81.

Hewitt, J., Evans, J. J., and Dritchel, B. (2000). Improving planning skills in people with traumatic brain injury through the use of an autobiographical episodic memory cueing procedure. Paper presented at the Autumn Meeting of the British Neuropsychological Society, 23 November, Nottingham, UK.

Hickin, J., Herbert, R., Best, W., Howard, D., and Osborne, F. (in press). Efficacy of treatment: effects on word retrieval and conversation. In *The aphasia therapy file* (eds S. Byng, K. Swinburn and C. Pound), Hove: Psychology Press.

Hickox, A. and Sunderland, A. (1992). Questionnaire and checklist approaches to assessment of everyday memory problems. In *A Handbook of Neuropsychological Assessment* (eds J. R. Crawford, D. M. Parker *et al.*). Hillsdale, NJ: Lawrence Erlbaum Associates.

High, W. M., Jr, Boake, C., and Lehmkuhl, L. D. (1995). Critical analysis of studies evaluating the effectiveness of rehabilitation after traumatic brain injury. *Journal of Head Trauma Rehabilitation,* **10**, 14–26.

Hilari, K. and Byng, S. (2001). Measuring quality of life in people with aphasia: the stroke specific quality of life scale. *International Journal of Language and Communication Disorders,* **36**, (Suppl.), 86–91.

Hilari, K., Wiggins, R. D., Roy, P., Byng, S., and Smith, S. C. (2003a). Predictors of health-related quality of life (HRQL) in people with chronic aphasia, *Aphasiology,* **17**, 365–81.

Hilari, K., Byng, S., Lamping, D. L., and Smith, S. C. (2003b). Stroke and Aphasia Quality of Life Scale-39 (SAQOL-39): Evaluation of acceptability, reliability and validity. *Stroke,* **34**, 1944–50.

Hill, R. D., Evankovich, K. D., Sheikh, J. I., and Yesavage, J. A. (1987). Imagery mnemonic training in a patient with primary degenerative dementia. *Psychology and Aging,* **2**, 204–5.

Hillis, A. E. (1993). The role of models of language processing in rehabilitation of language impairments. *Aphasiology,* **7**, 5–26.

Hillis, A. E. (1994). Contributions from cognitive analyses. In *Language intervention strategies in adult aphasia* (ed. R. Chapey), 3rd edn, pp. 207–19. Baltimore, MD: Williams and Wilkins.

Hillis, A. E. (1998). Treatment of naming disorders: new issues regarding old therapies. *Journal of the International Neuropsychological Society,* **4**, 648–60.

Hillis, A. E. (2002). *Adult language disorders: integration of cognitive neuropsychology, neurology, and rehabilitation.* New York: Psychology Press.

Hillis, A. (2002). *The handbook of adult language disorders.* New York: Psychology Press.

Hillis, A. E. and Caramazza, A. (1995). Converging evidence for the interaction of semantic and sublexical phonological information in accessing lexical representations for spoken output. *Cognitive Neuropsychology,* 12, 187–227.

Hillis, A. E. and Caramazza, A. (1995). 'I know it but I can't write it': Selective deficits in long and short-term memory. In *Broken memories: neuropsychological case studies* (ed. R. Campbell), pp. 344–65. Oxford: Blackwell Publishing.

Hillis, A. E. and Heidler, J. (2002). Mechanisms of early aphasia recovery: evidence from MR perfusion imaging. *Aphasiology,* 16, 885–96.

Hillis, A., Rapp, B., Romani, C., and Caramazza, A. (1990). Selective impairment of semantics in lexical processing. *Cognitive Neuropsychology,* 7, 191–243.

Hillis, A. E., Work, M., Barker, P. B., Jacobs, M. A., Breese, E. L., and Maurer, K. (2004). Re-examining the brain regions crucial for orchestrating speech articulation. *Brain,* 127, 1479–87.

Hinckley, J. J., Patterson, J. P., and Carr, T. H. (2001). Differential effects of context- and skill-based treatment approaches: Preliminary findings. *Aphasiology,* 15, 463–76.

Hinton, G. E., McClelland, J. L., and Rumelhart, D. E. (1990). Distributed representations. In *Philosophy of artificial intelligence* (ed. M. Boden), pp. 248–80. Oxford: Oxford University Press.

Hodges, J. R. and Patterson, K. (1995). Is semantic memory consistently impaired early in the course of Alzheimer's disease? Neuroanatomical and diagnostic implications. *Neuropsychologia,* 33, 441–59.

Hodges, J. R., Patterson, K., Oxbury, S., and Funnell, E. (1992). Semantic dementia – progressive fluent aphasia with temporal-lobe atrophy. *Brain,* 115, 1783–806.

Hoen B., Thelander, M., and Worsley, J. (1997). Improvement in psychological well-being of people with aphasia and their families: evaluation of a community based programme. *Aphasiology,* 11, 681–91.

Holland, A.L. (1980). *Communicative abilities in daily living.* Baltimore, MD: University of Press

Holland, A. (1991). Pragmatic aspects of intervention in aphasia. *Journal of Neurolinguistics,* 6, 197–211.

Holland, A. L. (1998). Functional outcome assessment of aphasia following left hemisphere stroke. *Seminars in Speech and Language,* 19, 249–59.

Holland, A. L., Frattali, C. M., and Fromm, D. (1998). *Communication activities of daily living,* 2nd edn. Austin, TX: Pro Ed.

Holland, A. L., Fromm, D. S., DeRuyter, F., and Stein, M. (1996). Treatment efficacy: aphasia. *Journal of Speech and Hearing Research,* 39, S27–S36.

Hopper, T., Holland, A., and Rewega, M. (2002). Conversational coaching: treatment outcomes and future directions. *Aphasiology,* 16, 745–62.

Horwitz, R. I., Viscoli, C. M., Clemens, J. D., and Sadock, R. T. (1990). Developing improved observational methods for evaluating therapeutic effectiveness. *American Journal of Medicine* 89, 630–8.

Howard, D. (1986). Beyond randomised controlled trials: the case for effective case studies of the effects of treatment in aphasia. *The British Journal of Disorders of Communication,* 21, 89–102.

Howard, D. (1995). Lexical anomia – or the case of the missing lexical entries. *Quarterly Journal of Experimental Psychology Section A – Human Experimental Psychology,* 48, 999–1023.

Howard, D. (1997). Language in the human brain. In *Cognitive neuroscience* (ed. M. D. Rugg), pp. 277–304. Hove: Psychology Press.

Howard, D. (2000). Cognitive neuropsychology and aphasia therapy: the case of word retrieval. In *Acquired neurogenic communication disorders: A clinical perspective* (ed. I. Papathanasiou), pp. 76–99. London: Whurr.

Howard, D. and Franklin, S. E. (1988). *Missing the meaning?* Cambridge, MA: M.I.T. Press.

Howard, D. and Hatfield, F. M. (1987). *Aphasia therapy; historical and contemporary issues.* London; Lawrence Erlbaum Associates.

Howard, D. and Orchard-Lisle, V. M. (1984). On the origin of semantic errors in naming; evidence from the case of a global aphasic. *Cognitive Neuropsychology,* 1, 163–90.

Howard, D. and Patterson, K. E. (1992). *The Pyramids and Palm Trees Test.* Bury St Edmunds: Thames Valley Test Company.

Howard, D. and Smith, K. (2002). The effects of lexical stress in aphasic word production. *Aphasiology,* 16, 198–237.

Howard, D., Patterson, K. E., Franklin, S., Morton, J., and Orchard-Lisle, V. M. (1984). Variability and consistency in picture naming by aphasic patients. In *Advances in neurology, 42: progress in aphasiology* (ed. F. C. Rose). New York: Raven Press.

Howard, D., Patterson, K., Wise, R., Brown, W. D., Friston, K., Weiller, C., and Frackowiak, R. (1992). The cortical localization of the lexicons – positron emission tomography Evidence. *Brain,* 115, 1769–82.

Hummelsheim, H., Arnberger, S., and Mauritz, K. H. (1996). The influence of EMG-initiated electrical muscle stimulation on motor recovery of the centrally paretic hand. *European Journal of Neurology,* 3, 245–54.

Humphreys, G. W., Romani, C., Olson, A., Riddoch, M. J., and Duncan, J. (1994). *Nature,* 372, 357–9.

Hunt, J. (1999). Drawing on the semantic system: The use of drawing as a therapy medium. In *The aphasia therapy file* (eds S. Byng, K. Swinburn and C. Pound). Hove: Psychology Press.

Iguchi, Y., Hoshi, Y., and Hashimoto, I. (2001). Selective spatial attention induces short-term plasticity in human somatosensory cortex. *NeuroReport,* 12, 3133–36.

Ingraham, L. J. and Aiken, C. B. (1996). An empirical approach to determining criteria for abnormality in test batteries with multiple measures. *Neuropsychology* 6, 395–415.

Ip, R. Y., Dornan, J., Schentag, C. (1995). Traumatic brain injury: factors predicting return to work or school. *Brain Injury,* 9(5), 517–32.

Irle, E., Wowra, B., Kunert, H. J., Hampl, J., and Kunze, S. (1992). Memory disturbances following anterior communicating artery rupture. *Annals of Neurology,* 31, 473–80.

Irwin, W. H., Wertz, R. T., and Avent, J. R. (2002). Relationships among language impairment, functional communication and pragmatic performance in aphasia. *Aphasiology,* 16, 823–35.

Ivnik, R. J., Malec, J. F., Smith, G. E., Tangalos, E. G., and Peterson, R. C. (1996). Neuropsychological tests' norms above age 55: COWAT, BNT, MAE Token, WRAT-R Reading, AMNART, STROOP, TMT, and JLO. *The Clinical Neuropsychologist,* 10, 262–78.

Jackson, N. and Coltheart, M. (2001). *Routes to reading success and failure.* Hove: Psychology Press.

Jacobsen, C. F. (1936). Studies of cerebral function in primates: I. The functions of the frontal association area in monkeys. *Comparative Psychology Monographs,* 13, 3–60.

Jahanshahi, M. and Frith, C. (1998). Willed action and its impairments. *Cognitive Neuropsychology,* 15, 483–533.

James, W. (1890). *The principles of psychology.* New York: Holt.

Jastreboff, P. J. (1990). Phantom auditory perception (tinnitus): Mechanisms of generation and perception. *Neuroscience Research,* 8, 221–54.

Jenkins, W. M. and Merzenich, M. M. (1987). Reorganization of neocortical representations after brain injury: A neurophysiological model of the bases of recovery from stroke. *Progress in Brain Research,* 71, 249–66.

Jenkins, W. M. and Merzenich, M. M. (1992). Cortical representational plasticity: some implications for the bases of recovery from brain damage. In *Neuropsychological rehabilitation* (ed. E. Poeppel), pp. 20–35. Berlin: Springer Verlag.

Johannsen-Horbach, H., Wenz, C., Funfgeld, M., Herrmann, M., and Wallesch, C. (1993). Psychosocial aspects on the treatment of adult aphasics and their families: A group therapy approach in Germany. In *Aphasia treatment world perspectives* (eds A. Holland and M. Forbes). London: Chapman and Hall.

John, E. R. (1972). Switchboard versus statistical theories of learning and memory. *Science,* 177, 850–64.

John, A. and Enderby, P. (2000). Reliability of speech and language therapists using therapy outcome measures. *International Journal of language and Communication Disorders,* 35, 287–302.

Johnston, M. (1997). Representations of disability. In *Perceptions of health and illness* (eds K. J. Petrie and J. A. Weinman), pp. 189–212. Amsterdam: Harwood Academic.

Johnstone, B. and Callaghan, T. S. (1996). Neuropsychological evaluation of traumatic brain injury in the United States: A Critical Analysis. In *Recovery after Traumatic Brain Injury* (eds B.P. Uzzell and H. H. Stonnington). Mahwah, NJ: Lawrence Erlbaum Associates.

Johnstone, B. and Frank, R. G. (1995). Neuropsychological assessment in rehabilitation: Current limitations and applications. *NeuroRehabilitation,* 5, 75–86.

Jones, E. (1986). Building the foundations for sentence production in a non-fluent aphasic. *British Journal of Disorders of Communication,* 21, 63–82.

Joseph, P., Darringrand, B., Koleck M., Mazaux J., de Seze M. P., de Seze M., and Dutheil, S. (2000). An evaluation of the aphasic patient's communication skills in daily life situations. *Journal of Neurolinguistics*, 13, 241–327.

Josephsson, S., Bäckman, L., Borell, L., Bernspang, B., Nygard, L., and Ronnberg, L. (1993). Supporting everyday activities in dementia: an intervention study. *International Journal of Geriatric Psychiatry*, 8, 395–400.

Kagan, A. and Gailey, G. (1993). Functional is not enough: training conversational partners for aphasic adults. In *Aphasia Treatment World Perspectives* (eds A. Holland and M. Forbes). London: Chapman and Hall.

Kagan, A., Black, S., Duchan, J., Simmons-Mackie, N., and Square, P. (2001). Training volunteers as conversational partners using 'Supported Conversation for Adults with Aphasia' (SCA): A controlled trial. *Journal of Speech Language and Hearing Research*, 44, 624–38.

Kalra, L., Perez, I., Gupta, S., and Wittink, M. (1997). The influence of visual neglect on stroke rehabilitation. *STROKE*, 28, 1386–391.

Kandel, E. R. (1998). A new intellectual framework for Psychiatry. *American Journal of Psychiatry*, 155, 457–69.

Kandel, E. R., Schwartz J. H., and Jessell, T. M. (1995). *Essentials of neuroscience and behavior*. Stamford, CT: Appleton and Lange.

Kaplan, E., Goodglass, H., and Weintraub, S. (1983). *The Boston Naming Test*. Philadelphia: Lea and Febiger.

Kapur, N. (1994). The coin-in-the-hand test: a new 'bedside' test for the detection of malingering in patients with suspected memory disorders. *Journal of Neurology, Neurosurgery and Psychiatry*, 57, 385–6.

Kapur, S., Craik, F., Tulving, E., Wilson, A. A., Houle, S., and Brown G. M. (1994). Neuroanatomical correlates of encoding in episodic memory: levels of processing effect. *Proceedings of the National Academy of Sciences of the USA*, 91, 2008–11.

Karbe, H., Kessler, J., Herholz, K., Fink, G. R., Heiss, W. D. (1995). Long-term prognosis of poststroke aphasia studied with positron emission tomography. *Archives of Neurology*, 52, 186–90.

Karli, D. C., Burke, D. T., Kim, H. J., Calvanio, R., Fitzpatrick, M., Temple, D., MacNeil, M., Pesez, K., and Lepak, P. (1999). Effects of dopaminergic combination therapy for frontal lobe dysfunction in traumatic brain injury rehabilitation. *Brain Injury*, 13, 63–68.

Karlsson, I., Bråne, G., Melin, E., Nyth, A.-L., and Rybo, E. (1988). Effects of environmental stimulation on biochemical and psychological variables in dementia. *Acta Psychiatrica Scandinavica*, 77, 207–13.

Karlsson, T., Backman, L., Herlitz, A., Nilsson, L.-G., Winblad, B., and Osterlind, P.-O. (1989). Memory improvement at different stages of Alzheimer's disease. *Neuropsychologia*, 27, 737–42.

Kaschel, R., Della Sala, S., Cantagallo, A., Fahlböck, A., Laaksonen, R., and Kazen, M. (2002). Imagery mnemonics for the rehabilitation of memory: A randomised group controlled trial. *Neuropsychological Rehabilitation*, 12(2), 127–53.

Kay, J., Byng, S., Edmundson, A., and Scott, C. (1990). Missing the wood and the trees: A reply to David, Kertesz, Goodglass and Weniger. *Aphasiology*, 4, 115–22.

Kay, J., Lesser, R., and Coltheart, M. (1992). *PALPA: Psycholinguistic Assessments of Language Processing in Aphasia*. Hove: Lawrence Erlbaum Associates.

Kearns, K. P. (1993). Functional outcome: Methodological considerations. In *Clinical aphasiology* (ed. M. L. Lemme), Vol. 21. Austin, TX: Pro Ed.

Kearns, K. and Elman, R. (2001). Group therapy for aphasia: Theoretical and practical considerations. In *Language intervention strategies in aphasia and related neurogenic communication disorders* (ed. R. Chapey), 4th edn. Baltimore, MD: Lippincott, Williams and Wilkins.

Keith, M. S., Stanislav, S. W., and Wesnes, K. A. (1998). Validity of a cognitive computerised assessment system in brain-injured patients. *Brain Injury*, 12, 1037–43.

Kerner, M. J. and Acker, M. (1985). Computer delivery of memory retraining with head injured patients. *Cognitive Rehabilitation*, Nov/Dec, 26–31.

Kertesz, A. (1982). *The Western Aphasia Battery*, New York: Grune and Stratton.

Kertesz, A. (1988). Is there a need for standardized aphasia tests? Why, how, what and when to test aphasics. *Aphasiology*, 2, 313–18.

Kertesz, A. (1990). What should be the core of aphasia tests? (The authors promise but fail to deliver). *Aphasiology*, **4**, 97–101.

Kessels, R. P. and de Hann, E. H. (2003). Implicit learning in memory rehabilitation: a meta-analysis on errorless learning and vanishing cues methods. *Journal of Clinical Experimental Neuropsychology*, **25**, 805–14.

Kewman, D. G., Seigerman, C., Kinter, H., Chu, S., Henson, D., and Reeder, C. (1985). Simulation training of psychomotor skills: Teaching the brain-injured to drive. *Rehabilitation Psychology*, **30**, 11–27.

Khan, S., Khan, A., and Feyz, M. (2002). Decreased length of stay, cost savings and descriptive findings of enhanced patients care resulting from an integrated traumatic brain injury programme *Brain Injury*, **16**, 537–54.

Kim, H. J., Burke, D. T., Dowds, M. D., and George, J. (1999). Utility of a microcomputer as an external memory aid for a memory impaired head injury patient during in-patient rehabilitation, *Brain Injury*, **13**(2), 147–50.

Kinomura, S., Larsson, J., Gulyas, B., and Roland, P. E. (1996). Activation by attention of the human reticular formation and thalamic intralaminar nuclei. *Science*, **271**, 512–15.

Kinsbourne, M. (1993). Orientation bias model of unilateral neglect: Evidence from attentional gradients within hemispace. In *Unilateral neglect: Clinical and experimental studies* (eds I. H. Robertson and J. C. Marshall), pp. 63–86. Hillsdale, NJ: Lawrence Erlbaum Associates.

Kiran, S. and Thompson, C. K. (2002). Typicality of category exemplars in aphasia: evidence from reaction time and treatment data. *Brain and Language*, **79**, 27–31.

Kirkwood, A., Rozas, C., Kirkwood, J., Perez, F., and Bear, M. (1999). Modulation of long-term synaptic depression in visual cortex by acetylcholine and norepinephrine. *Journal of Neuroscience*, **19**, 1599–609.

Kirsch, N. L., Levine, S. P., Lajiness, R., Mossaro, M., Schneider, M., and Donders, J. (1988). *Improving functional performance with computerized task guidance systems*. Paper presented at the Proceeding of 11th Annual Conference on Rehabilitation Technology, Montreal, Canada.

Kitwood, T. (1997). *Dementia Reconsidered: the Person Comes First*. Buckingham: Open University Press.

Kleist, K. (1934). *Gehirnpathologie*. Leipzig: Barth,.

Kline, P. (1993). *The Handbook of Psychological Testing*. London: Routledge.

Klüver, H. and Bucy, P. C. (1937). 'Psychic blindness' and other symptoms following bilateral lobectomy in rhesus monkeys. *American Journal of Physiology*, **119**, 352–3.

Knight, C., Rutterford, N. A., Alderman, N., and Swan, L. J. (2002). Is accurate self-monitoring necessary for people with acquired neurological problems to benefit from the use of differential reinforcement methods? *Brain Injury*, **16**, 75–87.

Knowlton, B. J., Mangels, J. A., and Squire, L. R. (1996). A neostriatal habit learning systems in humans. *Science*, **273**, 1399–402.

Kolb, B. (1990). Recovery from occipital stroke: A self-report and an inquiry into visual processes. *Canadian Journal of Psychology*, **44**, 130–47.

Kolb, B. (1995). *Brain plasticity and behavior*. Mahwah, NJ: Lawrence Erlbaum Associates.

Kolb, B. (2002). Frontal lobe plasticity and behaviour. In *Principles of Frontal Lobe Function* (eds D. T. Stuss and R. K. Knight), pp. 541–56. New York: Oxford University Press.

Kolb, B. and Gibb, R. (1999). Neuroplasticity and recovery of function after brain injury. In *Cognitive neurorehabilitation* (eds D. T. Stuss, G. Winocur and I. H. Robertson), pp. 9–25. Cambridge: Cambridge University Press.

Koltai, D. C., Welsh-Bohmer, K. A., and Schmechel, D. E. (2001). Influence of anosognosia on treatment outcome among dementia patients. *Neuropsychological Rehabilitation*, **11**, 455–75.

Kopelman, M. D. (1992). Storage, forgetting and retrieval in the anterograde and retrograde amnesia of Alzheimer dementia. In *Memory Functioning in Dementia* (ed. L. Bäckman). Amsterdam: Elsevier Science Publishers BV.

Kopelman, M., Wilson, B., and Baddeley, A. (1990). *The Autobiographical Memory Interview*. Bury St Edmunds: Thames Valley Test Company.

Korsakow, S. S. (1890). Über eine besondere Form psychischer Störung, combinirt mit multipler Neuritis. *Archiv für Psychiatrie und Nervenkrankheiten*, **21**, 669–704.

Kozlowski, D. A., James, D. C., and Schallert, T. (1996). Use-dependent exaggeration of neuronal injury after unilateral sensorimotor cortex lesions. *Journal of Neuroscience*, **16**, 4776–86.

Kraus, M. F. and Maki, P. (1997). The combined use of amantadine and l-dopa/cardiopa in the treatment of chronic brain injury. *Brain Injury,* **11**, 455–60.

Kreutzer, J. S., Seel, R. T., and Marwitz, J. H. (1999). *Neurobehavioral Functioning Inventory.* San Antonio, TX: The Psychological Corporation.

Kroll, N. E. A., Markowitsch, H. J., Knight, R., and von Cramon, D. Y. (1997). Retrieval of old memories – the temporo-frontal hypothesis. *Brain,* **120**, 1377–99.

Kunz, R. and Oxman, A. D. (1998). The unpredictability paradox: review of empirical comparisons of randomized and non-ramdomised clinical trials. *BMJ,* **317**, 1185–90.

Laakso, M. (2000). Self-initiated repair by aphasic speakers in home and aphasia therapy conversations. *Journal of Neurolinguistics,* **13**, 258–60.

Laberge, D. (2000). Networks of attention. In *The new cogntitve neurosciences* (ed. M. S. Gazzaniga), pp. 711–24. Cambridge, MA: MIT Press.

Ladavas, E., Berti, A., Ruozzi, E., and Barboni, F. (1997). Neglect as a deficit determined by an imbalance between multiple spatial representations. *Experimental Brain Research,* **116**, 493–500.

Lambon, Ralph, M. A., Graham, K. S., Ellis, A. W., and Hodges, J. R. (1998). Naming in semantic dementia – what matters? *Neuropsychologia,* **36**, 775–84.

Larrabee, G. J. and Crook, T. H. (1996). The ecological validity of memory testing procedure: Developments in the assessment of everyday memory. In *Ecological Validity of Neuropsychological Testing* (eds R. D. Sbordone and C. J. Long). Florida: GR Press/St Lucie Press.

Lashley, K. S. (1938). Factors limiting recovery after central nervous lesion. *Journal of Nervous and Mental Disease,* **88**(6), 733–55.

Lashley, K. S. (1950). *In search of the engram.* Society for Experimental Biology, Symposium No. 4, 454–82.

Lavie, N. (1995). Perceptual load as a necessary condition for selective attention. *Journal of Experimental Psychology: Human Perception and Performance,* **21**, 451–68.

Lawson, M. J. and Rice, D. N. (1989). Effects of training in use of executive strategies on a verbal memory problem resulting from closed head injury. *Journal of Clinical and Experimental Neuropsychology,* **11**, 842–54.

Lawson, R. and Fawcus, M. (1999). Increasing effective communication using a total communication approach. In *The aphasia therapy file* (eds S. Byng, K. Swinburn and C. Pound). Hove: Psychology Press.

Le Dorze, G. and Brassard, C. (1995). A description of the consequences of aphasia on aphasic persons and their relatives and friends based on the WHO model of chronic diseases. *Aphasiology,* **9**, 239–55.

Leff, A., Crinion, J., Scott, S., Turkheimer, F., Howard, D., and Wise, R. (2002). A physiological change in the homotopic cortex following left posterior temporal lobe infarction. *Annals of Neurology,* **51**, 553–8.

Leischner, A. and Lynk, H. A. (1967). Neure Erfahrungen mit der Behandlung von Aphasien. *Nervenartz,* **38**, 199–205.

Lendrem, W. and Lincoln, N. B. (1985). Spontaneous recovery of language in patients with aphasia between 4 and 34 weeks after stroke. *Journal of Neurology, Neurosurgery and Psychiatry,* **48**, 743–8.

Lennon, S. (1994). Behavioural rehabilitation of unilateral neglect. In *Cognitive neuropsychology and cognitive rehabilitation* (eds M. J. Riddoch and G. W. Humphreys), pp. 187–203. Hove: Lawrence Erlbaum Associates.

Lesser, R. and Algar, L. (1995). Towards combing the cognitive neuropsychological and the pragmatic in aphasia therapy. *Neuropsychological Rehabilitation,* **5**, 67–92.

Levelt, W. J. M., Roelofs, A., and Meyer, A. S. (1999). A theory of lexical access in speech production. *Behavioral and Brain Sciences,* **22**, 1–45.

Levin, H. S., High, W. M., and Goethe, K. E. (1987). The neurobehavioral rating scale: assessment of the sequelae of head injury by the clinician. *Journal of Neurology, Neurosurgery and Psychiatry,* **50**, 183–93.

Levin, H. S., O'Donnell, V. M., and Grossman, R. G. (1979). The Galveston Orientation and Amnesia Test. A practical scale to assess cognition after head injury. *Journal of Nervous and Mental Disease,* **167**, 675–84.

Levine, B., Robertson, I. H., Clare, L., Carter, G., Hong, J., Wilson, B. A., Duncan, J., and Stuss, D. T. (2000). Rehabilitation of executive functioning: an experimental-clinical validation of Goal Management Training. *Journal of the International Neuropsychological Society,* **6**, 299–312.

Levine, B., Black, S. E., Cabeza, R., Sinden, M., Mcintosy, A. R., Toth, J. P., Tulving, E., and Stuss, D. T. (1998). Episodic memory and the self in a case of retrograde amnesia. *Brain*, **121**, 1951–73.

Levine, B., Dawson, D., Boutet, I., Schwartz, M. L., and Stuss, D. T. (2000). Assessment of strategic self-regulation in traumatic brain injury: Its relationship to injury severity and psychosocial outcome. *Neuropsychology*, **14**, 491–500.

Levita, E. (1978). Effects of speech therapy on aphasics' responses to the Functional Communication Profile. *Perceptual and Motor Skills*, **47**, 151–4.

Lewis, F. D., Nelson, J., Nelson, C., and Reusink, P. (1988). Effects of three feedback contingencies on the socially inappropriate talk of a brain-injured adult. *Behavior Therapy*, **19**, 203–11.

Lezak, M. D. (1995). *Neuropsychological Assessment*. New York: Oxford University Press.

Lhermitte, F. (1986). Human autonomy and the frontal lobes. Part II: patient behaviour and social situations: the environmental dependency syndrome. *Annals of Neurology*, **19**, 335–43.

Lichtheim, L. (1885). Ueber Aphasie. *Deutsches Archiv fur klinische Medizin*, 36, 204–68. Translated as On aphasia (1885). *Brain*, **7**, 433–85.

Liepert, J., Bauder, H., Wolfgang, H. R., Miltner, W. H., Taub, E., and Weiller, C. (2000). Treatment-induced cortical reorganisation after stroke in humans. *Stroke*, **31**, 1210–16.

Lincoln, N. B., Drummond, A. E. R., and Berman, P. (1997). Perceptual impairment and its impact on rehabilitation outcome. *Disability and Rehabilitation*, **19**, 231–34.

Lincoln, N. B., Drummond, A. E. R., Edmans, J. A., Yeo D., and Willis, D. (1998). The Rey Figure Copy as a screening instrument for perceptual deficits after stroke. *British Journal of Occupational Therapy*, **61**, 1: 33–35.

Lincoln, N. B., Majid, M. J., and Weyman, N. (2001). Cognitive rehabilitation for attention deficts following stroke (Cochrane Review). In *The Cochrane Library*, **2**, Oxford: Update Software.

Lincoln, N., Mulley, G., Jones, A., McGuirk, E., Lendrem, W., and Mitchell, J. (1984). Effectiveness of speech therapy for aphasic stroke patients. *Lancet*, **1**, 1197–200.

Lincoln, N. B., McGuirk, E., Mulley, G. P., Lendrem, W., Jones, A. C., and Mitchell, J. R. A. (1984). Effectiveness of speech therapy for aphasic stroke patients: A randomized controlled trial. *Lancet*, **1**, 1197–200.

Lincoln, N. B., Willis D., Philips S. A., Juby L. C., and Berman, P. (1996). Comparison of rehabilitation practice on hospital wards for stroke patients. *Stroke*, **27**, 18–23.

Lindsay, J. and Wilkinson, R. (1999). Repair sequences in aphasic talk: a comparison of aphasic-speech and language therapist and aphasic-spouse conversations. *Aphasiology*, **13**, 305–25.

Lipinska, B., Bäckman, L., Mantyla, T., and Viitanen, M. (1994). Effectiveness of self-generated cues in early Alzheimer's disease. *Journal of Clinical and Experimental Neuropsychology*, **16**, 809–19.

Little, A. G., Volans, P. J., Hemsley, D. R., and Levy, R. (1986). The retention of new information in senile dementia. *British Journal of Clinical Psychology*, **25**, 71–72.

Liu, K. P. Y., Chan, C. C. H., Lee, T. M. C., Li, L. S. W., and Hui-Chan, C. W. Y. (2002). Self-regulatory learning and generalization for people with brain inury. *Brain Injury*, **16**, 817–24.

Lock, S., Wilkinson, R., and Bryan, K. (2001b). *SPPARC Supporting partners of people with aphasia in relationships and conversations*, Bicester: Winslow Press.

Lock, S., Wilkinson, R., Bryan, K., Maxim, J., Edmundson, A., Bruce, C., and Moir, D. (2001a). Supporting partners of people with aphasia in relationships and conversation (SPPARC). *International Journal of Language and Communication Disorders*, Supplement, 25–30.

Lomas, J., Pickard, L., Bester, S., Elbard, H., Finlayson, A., and Zoghaib, C. (1989). The Communicative Effectiveness Index: Development and psychometri c evaluation of a functional communication measure for adult aphasia. *Journal of Speech and Hearing Disorders*, **54**, 113–24.

Lord, S. E., Wade, D. T., and Halligan, P. W. (1998). A comparison of two physiotherapy treatment approaches to improve walking in multiple sclerosis: a pilot randomised controlled trial. *Clinical Rehabilitation*, **12**, 477–86.

Loya, G. J. (2000). Efficacy of memory rehabilitation among adolescent and adult traumatic brain injury survivors: a meta-analysis. Unpublished doctoral dissertation, University of Nebraska.

Lucchelli, F., Muggia S., and Spinnler, H. (1995). The 'Petites Madeleines' phenomenon in two amnesic patients. Sudden recovery of forgotten memories. *Brain*, **118**, 167–83.

Luria, A. R. (1948/1963). *Restoration of function after brain trauma* (in Russian). Moscow: Academy of Medical Science (Pergamon), London.

Luria, A. R. (1963). *Restoration of function after brain injury* (B. Haigh, trans.). New York: MacMillan.

Luria, A. R. (1966). *Higher Cortical Functions in Man.* London, Tavistock.

Luria, A. R. (1972). *The man with the shattered world.* New York: Basic Books.

Luria, A. R., Naydin, V. L., Tsvetkova L. S., and Vinarskaya, E. N. (1969). Restoration of higher cortical function following local brain damage. In *Handbook of clinical neurology* (eds P. J. Vinken and G. W. Bruyn), vol. 3, pp. 368–433. Amsterdam: North-Holland.

Luria, A. R. and Homskaya, E. D. (1964). Disturbance in the regulative role of speech with frontal lobe lesions. In *The Frontal Granular Cortex and Behavior*J. (eds M. Warren and K. Akert), pp. 353–71. New York: McGraw-Hill.

Lustig, A. and Tompkins, C. (2002). A written communication strategy for a speaker with aphasia and apraxia of speech: treatment outcomes and social validity. *Aphasiology,* **16,** 507–21.

Lyon, J. (1989). Communicative partners: their value in re-establishing communication with aphasic adults. In *Clinical aphasiology conference proceedings* (ed. T. Prescott), **18,** 1–17. San Diego: College Hill Press.

Lyon, J. (1995). Drawing: its value as a communication aid for adults with aphasia. *Aphasiology,* **9,** 33–50.

Lyon, J. (1998). Treating real life functionality in a couple coping with severe aphasia. In *Approaches to the treatment of aphasia* (eds N. Helm-Estabrooks and A. Holland). San Diego: Singular Publishing Group.

Lyon, J. G., Cariski, D., Keisler, L., Rosenbek, J., Levine, R., Kumpula, J., Ryff, C., Coyne, S., and Blanc, M. (1997). Communication partners: Enhancing participation in life and communication for adults with aphasia in natural settings. *Aphasiology,* **11,** 693–708.

Mackenzie, C. (1991). An aphasia group intensive efficacy study. *British Journal of Disorders of Communication,* **26,** 275–91.

MacKinnon, D. F. and Squire, L. R. (1989). Autobiographical memory and amnesia. *Psychobiology,* **17,** 247–56.

MacLennan, D. L., Nicholas, L. E., Morley, G. K., and Brookshire, R. H. (1991). The effects of bromocriptine on speech and language function in a man with transcortical motor aphasia. *Clinical Aphasiology,* **21,** 145–55.

Majid, M. J., Lincoln, N. B., and Weyman, N. (2001). Cognitive rehabilitation for memory deficits following stroke (Cochrane Review). In *The Cochrane Library,* **2,** Oxford: Update Software.

Malec, J. F. (2001). Impact of comprehensive day treatment on societal participation for persons with acquired brain injury. *Archives of Physical Medicine and Rehabilitation,* **82,** 885–95.

Malec, J. F. and Basford, J. S. (1996). Post-acute brain injury rehabilitation. *Archives of Physical Medicine and Rehabilitation,* **77,** 198–207.

Malec, J. F. and Degiorgio, L. (2002). Characteristics of successful and unsuccessful completers of 3 postacute brain injury rehabilitation pathways. *Archives of Physical Medicine and Rehabilitation,* **83,** 1759–64.

Malloy, P., Bihrle, A., Duffy, J., and Cimino, C. (1993). The orbitomedial frontal syndrome. *Archives of Clinical Neuropsychology,* **8,** 185–201.

Manchester, D., Hodgkinson, A., and Casey, T. (1997). Prolonged severe behavioural disturbance following traumatic brain injury: what can be done? *Brain Injury,* **11,** 605–17.

Maneta, A., Marshall, J., and Lindsay, J. (2001). Direct and indirect therapy for word sound deafness. *International Journal of Language and Communication Disorders,* **36,** 91–106.

Manly, T. (2002). Cognitive rehabilitation for unilateral neglect: review. *Neuropsychological Rehabilitation,* **12,** 289–310.

Manly, T., Hawkins, K., Evans, J. J., Woldt, K., and Robertson, I. H. (2002). Rehabilitation of executive function: facilitation of effective goal management on complex tasks using periodic auditory alerts. *Neuropsychologia,* **40,** 271–81.

Manly, T., Lewis, G. H., Robertson, I. H., Watson, P. C., and Datta, A. K. (2002b). Coffee in the cornflakes: Time-of-day as a modulator of executive response control. *Neuropsychologia,* **40,** 1–6.

Manochiopinig, S., Sheard, C., and Reed, V. A. (1992). Pragmatic assessment in adult aphasia: A clinical review. *Aphasiology,* **6,** 519–33.

Marcel, A. J. (1980). Conscious and preconscious recognition of polysemous words: Locating the effects of prior verbal contexts. In *Attention and performance VII* (ed. R. S. Nickerson). Hillsdale NJ: Lawrence Erlbaum Associates.

Marie, P. (1906). Revision de la question de l'aphasie: la troisieme circonvolution frontale gauche ne joue aucun role special dans la fonction du langage. *Semaine Medicale*, **26**, 241–7.

Markowitsch, H. J. (1984). Can amnesia be caused by damage of a single brain structure? *Cortex*, **20**, 27–45.

Markowitsch, H. J. (1988). Diencephalic amnesia: a reorientation towards tracts? *Brain Research Reviews*, **13**, 351–70.

Markowitsch, H. J. (ed.) (1990). *Transient global amnesia and related disorders*. Toronto: Hogrefe and Huber Publs.

Markowitsch, H. J. (1992). *Intellectual functions and the brain*. Toronto: Hogrefe and Huber Publs.

Markowitsch, H. J. (1995). Which brain regions are critically involved in the retrieval of old episodic memory? *Brain Research Reviews*, **21**, 117–27.

Markowitsch, H. J. (1996). Organic and psychogenic retrograde amnesia: two sides of the same coin? *Neurocase*, **2**, 357–71.

Markowitsch, H. J. (1998). Cognitive neuroscience of memory. *Neurocase*, **4**, 429–35.

Markowitsch, H. J. (1999). Functional neuroimaging correlates of functional amnesia. *Memory*, **7**, 561–83.

Markowitsch, H. J. (2000a). Repressed memories. In *Memory, consciousness, and the brain: the Tallinn conference* (ed. E. Tulving), pp. 319–30. Philadelphia, PA: Psychology Press.

Markowitsch, H. J. (2000b). Memory and amnesia. In *Principles of cognitive and behavioral neurology* (ed. M.-M. Mesulam), pp. 257–93. New York: Oxford University Press.

Markowitsch, H. J. (2001). Amnesia, transient and psychogenic. In *International encyclopedia of the social and behavioral sciences* (eds N. J. Smelser and P. B. Baltes), *Vol. 1: Behavioral and cognitive neuroscience*; pp. 467–71. Oxford: Elsevier Science.

Markowitsch, H. J. (2002). Functional retrograde amnesia – mnestic block syndrome. *Cortex*, **38**, 651–4.

Markowitsch, H. J. (2003a). Autonoëtic consciousness. In *The self in neuroscience and psychiatry* (eds A. S. David and T. Kircher), pp. 180–96. Cambridge: Cambridge University Press.

Markowitsch, H. J. (2003b). Functional amnesia. *NeuroImage*, **20**, S132–8.

Markowitsch, H. J., Calabrese P., Neufeld H., Gehlen W., and Durwen, H. F. (1999a). Retrograde amnesia for famous events and faces after left fronto-temporal brain damage. *Cortex*, **35**, 243–52.

Markowitsch, H. J., Calabrese, P., Würker, M. *et al.* (1994). The amygdala's contribution to memory – a PET-study on two patients with Urbach-Wiethe disease. *NeuroReport*, **5**, 1349–52.

Markowitsch, H. J., Kalbe, E., Kessler, J., von Stockhausen, H.-M., Ghaemi, M., and Heiss, W.-D. (1999b). Short-term memory deficit after focal parietal damage. *Journal of Clinical and Experimental Neuropsychology*, **21**, 784–96.

Markowitsch, H. J., Kessler, J., Kalbe, E., and Herholz, K. (1999c). Functional amnesia and memory consolidation. A case of persistent anterograde amnesia with rapid forgetting following whiplash injury. *Neurocase*, **5**, 189–200.

Markowitsch, H. J., Kessler, J., Russ, M. O., Frölich, L., Schneider, B., and Maurer, K. (1999d). Mnestic block syndrome. *Cortex*, **35**, 219–30.

Markowitsch, H. J., Kessler, J., Schramm, U., and Frölich, L. (2000a). Severe degenerative cortical and cerebellar atrophy and progressive dementia in a young adult. *Neurocase*, **6**, 357–64.

Markowitsch, H. J., Kessler, J., Van der Ven, C., Weber-Luxenburger, G., and Heiss, W.-D. (1998). Psychic trauma causing grossly reduced brain metabolism and cognitive deterioration. *Neuropsychologia*, **36**, 77–82.

Markowitsch, H. J., Kessler, J., Weber-Luxenburger, G., Van der Ven, C., and Heiss, W.-D. (2000b). Neuroimaging and behavioral correlates of recovery from 'mnestic block syndrome' and other cognitive deteriorations. *Neuropsychiatry, Neuropsychology, and Behavioral Neurology*, **13**, 60–6.

Markowitsch, H. J., Vandekerckhove, M. M. P., Lanfermann, H., and Russ, M. O. (2003). Engagement of lateral and medial prefrontal areas in the ecphory of sad and happy autobiographical memories. *Cortex*, **39**, 643–66.

Markowitsch, H. J., von Cramon, D. Y., and Schuri, U. (1993). The mnestic performance profile of a bilateral diencephalic infarct patient with preserved intelligence and severe amnesic disturbances. *Journal of Clinical and Experimental Neuropsychology*, **14**, 627–52.

Markowitsch, H. J., Weber-Luxenburger, G., Ewald, K., Kessler, J., and Heiss, W.-D. (1997). Patients with heart attacks are not valid models for medial temporal lobe amnesia. A neuropsychological and FDG-PET study with consequences for memory research. *European Journal of Neurology*, 4, 178–84.

Marks, M., Taylor, M., and Rusk, H. A. (1957). Rehabilitation of the aphasic patient: a summary of three years' experience in a rehabilitation setting. *Archives of Physical Medicine and Rehabilitation* 38, 219–26.

Marr, D. (1982). *Vision*. San Francisco: Freeman.

Marsh, N. V. and Kersel, D. A. (1993). Screening tests for visual neglect following stroke. *Neuropsychological Rehabilitation*, 3, 245–57.

Marshall, J. (1999). Doing something about a verb impairment: Two therapy approaches. In *The aphasia therapy file* (eds S. Byng, K. Swinburn and C. Pound). Hove: Psychology Press.

Marshall, J. (2002). The assessment and treatment of sentence processing disorders: A review of the literature. In *The handbook of adult language disorders* (ed. A. Hillis). New York: Psychology Press.

Marshall, J., Chiat, S., Pring, T., Byng, S., and Black, M. (1998). *The sentence processing resource pack*. London: Winslow Press.

Marshall, R. C., Tompkins, C. A., and Phillips, D. S. (1980). Effects of scheduling on communicative assessment of aphasic patients. *Journal of Communication Disorders*, 13, 105–14.

Marshall, R. C., Tompkins, C., and Phillips, D. S. (1982). Improvement in treated aphasia: Examination of selected prognostic factors. *Folia Phoniatrica*, 34, 305–15.

Marshall, R., Wertz, R., Weiss, D., Aten, J., Brookshire, R., Garcia-Bunuel, L., Holland, A., Kurtzke, J., LaPointe, L., Millianti, F., Brannegan, R., Greenbaum, H., Vogel, D., Carter, J., Barnes, N., and Goodman, R. (1989). Home treatment for aphasic patients by trained non professionals. *Journal of Speech and Hearing Disorders*, 54, 462–70.

Martelli, M. (1999). Protocol for increasing initiation, decreasing adynamia. *Heads Up: RSS Newsletter*, 2–9.

Martin, S. and Pauly, F. (2000). Cognitive rehabilitation: An annotated bibliography. *Journal of Cognitive Rehabilitation*, 18, 6–15.

Martin, N. and Saffran, E. (1992). A computational account of deep dysphasia: Evidence from a single case study. *Brain and Language*, 43, 240–74.

Martin, N., Dell, G. S., Saffran, E. M., and Schwartz, M. F. (1994). Origins of paraphasias in deep dysphasia – testing the consequences of a decay impairment to an interactive spreading activation model of lexical retrieval. *Brain and Language*, 47, 609–60.

Martin, A., Wiggs, C. L., Lalonde, F., and Mack, C. (1994). Word retrieval to letter and semantic cues: a double dissociation in normal subjects using interference tasks. *Neuropsychologia*, 32, 1487–94.

Mateer, C. A. (1999). The rehabilitation of executive disorders. In *Cognitive Neurorehabilitation* (eds D. T. Stuss, G. Winocur and I. H. Robertson), pp. 314–332. Cambridge: Cambridge University Press.

Mateer, C. A. and Mapou, R. L. (1996). Understanding, evaluating, and managing attention disorders after traumatic brain injury. *Journal of Head Trauma Rehabilitation*, 11(2), 1–16.

Mateer, C. A., Sohlberg, M. M., and Crinean, J. (1987). Perceptions of memory functions in individuals with closed head injury. *Journal of Head Trauma Rehabilitation*, 2, 79–84.

Matthey, S. (1996). Modification of perseverative behaviour in an adult with anoxic brain damage. *Brain Injury*, 10, 219–27.

Mattingley, J. B., Robertson, I. H., and Driver, J. (1998). Modulation of covert visual attention by hand movement: Evidence from parietal extinction after right-hemisphere damage. *Neurocase*, 4, 245–53.

Mayer, E., Brown, V. J., Dunnett, S. B., and Robbins, T. W. (1992). Striatal graft-associated recovery of a lesion-induced performance deficit in the rat requires learning to use the transplant. *European Journal of Neuroscience*, 4, 119–26.

Mayes, A. R., Daum, I., Markowitsch, H. J., and Sauter, B. (1997). The relationship between retrograde and anterograde amnesia in patients with typical global amnesia. *Cortex*, 33, 197–217.

Mayes, A. and Warburg, R. (1992). Memory assessment in clinical practice and research. In *A Handbook of Neuropsychological Assessment* (eds J. R. Crawford, D. M. Parker, *et al.*). Hillsdale, NJ: Lawrence Erlbaum Associates.

Mazaux, J. M. and Richer, E. (1998). Rehabilitation after traumatic brain injury in adults. *Disability and Rehabilitation*, 20, 435–47.

Mazaux, J. M., Masson, F., Levin, H. S., Alaoui, P., Maurette, P., and Barat, M. (1997). Long-term neuropsychological outcome and loss of social autonomy after traumatic brain injury. *Archives of Physical Medicine and Rehabilitation*, **78**, 1316–20.

Mazzoni, M., Vista, M., Geri, E., Avila, L., Bianchi, F., and Moretti, P. (1995). Comparison of language recovery in rehabilitated and matched, non-rehabilitated aphasic patients. *Aphasiology*, **9**, 553–63.

McCandliss, B. D., Fiez, J., Protopapas, A., Conway, M., and McClelland, J. (2002). Success and failure in teaching the [r]-[l] contrast to Japanese adults: tests of a Hebbian model of plasticity and stabilization in spoken language perception. *Cognitive, Affective and Behavioral Neuroscience*, **2**, 89–108.

McCarthy, R. and Warrington, E. K. (1984). A two-route model of speech production: evidence from aphasia. *Brain*, **107**, 463–85.

McClelland, J. L. (2002). Neuroplasticity and recovery of function. Paper presented at the NIDCD workshop on the role of neuroimaging in the study of aphasia recovery and rehabilitation: research needs and opportunities. Bethesda, MD; May **13**, 2002.

McClelland, J. L., McNaughton, B. L., and O'Reilly, R. C. (1995). Why there are complementary learning systems in the hippocampus and neocortex: insights from the successes and failures of connectionist models of learning and memory. *Psychology Review*, **102**, 419–57.

McCormack, J. and Greenhalgh, T. (2000). Seeing what you want to see in randomized controlled trials: versions and perversions of UKPDS data. *BMJ* **320**, 1720–3.

McDowell, S., Whyte, J., and D'Esposito, M. (1998). Differential effects of a dopaminergic agonist on prefrontal function in traumatic brain injury patients. *Brain*, **121**, 1155–64.

McGaugh, J. L. (2000). Memory – a century of consolidation. *Science*, **287**, 248–51.

McGaugh, J. L. (2002). Memory consolidation and the amygdala: a systems perspective. *Trends in Neurosciences*, **25**, 456–61.

McKenna, P. and Warrington, E. K. (1980). *The Graded Naming Test*. Windsor: Nelson.

McKinney, M., Blake, H., Treece, K., Lincoln, N. B., Playford, E. D., and Gladman, J. R. F. (2002). Evaluation of cognitive assessment in stroke rehabilitation. *Clinical Rehabilitation*, **16**, 129–136.

McKitrick, L. A. and Camp, C. J. (1993). Relearning the names of things: the spaced-retrieval intervention implemented by a caregiver. *Clinical Gerontologist*, **14**, 60–2.

McLaughlin, A. M. and Peters, S. (1993). Evaluation of an innovative cost-effective programme for brain injury patients: response to a need for flexible treatment planning. *Brain Injury*, **7**, 71–5.

McLellan, D. L. (1991). Functional recovery and the principles of disability medicine. In *Clinical Neurology* (eds M. Swash and J. Oxbury), Vol. **1**, pp. 768–90. London: Churchill Livingstone.

McLeod, P. D. (1978). Does probe RT measure central processing demand? *Quarterly Journal of Experimental Psychology*, **30**, 83–9.

McMillan, T. M. and Greenwood, R. J. (1993). Models of rehabilitation programmes for the brain-injured adult – II: Model services and suggestions for change in the UK. *Clinical Rehabilitation*, **7**, 346–55.

McMillan, T., Robertson, I., Brock, D., and Chorlton, L. (2002). Brief mindfulness training for attentional problems after traumatic brain injury: A randomized control treatment trial. *Neuropsychological Rehabilitation*, **12**(2), 117–25.

Mehta, M. A., Sahakian, B. J., and Robbins, T. W. (2001). Comparative psychopharmcology of methlyphenidate and related drugs in human volunteers, patients with ADHD and experimental animals. In *Stimulant Drugs and ADHD: Basic and Clinical Neuroscience* (eds M. V. Solanto, A. F. T. Arnsten and F. X. Castellanos), pp. 303–31. Oxford: Oxford University Press.

Meichenbaum, D. (1974). Self-instruction strategy training: a cognitive prosthesis for the aged. *Human Development*, **17**, 273–80.

Meichenbaum, D. H. and Goodman, J. (1971). Training impulsive children to talk to themselves: A means of developing self-control. *Journal of Abnormal Psychology*, **77**, 115–26.

Meikle, M., Wechsler, E., Tupper, A., Benenson, M., Butler, J., Mulhall, D., and Stern, G. (1979). Comparative trial of volunteer and professional treatments of dysphasia after stroke. *BMJ*, **2**, 87–9.

Mercer, B., Wapner, W., Gardner, H., and Benson, D. F. (1977). A study of confabulation. *Archives of Neurology*, **34**, 429–33.

Mercier, L., Audet, T., Herbert, R., Rochette, A., and Dubois, M. F. (2001). Impact of motor, cognitive and perceptual disorders on ability to perform activities of daily living after stroke. *Stroke*, **32**, 2602–8.

Merzenich, M. M., Kaas, J. H., Wall, J.T., Nelson, R. J., Sur, M., and Felleman, D. (1983). Topographic reorganization of somatosensory cortical areas 3b and 1 in adult monkeys following restricted deafferentation. *Neuroscience*, **8**, 33–55.

Mesulam, M. (1986). Editorial: Frontal cortex and behaviour. *Annals of Neurology*, **19**, 320–25.

meta-analysis. *Journal of the International Neuropsychological Society*.

Meyers, J. E. and Meyers, K. R. (1995). *Rey Complex Figure Test and Recognition Trial*. San Antonio, TX: The Psychological Corporation.

Michon, J. A. (1979). *Dealing with danger*. Internal report Traffic Research Centre, State University Groningen.

Middleton, D. K., Lambert, M. J., and Seggar, L. B. (1991). Neuropsychological rehabilitation: Microcomputer-assisted treatment of brain-injured adults. *Perceptual and Motor Skills*, **72**, 527–30.

Milders, M. V., Berg, I. J., and Deelman, B. G. (1995). Four-year follow-up of a controlled memory training study in closed head injured patients. *Neuropsychological Rehabilitation*, 5(3), 223–38.

Millis, S. R. and Kler, S. (1995). Limitations of the Rey Fifteen-Item Test in the detection of malingering. *The Clinical Neuropsychologist*, **9**, 241–4.

Mills, C. K. (1904). Treatment of aphasia by training. *Journal of the American Medical Association*, **43**, 1940–9.

Mills, V. M., Cassidy, J. W., and Katz, D. I. (1997). *Neurologic rehabilitation: A guide to diagnosis, prognosis, and treatment planning*. Malden, MA: Blackwell Science.

Milner, A. D. and Goodale, M. A. (1995). *The visual brain in action*. New York: Oxford University Press.

Miltner, W. H., Bauder, H., Sommer, M., Dettmers, C., and Taub, E. (1999). Effects of constraint-induced movement therapy on patients with chronic motor deficits after stroke: a replication. *Stroke*, **30**(3), 586–92.

Mirsky, A. F. (1989). The neuropsychology of attention: Elements of a complex behavior. In *Integrating theory and practice in clinical neuropsychology* (ed. E. Perenman), pp. 75–91. Hillsdale, NJ: Lawrence Erlbaum Associates.

Mirsky, A. F., Anthony, B. J., Duncan, C. C., Ahearn, M. B., and Kellam, S. G. (1991). Analysis of the elements of attention: A neuropsychological approach. *Neuropsychology Review*, **2**, 109–45.

Mishkin, M. and Petri, H. L. (1984). Memories and habits: Some implications for the analysis of learning and retention. In *Neuropsychology of memory* (eds L. R. Squire and N. Butters), pp. 287–96. New York: Guilford Press.

Mitchum, C. C. and Berndt, R. S. (1995). The cognitive neuropsychological approach to treatment of language disorders. *Neuropsychological Rehabilitation*, **5**, 1–16.

Miyake, A., Friedman, N. P., Emerson, M. J., Witzki, A. H., Howerter, A., and Wager, T. D. (2000). The unity and diversity of executive functions and their contributions to complex 'frontal lobe' tasks: a latent variable analysis. *Cognitive Psychology*, **41**, 49–100.

Mohr, J. P. (1976). Broca's area and Broca's aphasia. In *Studies in neurolinguistics* (ed. H. A. Whitaker), Vol. 1, pp. 201–35. New York: Academic Press.

Montgomery, E. B. and Turkstra, L. S. (2003). Evidence-based medicine: Let's be reasonable. *Journal of Medical Speech-Language Pathology*, **11**(2), ix–xii.

Moore, C. J. and Price, C. J. (1999). Three distinct ventral occipitotemporal regions for reading and object naming. *Neuroimage*, **10**, 181–92.

Morris, R. G. (1996). The neuropsychology of Alzheimer's disease and related dementias. In *Handbook of the Clinical Psychology of Ageing* (ed. R. T. Woods). Chichester: John Wiley and Sons Ltd.

Morton, J. (1969). The interaction of information in word recognition. *Psychological Review*, **76**, 165–78.

Morton, J. and Bekerian, D. A. (1986). *Three Ways of Looking at Memory. Advances in Cognitive Sciences I*, pp. 43–71. Chichester: Ellis Horwood Ltd.

Morton, J. and Patterson, K. E. (1980). A new attempt at an interpretation, or an attempt at a new interpretation. In *Deep dyslexia* (ed. J. C. Marshall), pp. 91–118. London: Routlege and Kegan Paul.

Moscovitch, M. and Melo, B. (1997). Strategic retrieval and the frontal lobes: evidence from confabulation and amnesia. *Neuropsychologia*, **35**, 1017–34.

Mountain, M. A. and Snow, W. G. (1993). Wisconsin Card Sorting Test as a measure of frontal pathology: A review. *The Clinical Neuropsychologist*, **7**, 108–18.

Mummery, C. J., Ashburner, J., Scott, S. K., and Wise, R. J. S. (1999). Functional neuroimaging of speech perception in six normal and two aphasic subjects. *Journal of the Acoustical Society of America,* **106**, 449–57.

Mummery, C. J., Patterson, K., Hodges, J. R., and Price, C. J. (1998). Functional neuroanatomy of the semantic system: Divisible by what? *Journal of Cognitive Neuroscience,* **10**, 766–77.

Murray, L. L. and Chapey, R. (2001). Assessment of language disorders in adults. In *Language intervention strategies in aphasia and related neurogenic communication disorders* (ed. R. Chapey), 4th edn, pp. 55–126. Philadelphia: Lippincott, Williams and Wilkins.

Murre, J. M. J. and Robertson, I. H. (1995). Self-repair in neural networks: A model for recovery from brain damage. *European Journal of Neuroscience Supplement,* **8**, 155.

Musso, M., Weiller, C., Kiebel, S. *et al.* (1999). Training-induced brain-plasticity in aphasia. *Brain,* **122**, 1781–90.

Naccache, L. and Dehaene, S. (2001). The priming method: imaging unconscious repetition priming reveals an abstract representation of number in the parietal lobes. *Cerebral Cortex,* **11**, 966–74.

Naesser, M., Hugo, T., Kobayashi, M., Martin, P., Nicholas, M., Baker, E., and Pascual-Leone, A. (2002). *Modulation of Cortical Areas with Repetitive Transcranial Magnetic Stimulation to Improve Naming in Nonfluent Aphasia.* Paper presented at the NeuroImage Human Brain Mapping 2002 Meeting, Sendai, Japan.

Najenson, T., Groswasser, Z., Mendelson, L., and Hackett, P. (1980). Rehabilitation outcome of brain damaged patients after severe head injury. *International Rehabilitation Medicine,* **2**, 17–22.

Nakada, T. and Tasaka, N. (2001). Human brain imaging in the upright position. *Neurology,* **57**, 1720–2.

National Institutes of Health (1999). Rehabilitation of persons with traumatic brain injury. *Journal of the American Medical Association,* **282**, 974–83.

National Institutes of Health (NIH) Consensus Development Panel on Rehabilitation of Persons with Brain Injury (1998, October). *Consensus Conference: Rehabilitation of Persons with Brain Injury* [Online]. Available: http://www.odp.od.nih.gov/consensus/.

Nauta, W. J. H. (1979). Expanding borders of the limbic system concept. In *Functional neurosurgery* (eds T. Rasmussen and R. Marino), pp. 7–23. New York: Raven Press.

Neilson, J. (1946). *Agnosia, apraxia, aphasia.* New York: Hafner.

Neistadt, M. E. (1992). Occupational therapy treatments for constructional deficits. *American Journal of Occupational Therapy,* **46**, 141–48.

Nelson, E., Wasson, J., Kirk, J., Keller, A., Clark, D., Dietrich, A., Stewart, A., and Zubkoff, M. (1987). Assessment of function in routine clinical practice: Description of the COOP Chart method and preliminary findings. *Journal of Chronic Disease,* **40**, 55S–63S.

Nelson, H. E. (1976). A modified card sorting test sensitive to frontal lobe defects. *Cortex,* **12**, 313–24.

Nelson, H. E. and Willison, J. (1991). *National Adult Reading Test manual.* Windsor: NFER-Nelson.

Newcombe, F. (2002). An overview of neuropsychological rehabilitation: a forgotten past and a challenging future. In *Cognitive rehabilitation: A clinical neuropsychological approach* (eds W. Brower, E. van Zomeren, I. Berg, A. Bouma and E. de Haan), pp. 23–51. Amsterdam: Boom.

Nickels, L. (1992). *Spoken word production and its breakdown in aphasia.* Hove: Psychology Press.

Nickels, L. A. (1997). *Spoken word production and its breakdown in aphasia.* Hove: Psychology Press.

Nickels, L. A. (2002). Therapy for naming disorders: Revisiting, revising and reviewing. *Aphasiology,* **16**, 935–80.

Nickels, L. and Howard, D. (1995). Phonological errors in aphasic naming; comprehension, monitoring and lexicality. *Cortex,* **31**, 209–37.

Nickels, L. A. and Howard, D. (2000). When the words won't come: relating impairments and models of spoken word production. In *Aspects of Language Production* (ed. L. R. Wheeldon), pp. 115–42. Hove: Psychology Press.

Nielson, J. M. (1946). *Aphasia, apraxia, agnosia: their value in cerebral localization.* (Second edition). New York: Paul B. Hoeber.

Niemann, H., Ruff, R. M., and Baser, C. A. (1990). Computer assisted attention retraining in head injured individuals: A controlled efficacy study of an out-patient program. *Journal of Consulting and Clinical Psychology,* **58**, 811–17.

Nies, K. J. (2002). Cognitive and emotional changes associated with mesial orbito-frontal damage: assessment and implications or treatment. *Neurocase*, **5**, 313–24.

NIH Consensus Development Panel on Rehabilitation of Persons with Traumatic Brain Injury. (1999). Rehabilitation of persons with TBI. *JAMA*, **282**, 974–83.

Noppeney, U. and Price, C. J. (2002). A PET study of stimulus- and task-induced semantic processing. *Neuroimage*, **15**, 927–35.

Noppeney, U. and Price, C. J. (2003). Functional imaging of the semantic system: Retrieval of sensory-experienced and verbally learned knowledge. *Brain and Language*, **84**, 120–33.

Norman, D. A. and Shallice, T. (1986). Attention to action: Willed and automatic control of behavior. In *Consciousness and self regulation: Advances in research and theory* (eds R. Davidson, G. Schwartz and D. Shapiro), Vol. 4, pp. 1–18. New York: Plenum Press.

Norman, D. and Shallice, T. (1986). Attention to action. In *Consciousness and Self-Regulation* (eds R. J. Davidson, G. E. Schwartz and D. Shapiro), pp. 1–18. New York: Plenum Press.

Novack, T. A., Caldwell, S. G., Duke, L. W., Bergquist, T. F., and Gage, R. J. (1996). Focused versus unstructured intervention for attention deficits after traumatic brain injury. *Journal of Head Trauma Rehabilitation*, **11**(3), 52–60.

Nudo, R. J., Barbay, S., and Kleim, J. A. (2000). Role of neuroplasticity in functional recovery after stroke. In *Cerebral reorganization of function after brain damage* (eds H. S. Levin and J. Grafman), pp. 168–97. Oxford: Oxford University Press.

Nudo, R. J., Wise, B. M., SiFuentes, F., and Milliken, G. W. (1996). Neural substrates for the effects of rehabilitative training on motor recovery after ischemic infarct. *Science*, **272**, 1791–4.

O'Carroll, R. (1995). The assessment of premorbid ability: A critical review. *Neurocase*, **1**, 83–9.

O'Carroll, R. E., Egan, V., and MacKenzie, F. (1994). Assessing cognitive estimation. *British Journal of Clinical Psychology*, **33**, 193–7.

O'Connell, M. E., Mateer, C. A., and Kerns, K. A. (2003). Prosthetic systems for addressing problems with initiation: Guidelines for selection, training, and measuring efficacy. *NeuroRehabilitation*, **18**, 9–20.

O'Hara, C., Harrell, M., Bellingrath, E., and Lisicia, K. (1993). *Cognitive Symptom Checklists*. Odessa, FL: Psychological Assessment Resources, Inc.

Obonsawin, M. C., Crawford, J. R., Page, J., Chalmers, P., Cochrane, R., Low, G., and Marsh, P. (2002). Performance on tests of frontal lobe function reflect general intellectual ability. *Neuropsychologia*, **40**, 970–7.

Ochipa, C., Rothi, L. J. G., and Heilman, K. M. (1992). Conceptual apraxia in Alzheimer's disease. *Brain*, **115**, 1061–71.

Office of Technology Assessment (1978). *Assessing the efficacy and safety of medical technologies*, OTA-H-75. Washington, DC: US Government Printing Office.

Ogden, J. A. (2000). Neurorehabilitation in the third millenium: New roles for our environment, behaviors and mind in brain damage and recovery? *Brain and Cognition*, **42**, 110–12.

Ohyama, M., Senda, M., Kitamura, S. *et al.* (1996). Role of the nondominant hemisphere and undamaged area during word repetition in poststroke aphasics. A PET activation study. *Stroke*, **27**, 897–903.

Ojemann, G. A. (1991). Cortical organisation of language. *Journal of Neuroscience*, **11**, 2281–7.

Okada, K., Kobayashi, S., Yamagata, S., Takahashi, K., and Yamaguchi, S. (1997). Poststroke apathy and regional cerebral blood flow. *Stroke*, **28**, 2437–41.

Owen, A. M., Downes, J. J., Sahakian, B. J., Polkey, C. E., and Robbins, T. W. (1990). Planning and spatial working memory following frontal lobe lesions in man. *Neuropsychologia*, **28**, 757–66.

Page, S. J., Levine, P., Sisto, S., Bond, Q., and Johnston, M. V. (2002). Stroke patients' and therapists' opinions of constraint-induced movement therapy. *Clinical Rehabilitation*, **16**, 55–60.

Paolucci, S., Antonucci, G., Grasso, M. G., and Pizzamiglio, L. (2001.). The role of unilateral spatial neglect in rehabilitation of right brain-damaged ischaemic stroke patients: a matched comparison. *Arch Phys Med Rehabil*, **82**, 743–49.

Papagno, C. and Baddeley, A. D. (1997). Confabulation in a dysexecutive patient: implication for models of retrieval. *Cortex*, **33**, 743–52.

Papez, J. W. (1937). A proposed mechanism of emotion. *Archives of Neurology and Psychiatry*, **38**, 725–43.

Parasuraman, R. (ed.) (1998). *The attentive brain.* Cambridge, MA: MIT Press.

Paré, D. (2003). Role of the basolateral amygdala in memory consolidation. *Progress in Neurobiology,* **70**, 409–20.

Parente, R. and Stapleton, M. (1999). Development of a cognitive strategies group for vocational training after traumatic brain injury. *Neurorehabilitation,* **13**, 13–20.

Park, N. W. and Barbuto, E. (2004). *Effects of dual task on encoding and production of naturalistic actions.* Paper presented at the International Neuropsychological Society, Baltimore, MD.

Park, N. W. and Ingles, J. L. (2001). Effectiveness of attention rehabilitation after acquired brain injury: A meta-analysis. *Neuropsychology,* **15**(2), 199–210.

Park, N. W., Chung, J., and Barbuto, E. (2004). *Investigation of the cognitive processes underlying the encoding of naturalistic actions.* Paper presented at the 32nd Annual Meeting of the International Neuropsychological Society, Baltimore, MD.

Park, N. W., Proulx, G. B., and Towers, W. M. (1999). Evaluation of the Attention Process Training programme. *Neuropsychological Rehabilitation,* **92**, 135–54.

Parker, D. M. and Crawford, J. R. (1992). Assessment of frontal lobe function. In *A handbook of neuropsychological assessment* (eds J. R. Crawford, D. M. Parker and W. W. McKinlay), pp. 267–91, London: Lawrence Erlbaum Associates.

Parker, C. J., Gladman, J. R. F., Drummond, A. E. R., Dewey, M. E., Lincoln, N. B., Barer, D., Logan, P. A., Radford K. A. on behalf of the TOTAL study group (2001). A multi-centre randomised controlled trial of leisure therapy and conventional occupational therapy after stroke. *Clinical Rehabilitation,* **15**, 42–52.

Parr S., Byng, S. and Gilpin, S. (1997). *Talking about aphasia: Living with loss of language after stroke.* Buckingham: Open University Press.

Pashler, H. (1998). *The psychology of attention.* Cambridge, MA: MIT Press.

Passingham, R. E., Stephan, K. E., and Kötter, R. (2002). The anatomical basis of functional localization in the cortex. *Nature Reviews Neuroscience,* **3**, 606–16.

Passingham, R. (1993). *The Frontal Lobes and Voluntary Action.* Oxford: Oxford University Press.

Passingham, R. E. (1996). Attention to action. *Proceedings of the Royal Society of London,* B **351**, 1473–9.

Patel, M. D., Coshall C., Rudd A. G., and Wolfe C. D. A. (2002). Cognitive impairment after stroke: clinical determinants and its associations with long-term stroke outcomes. *Journal of the American Geriatric Society,* **50**, 700–6.

Patterson, K. E., and Shewell, C. (1987). Speak and spell: Dissociations and word-class effects. In *The cognitive neuropsychology of language* (ed. G. Sartori) pp. 273–94. Hillsdale, NJ: Lawrence Erlbaum Associates.

Patterson, K. E., Lambon, E., and Ralph, M. A. (1999). Selective disorders of reading? *Current Opinion in Neurobiology,* **9**, 235–9.

Pedersen, P. M., Jorgensen, H. S., Nakayama, H., Raaschou, H. O., and Olsen, T. S. (1995). Aphasia in acute stroke: incidence, determinants and recovery. Annals of Neurology, **38**, 659–66.

Pederson, P. M., Jorgensen, H. S., Nakayama, H., Raaschou, H. O., and Olsen, T. S. (1996). Aphasia in acute stroke: Incidence, determinants, and recovery. Reply. *Annals of Neurology,* **40**, 130.

Penades, R., Boget, T., Lomena, F. *et al.* (2002). Could the hypofrontality pattern in schizophrenia be modified through neuropsychological rehabilitation? *Acta Psychiatrica Scandinavica,* **105**, 202–8.

Penman, T. (1999). Breaking down the barriers. *Bulletin of the Royal College of Speech and Language Therapists,* August, 14–15.

Perkins, L., Crisp, J., and Walshaw, D. (1999). Exploring conversation analysis as an assessment tool for aphasia: the issue of reliability. *Aphasiology,* **13**, 259–81.

Perret, E. (1974). The left frontal lobe of man and the suppression of habitual responses in verbal categorical behaviour. *Neuropsychologia,* **12**, 323–30.

Perry, R. J. and Hodges, J. R. (1999). Attention and executive deficits in Alzheimer's disease: a critical review. *Brain,* **122**, 383–404.

Petersen, S. E., Fox, P. T., Posner, M. I., Mintun, M., and Raichle, M. E. (1988). Positron emission tomographic studies of the cortical anatomy of single-word processing. *Nature,* **331**, 585–9.

Petersen, S. E., Fox, P. T., Posner, M. I., Mintun, M., and Raichle, M. E. (1989). Positron emission tomographic studies of the processing of single words. *Journal of cognitive Neuroscience,* **1**, 153–70.

Petrides, M. (1994). Frontal lobes and working memory: evidence from investigations of the effects of cortical excisions in nonhuman primates. In *Handbook of Neuropsychology* (eds F. Boller and J. Grafman), Vol. **9**, pp. 59–82.

Petrides, M. (1998). Specialized systems for the processing of mnemonic information within the primate frontal cortex. In *The Prefrontal Cortex: Executive and Cognitive Functions* (eds A. C. Roberts, T. W. Robbins and L. Weiskrantz), pp. 103–16. Oxford: Oxford University Press.

Petrides, M. and Milner, B. (1982). Deficits on subject-ordered tasks after frontal- and temporal-lobe lesions in man. *Neuropsychologia*, **20**, 249–62.

Petty, R. G., Bonner, D., Mouratoglou, V., and Silverman, M. (1996). Acute frontal lobe syndrome and dyscontrol associated with bilateral caudate nucleus infarctions. *British Journal of Psychiatry*, **168**, 237–40.

Piaget, J. (1952). *The Origins of Intelligence in Children*. New York: International Universities Press, Inc.

Piatt, A. L., Fields, J. A., Paolo, A. M., and Troster, A. I. (1999). Action (verb naming) fluency as an executive measure: Convergent and divergent evidence. *Neuropsychologia*, **37**, 1499–503.

Pick, A. (1906). Ueber einen weiteren Symptomenkomplex im Rahmen der Dementia senilis, bedingt durch umschriebene stärkere Hirnatrophie (gemischte Apraxie). *Monatsschrift für Psychiatrie and Neurologie*, **19**, 97–108.

Pickersgill, M. J. and Lincoln, N. B. (1983). Prognostic indicators and the pattern of recovery of communication in aphasic stroke patients. *Journal of Neurology, Neurosurgery and Psychiatry*, **46**, 130–9.

Picton, T. W., Alain, C., and McIntosh, A. R. (2002). The theatre of the mind: Physiological studies of the human frontal lobes. In *Principles of Frontal Lobe Function* (eds D. T. Stuss and R. K. Knight), pp. 109–26. New York: Oxford University Press.

Piefke, M., Weiss, P. H., Zilles, K., Markowitsch, H. J., and Fink, G. R. (2003). Differential remoteness and emotional tone modulate the neural correlates of autobiographical memory. *Brain*, **126**, 650–68.

Pierce, S. R. and Buxbaum, L. J. (2002). Treatments of unilateral neglect: a review. *Arch Phys Med Rehabil*, **83**, 256–68.

Plaut, D. (1996). Relearning after damage in connectionist networks: toward a theory of rehabilitation. *Brain and Language*, **52**, 25–82.

Plaut, D. C. (1997). Structure and function in the lexical system: Insights from distributed models of word reading and lexical decision. *Language and Cognitive Processes*, **12**, 765–805.

Plaut, D. C. and Shallice, T. (1993). Deep dyslexia: a case study in connectionist neuropsychology. *Cognitive Neuropsychology*, **10**, 377–500.

Plaut, D. C., McClelland, J. L., Seidenberg, M. S., and Patterson, K. (1996). Understanding normal and impaired word reading: Computational principles in quasi-regular domains. *Psychological Review*, **103**, 56–115.

Poeck, K., Huber, W., and Willmes, K. (1989). Outcome of intensive language treatment in aphasia. *Journal of Speech and Hearing Disorders*, **54**, 471–9.

Polster, M. and Rapcsak, S. (1996). Representations in learning new faces: Evidence from prosopagnosia. *Journal of the International Neuropsychological Society*, **2**, 240–8.

Ponsford, J. and Kinsella, G. (1991). The use of a rating scale of attentional behaviour. *Neuropsychological Rehabilitation*, **1**, 241–58.

Ponsford, J. L. and Kinsella, G. (1988). Evaluation of a remedial programme for attentional deficits following closed-head injury. *Journal of Clinical and Experimental Neuropsychology*, **10**, 693–708.

Ponsford, J., Sloan, W., and Snow, P. (1995). *Traumatic brain injury: Rehabilitation for everyday adaptive living*. Hove: Lawrence Erlbaum Associates.

Poppelreuter, W. (1917, translated by J. Zihl with the assistance of L. Weinkrantz) (1990). *Disturbances of lower and higher visual capacities caused by occipital damage: With special reference to the psychopathological, pedagogical, industrial, and social implications*. Oxford: Oxford University Press.

Porch, B. (1967). *The Porch Index of Communicative Ability: Theory and Development, vol 1*. Palo Alto, CA: Consulting Psychologists Press.

Porch, B. E. (1967). *Porch index of communicative ability, Vol. 2: Administration, scoring and interpretation*, 3rd edn. Palo Alto, CA: Consulting Psychologists Press.

Porch, B. E. (1981). *Porch index of communicative ability*. Palo Alto, CA: Consulting Psychologists Press.

Posner, M. I. (1993). Interaction of arousal and selection in the posterior attention network. In *Attention: Selection, awareness and control* (eds A. Baddeley and L. Weiskrantz), pp. 390–405. Oxford: Clarendon Press.

Posner, M. I. and Badgaiyan, R. D. (1998). Attention and neural networks. In *Fundamentals of neural network modelling* (eds R. W. Parks, D. S. Levine and D. L. Long), pp. 61–76. Cambridge, MA: MIT Press.

Posner, M. I. and Dehaene, S. (2000). Attentional networks. In *Cognitive neuroscience: A reader* (ed. M. S. Gazzaniga). Oxford: Blackwell Publishing Ltd.

Posner, M. I. and Petersen, S. E. (1990). The attentional system of the human brain. *Annual Review of Neuroscience*, **13**, 25–42.

Posner, M. I., Petersen, S. E., Fox, P. T., and Raichle, M. E. (1988). Localization of cognitive operations in the human-brain. *Science*, **240**, 1627–31.

Posner, M. I., Snyder, C. R. R., and Davidson, B. J. (1980). Attention and the detection of signals. *Journal of Experimental Psychology: General*, **109**, 160–74.

Posner, M. I.,Walker, J. A., Freidrick, F. J., and Rafal, R. D. (1984). Effects of parietal injury on covert orienting of visual attention. *Journal of Neuroscience*, **4**, 1863–74.

Post, M. W. M., de Witte, L. P., and Schrijvers, A. J. P. (1999). Quality of life and the ICIDH: towards an integrated conceptual model for rehabilitation outcomes research. *Clinical Rehabilitation*, **13**, 5–15.

Pound, C. (1998). Therapy for life: finding new paths across the plateau. *Aphasiology*, **12**, 222–7.

Pound, C., Parr, S., Lindsay J., and Woolf, C. (2000). *Beyond Aphasia: Therapies for Living with Communication Disability*. Bicester: Winslow Press.

Powell, J., Heslin, J., and Greenwod, R. (2002). Community based rehabilitation after severe traumatic brain injury: a randomized controlled trial. *Journal of Neurology, Neurosurgery and Psychiatry*, **72**, 193–202.

Powell, J. H., al-Adawi, S., Morgan, J., and Greenwood, R. J. (1996). Motivational deficits after brain injury: effects of bromocriptine in 11 patients. *Journal of Neurology, Neurosurgery and Psychiatry*, **60**, 416–21.

Powell, J. M., Temkin, N. R., Machamer, J. E., and Dikmen, S. S. (2002). Nonrandomized studies of rehabilitation for traumatic brain injury: can they determine effectiveness? *Archives of Physical Medicine and Rehabilitation*, **83**, 1235–44.

Prada, G. and Tallis, R. C. (1995). Treatment of neglect syndrome in stroke patients using a contingency electrical stimulator. *Clinical Rehabilitation*, **9**, 304–13.

Pressly, M. (1993). Teaching cognitive strategies to brain injured clients: the good information processing perspective. *Seminars in Speech and Language*, **14**, 1–17.

Pribram, K. H. (1971). *Languages of the brain. Experimental paradoxes and principles in neuropsychology*. Englewood Cliffs, NJ: Prentice-Hall.

Price, C. J. (2000). The anatomy of language: contributions from functional neuroimaging. *Journal of Anatomy*, **197**, 335–59.

Price, C. J. and Friston, K. J. (2002). Functional imaging studies of neuropsychological patients: Applications and limitations. *Neurocase*, **8**, 345–54.

Price, C. J., Wise, R. J. S., Warburton, E. A., Moore, C. J., Howard, D., Patterson, K., Frackowiak, R. S. J., and Friston, K. J. (1996). Hearing and saying – The functional neuro-anatomy of auditory word processing. *Brain*, **119**, 919–31.

Price, C. J., Wise, R. J. S., Watson, J. D. G., Patterson, K., Howard, D., and Frackowiak, R. S. J. (1994). Brain activity during reading – the effects of exposure duration and task. *Brain*, **117**, 1255–69.

Prigatano, G. P. (1986a). Higher cerebral deficits: History of methods of assessment and approaches to rehabilitation: Part I. *BNI Quarterly*, **2**(4), 9–17.

Prigatano, G. P. (1986b). Higher cerebral deficits: History of methods of assessment and approaches to rehabilitation: Part II. *BNI Quarterly*, **2**(3), 15–26.

Prigatano, G. P. (1991). Disturbances of self-awareness of deficit after traumatic brain injury. In *Awareness of Deficit After Brain Injury: Clinical and Theoretical Issues* (eds G. P. Prigatano and D. L. Schacter). New York: Oxford University Press.

Prigatano, G. P. (1995). Personality and social aspects of memory rehabilitation. In *Handbook of memory disorders* (eds A. D. Baddeley, B. A. Wilson and F. N. Watts), pp. 603–14. Chichester: John Wiley and Sons.

Prigatano, G. P. (1999). *Principles of neuropsychological rehabilitation.* New York: Oxford University Press.

Prigatano, G. P. (2001). Rehabilitation of higher cerebral functions and the patient's personality. *BNI Quarterly,* **17**(2), 21–9.

Prigatano, G. P. and Kime, S. K. (2003). What do brain dysfunctional patients report following memory compensation training? *Neurorehabilitation,* **18**, 47–55.

Prigatano, G. P. and Pliskin, N. (eds) (2003). *Clinical Neuropsychology and Cost Outcome Research: A Beginning,* New York: Psychology Press (First book in NAN Book Series).

Prigatano, G. P. and Weinstein, E. A. (1996). Edwin A. Weinstein's contributions to neuropsychological rehabilitation. *Neuropsychological rehabilitation,* **6**(4), 305–26.

Prigatano, G. P., Fordyce, D. J., Zeiner, H. K., Roueche, J. R., Pepping, M., and Wood, B. C. (1984). Neuropsychological rehabilitation after closed head injury in young adults. *Journal of Neurology, Neurosurgery and Psychiatry,* **47**, 505–13.

Prigatano, G. P., Fordyce, D. J., Zeiner, H. K., Roueche, J. R., Pepping, M., and Wood, B. C. (1986). *Neuropsychological rehabilitation after brain injury.* Baltimore: The Johns Hopkins University Press.

Prigatano, G. P., Ziegler, L., and Rosenstein, L. (2003). The clinical neuropsychological examination: Its scope, cost, and healthcare value. In *Clinical neuropsychology and cost outcome research: A beginning* (eds G. P. Prigatano and N. Pliskin). New York: Psychology Press.

Pring, T. (1986). Evaluating the effects of speech therapy for aphasics: developing single case methodology. *The British Journal of Disorders of Communication,* **21**, 103–16.

Prins, R. S., Schoonen, R., and Vermeulen, J. (1989). Efficacy of two different types of speech therapy for aphasic stroke patients. *Applied Psycholinguistics,* **10**, 85–123.

Pritchard, D. A. (1998). *The Tests of Neuropsychological Malingering.* New York: CRC Press.

Quayhagen, M. P., Quayhagen, M., Corbeil, R. R., Hendrix, R. C., Jackson, J. E., Snyder, L., and Bower, D. (2000). Coping with dementia: evaluation of four nonpharmacologic interventions. *International Psychogeriatrics,* **12**, 249–65.

Quayhagen, M. P., Quayhagen, M., Corbeil, R. R., Roth, P. A., and Rodgers, J. A. (1995). A dyadic remediation program for care recipients with dementia. *Nursing Research,* **44**, 153–59.

Ramachandran, V. S., Stewart, M., and Rogers-Ramachandran, D. C. (1992). Perceptual correlates of massive cortical reorganisation. *NeuroReport,* **3**, 583–86.

Rath, J. F., Simon D., Langenbahn, D. M., Sherr, L., and Diller, L. (2003). Group treatment of problem solving deficits in outpatients with traumatic brain injury: a randomized outcome study. *Neuropsychological Rehabilitation,* **13**, 461–88.

Rattok, J., Ben-Yishay, Y., Ezrachi, O. *et al.* (1992). Outcome of different treatment mixes in a multidimensional neuropsychological rehabilitation program. *Neuropsychology,* **6**, 395–415.

Raymer, A. and Gonzalez, Rothi, L. (2002). Clinical diagnosis and treatment of naming disorders. In *The handbook of adult language disorders* (ed. A. Hillis) . Psychology Press: New York.

Rayner, H. and Marshall, J. (2003). Training volunteers as conversation partners for people with aphasia. *The International Journal of Language and Communication Disorders,* **38**, 149–64.

Reason, J. T. (1984). Lapses of attention in everyday life. In *Varieties of attention* (eds R. Parasuraman, R. Davies and J. Beatty), pp. 515–49. Orlando, FL: Academic Press.

Recanzone, G. H., Schreiner, C. E., and Merzenich, M. M. (1993). Plasticity in the frequency representation of primary auditory cortex. *Journal of Neuroscience,* **13**, 87–103.

Reifler, B. V. and Larson, E. (1990). Excess disability in dementia of the Alzheimer's type. In *Alzheimer's Disease Treatment and Family Stress* (eds E. Light and B. D. Lebowitz). New York: Hemisphere.

Reitan, R. M. and Wolfson, D. (1994). A selective and critical review of neuropsychological deficits and the frontal lobes. *Neuropsychology Review,* **4**, 161–98.

Rey, A. (1964). *L'examen clinique en psychologie.* Paris: Presses Universitaires de France.

Ribot, T. (1882). *Diseases of Memory.* D. Appleton and Co., New York.

Richardson, J. T. E. (1995). The efficacy of imagery mnemonics in memory remediation. *Neuropsychologia,* **33**(11), 1345–7.

Riddoch, M. J. and Humphreys, G. (1994a). *Cognitive neuropsychology and cognitive rehabilitation.* Hove: Lawrence Erlbaum Associates.

Riddoch, M. J. and Humphreys, G. (1994b). Cognitive Neuropsychology and cognitive rehabilitation: A marriage of equal partners? In *Cognitive neuropsychology and cognitive rehabilitation* (eds M. J. Riddoch and G. Humphreys), pp.1–15. Hove: Lawrence Erlbaum Associates.

Riddoch, M. J. and Humphreys, G. W. (1993). *BORB*: Birmingham Object Recognition Battery. Hove: Psychology Press.

Rizzolati, G., Riggio, L., and Sheliga, B. M. (1994). Space and selective attention. In *Attention and performance XV, Conscious and non-conscious information processing* (eds C. Umilta and M. Moscovitch), pp. 231–66. Cambridge, MA: MIT Press.

Robbins, T. W. (1998). Dissociating executive functions of the prefrontal cortex. In *The Prefrontal Cortex: Executive and Cognitive Functions* (eds A. C. Roberts, T. W. Robbins and L. Weiskrantz), pp. 117–30. Oxford: Oxford University Press.

Roberts, W. A. (2002). Are animals stuck in time? *Psychological Bulletin,* **128,** 473–89.

Robertson, I. H. (1994). Editorial: Methodology in neuropsychological rehabilitation research. *Neuropsychological Rehabilitation, 4,* 1–6.

Robertson, I. H. (1996). *Goal Management Training: A Clinical Manual.* Cambridge: PsyConsult.

Robertson, I. H. (1999). The Rehabilitation of Attention. In *Cognitive Neurorehabilitation* (eds D. T. Stuss, G. Winocur and I. H. Robertson), pp. 302–313. Cambridge: Cambridge University Press.

Robertson, I. H. (1999). Setting goals for cognitive rehabilitation. *Current Opinion in Neurology,* **12,** 703–08.

Robertson, I. H. and Halligan, P. W. (1999). *Spatial neglect. A clinical handbook for diagnosis and treatment.* Hove: Psychology Press.

Robertson, I. H. and Heutink, J. (2002). Rehabilitation of unilateral neglect. In *Cognitive rehabilitation – a clinical neuropsychological approach* (eds W. H. Brouwer, A. H. van Zomeren *et al.*). Amsterdam: Boom.

Robertson, I. H. and Manly, T. (1999). Sustained attention deficits in time and space. In *Attention, space and action* (eds G. W. Humphreys, J. Duncan and A. Treisman). Oxford: Oxford University Press.

Robertson, I. H. and Murre, J. M. J. (1999). Rehabilitation of brain damage: Brain plasticity and principles of guided recovery. *Psychological Bulletin,* **125,** 544–75.

Robertson, I. H. and North, N. (1994). One hand is better than two: Motor extinction of left hand advantage in unilateral neglect. *Neuropsychologia, 32,* 1–11.

Robertson, I. H., Hogg, K., and McMillan, T. M. (1998). Rehabilitation of unilateral neglect: improving function by contralesional limb activation. *Neuropsychological Rehabilitation, 8,* 19–29.

Robertson, I. H., Manly, T., Andrade, J., Baddeley, B. T., and Yiend, J. (1997). 'Oops!': Performance correlates of everyday attentional failures in traumatic brain injured and normal subjects. *Neuropsychologia, 35,* 747–58.

Robertson, I. H., Mattingley, J. B., Rorden, C., and Driver, J. (1998b). Phasic alerting of neglect patients overcomes their spatial deficit in visual awareness. *Nature, 395*(10), 169–72.

Robertson, I. H., McMillan, T. M., MacLeod, E., and Brock, D. (2002). Rehabilitation by Limb Activation Training (LAT) reduces impairment in unilateral neglect patients: A single-blind randomised control trial. *Neuropsychological Rehabilitation, 12,* 439–54.

Robertson, I. H., North, N., and Geggie, C. (1992). Spatio-motor cueing in unilateral neglect: Three single case studies of its therapeutic effectiveness. *Journal of Neurology, Neurosurgery and Psychiatry, 55,* 799–805.

Robertson, I. H., Ridgeway, V., Greenfield, E., and Parr, A. (1997). Motor recovery after stroke depends on intact sustained attention: A two-year follow-up study. *Neuropsychology, 11,* 290–5.

Robertson, I. H., Tegner, R., Tham, K., Lo, A., and Nimmo-Smith, I. (1995). Sustained attention training for unilateral neglect: theoretical and rehabilitation implications. *Journal of Clinical and Experimental Neuropsychology, 17,* 416–30.

Robertson, I. H., Ward, T., Ridgeway V., and Nimmo-Smith, I. (1994). *The Test of Everyday Attention.* Bury St. Edmunds: Thames Valley Test Company.

Robey, R. R. (1994). The efficacy of treatment for aphasic persons: A meta-analysis. *Brain and Language, 47,* 582–608.

Robey, R. R. (1998). A meta-analysis of clinical outcomes in the treatment of aphasia. *Journal of Speech, Language, and Hearing Research, 41,* 172–87.

Robey, R. (2001). CEU part III: Evidence-based practice. *ASHA Special Interest Division 2 Newsletter,* **11**(1), 10–5.

Robey, R. R., Schultz, M. C., Crawford, A. B., and Sinner, C. A. (1999). Single subject clinical-outcome research: designs, data, effect sizes, and analyses. *Aphasiology, 13*, 445–73.

Robson, J., Marshall, J., Chiat, S., and Pring, T. (2001). Enhancing communication in jargon aphasia: a small group study of writing therapy. *International Journal of Language and Communication Disorders, 36*, 471–88.

Robson, J., Pring, T., Marshall, J., Morrison, S., and Chiat, S. (1998). Written communication in undifferentiated jargon aphasia: a therapy study. *International Journal of Language and Communication Disorders, 33*, 305–28.

Rogers, M., Alarcon, N., and Olswang, L. (1999). Aphasia management considered in the context of the World Health Organisation model of disablements. *Physical Medicine and Rehabilitation Clinics of North America, 10*, 907–23.

Romijn, H. (1997). About the origin of consciousness. A new, multidisciplinary perspective on the relationship between brain and mind. *Proceedings van de Koningklijke Nederlandse Akadmie van Wetenschappen, 100*, 181–267.

Romijn, H. (2002). Are virtual photons the elementary carriers of consciousness? *Journal of Consciousness Studies, 9*, 61–81.

Rosenstein, L. D. and Price, R. F. (1994). Shaping a normal rate of eating using audiotaped pacing in conjunction with a token economy. *Neuropsychological Rehabilitation, 4*, 387–98.

Rosenthal, M., Griffith, E. R., Kreutzer, J. S., and Pentland, B. (eds) (1999). *Rehabilitation of the Adult and Child with Traumatic Brain Injury.* Philadelphia: F. A. Davis Company/Publishers.

Roskies, A. L., Fiez, J. A., Balota, D. A., Raichle, M. E., and Petersen, S. E. (2001). Task-dependent modulation of regions in the left inferior frontal cortex during semantic processing. *Journal of Cognitive Neuroscience, 13*, 829–43.

Ross, K. and Wertz, R. (1999). Comparison of impairment and disability measures for assessing severity of and improvement in aphasia. *Aphasiology, 13*, 113–24.

Ross, K. B. and Wertz, R. T. (2002). Relationships between language-based disability and quality of life in chronically aphasic adults. *Aphasiology, 16*, 791–800.

Ross, K. B. and Wertz, R. T. (2003). Quality of life with and without aphasia. *Aphasiology, 17*, 355–64.

Roth, M., Tym, E., Mountjoy, C. *et al.* (1986). CAMDEX. A standardised instrument for the diagnosis of mental disorder in the elderly with special reference to the early detection of dementia. *British Journal of Psychiatry, 149*, 698–709.

Rothi, L. J. G., Ochipa, C., and Heilman, K. M. (1997). A cognitive neuropsychological model of limb praxis and apraxia. In *Apraxia: The neuropsychology of action* (eds L. J. G. Rothi and K. M. Heilman), pp. 29–49. Hove: Psychology Press.

Roy, E. A. and Square, P. A. (1985). Common considerations in the study of limb, verbal, and oral apraxia. In *Neuropsychological studies of apraxia and related disorders* (ed. E. A. Roy), pp. 111–61. Amsterdam: North-Holland.

Royal College of Physicians (2002). *National Guidelines for Stroke.* London: Royal College of Physicians, Clinical Effectiveness and Evaluation Unit.

Rubenfield, G. D. (2001). Understanding why we agree on the evidence but disagree on the medicine. *Respiratory Care, 46*(12), 1442–9.

Ruchinskas, R. (2002). Rehabilitation therapists' recognition of cognitive and mood disorders in geriatric patients. *Arch. Phys Med. Rehabil, 83*, 609–12.

Ruff, R. M. and Niemann, H. (1990). Cognitive rehabilitation versus day treatment in head-injured adults: Is there an impact on emotional and psychosocial adjustment? *Brain Injury, 4*, 339–47.

Ruff, R. M., Baser, C. A., Johnston, J. W. *et al.* (1989). Neuropsychological rehabilitation: an experimental study with head-injured patients. *Journal of Head Trauma Rehabilitation, 4*(3), 20–36.

Ruff, R., Mahaffey, R., Engel, J., Farrow, C., Cox, D., and Karzmark, P. (1994). Efficacy study of THINKable in the attention and memory retraining of traumatically head-injured patients. *Brain Injury, 8*, 3–14.

Rumelhart, D. E., McClelland, J. L., and the PDP Research Group (1986). *Parallel distributed processing: Explorations in the microstructure of cognition. Volume 1: Foundations.* Cambridge, MA: Bradford Books/MIT Press.

Ruml, W. and Caramazza, A. (2000). An evaluation of a computational model of lexical access: Comment on Dell *et al.* (1997). *Psychological Review, 107*, 609–34.

Ruml, W., Caramazza, A., Shelton, J. R., and Chialant, D. (2000). Testing assumptions in computational theories of aphasia. *Journal of Memory and Language, 43*, 217–48.

Ryan, T. V. and Ruff, R. M. (1988). The efficacy of structured memory retraining in a group comparison of head trauma patients. *Archives of Clinical Neuropsychology, 3*, 165–79.

Ryff, C. (1989). Happiness is everything, or is it? Explorations on the meaning of well-being. *Journal of Personality and Social Psychology, 57*, 1069–81.

Sabel, B. A. (1997). Unrecognized potential of surviving neurons: Within-systems plasticity, recovery of function and the hypothesis of minimal residual structure. *The Neuroscientist, 3*, 366–70.

Sacchett, C., Byng, S., Marshall, J., and Pound, C. (1999). Drawing together: evaluation of a therapy programme for severe aphasia. *International Journal of Language and Communication Disorders, 34*, 265–89.

Sacchett, C. and Marshall, J. (1992). Functional assessment of communication: Implications for the rehabilitation of aphasic people: Reply to Carol Frattali. *Aphasiology, 6*, 95–100.

Sackett, D. L., Straus, S. E., Richardson, W. S., Rosenberg, W., and Haynes, R. B. (eds) (2000). *Evidence-based medicine. How to practice and teach EBM*. Edinburgh, London, New York: Churchill Livingstone.

Saffran, E. M., Berndt, R. S., and Schwartz, M. F. (1989). The quantitative analysis of agrammatic production: Procedure and data. *Brain and Language, 37*, 440–79.

Sahakian, B. J., Coull, J. J., and Hodges, J. R. (1994). Selective enhancement of executive function in a patient with dementia of the frontal lobe type. *Journal of Neurology, Neurosurgery and Psychiatry, 57*, 120–1.

Salazar, A. M., Warden, D. L., Schwab, K., Spector, J., Braverman, S., Walter, J., Cole, R., Rosner, M. M., Martin, E. M., Ecklund, J., and Elenberg, R. G. (2000). Cognitive rehabilitation for traumatic brain injury. A randomized trial. *Journal of the American Medical Association, 282*(23), 3075–81.

Salmon, D. P., and Fennema-Notestine, C. (1996). Implicit memory. In *The Cognitive Neuropsychology of Alzheimer-type Dementia* (ed. R. Morris) . Oxford: Oxford University Press.

Salmon, D. P., Heindel, W. C., and Butters, N. (1992). Semantic memory, priming and skill learning in Alzheimer's disease. In *Memory Functioning in Dementia* (ed. L. Bäckman). Amsterdam: Elsevier Science Publications BV.

Sands, E., Sarno, M. T., and Shankweiler, D. (1969). Long-term assessment of language function in aphasia due to stroke. *Archives of Physical Medicine and Rehabilitation, 50*, 202–6.

Sara, S. J. (2000). Retrieval and reconsolidation. Toward a neurobiology of remembering. *Learning and Memory, 7*, 73–84.

Sarno, M. T. (1969). *The Functional Communication Profile*. New York: Institute of Rehabilitation Medicine, NYU Medical Center.

Sarno, M. T. and Levita, E. (1971). Natural course of recovery in severe aphasia. *Archives of Physical Medicine and Rehabilitation, 52*, 175–8.

Sarno, M. T. and Levita, E. (1979). Recovery in treated aphasia in the first year post-stroke. *Stroke, 10*, 663–9.

Sarno, M. T., Silverman, M., and Sands, E. (1970). Speech therapy and language recovery in severe aphasia. *Journal of Speech and Hearing Research, 13*, 607–23.

Sarter, M. and Markowitsch, H. J. (1985). The amydala's role in human mnemonic processing. *Cortex, 21*, 7–24.

Sbordone, R. J. (1996). Ecological validity: Some critical issues for the neuropsychologist. In *Ecological validity of neuropsychological testing* (eds. R. D. Sbordone and C. J. Long). Florida: GR Press/St Lucie Press.

Schacter, D. L. and Buckner, R. I. (1998). Priming and the brain. *Neuron, 20*, 185–95.

Schacter, D. L. and Glisky, E. L. (1986). Memory remediation: restoration, alleviation and the acquisition of domain-specific knowledge. In *Clinical neuropsychology of intervention* (eds B. Uzzell and Y. Gross), pp. 257–82. Boston: Martinus Nijhoff.

Schank, R. C. (1982). *Dynamic Memory: A Theory of Reminding and Learning in Computers and People*. Cambridge: Cambridge University Press.

Scharf, B. (1998). Auditory attention: The psychoacoustical approach. In *Attention* (ed. H. Pashler). Hove: Psychology Press.

Scherzer, B. P. (1986). Rehabilitation following severe head trauma: Results of a three-year program. *Archives of Physical Medicine and Rehabilitation, 67*, 366–74.

Schindler, I., Kerkhoff, G., Karnath, H.-O., Keller, I., and Goldenberg, G. (2002). Neck muscle vibration induces lasting recovery in unilateral neglect. *Journal of Neurology, Neurosurgery and Psychiatry* **73**, 412–19.

Schmitter-Edgecombe, M., Fahy, J. F., Whelan, J. P., and Long, C. J. (1995). Memory remediation after severe closed head injury: Notebook training versus supportive therapy. *Journal of consulting and Clinical psychology*, **63**, 484–9.

Schnider, A., Ptak, R., von Deniken, C., and Remonda, L. (2000). Recovery from spontaneous confabulations parallels recovery of temporal confusion in memory. *Neurology*, **55**, 74–83.

Schoonen, R. (1991). The internal validity of efficacy studies: Design and statistical power in studies of language therapy for aphasics. *Brain and Language*, **41**, 446–64.

Schuell, H. (1965). *The Minnesota test for differential diagnosis of aphasia*. Minneapolis, MN: University of Minnesota Press.

Schulz, K. F., Chalmers, I., Hayes, R. J., and Altman, D. G. (1995). Empirical evidence of bias: dimensions of methodological quality associated with estimates of treatment effects in controlled trials. *Journal of the American Medical Association*, **273**, 408–12.

Schwartz, M. F., Buxbaum, L. J., Montgomery, M. W., Fitzpatrick-DeSalme, E., Hart, T., Ferraro, M. *et al.* (1999). Naturalistic action production following right hemisphere stroke. *Neuropsychologia*, **37**, 51–66.

Schwartz, M. F., Lee, S. S., Coslett, H. B., Montgomery, M. W., Buxbaum, L. J., Carew, T. G. *et al.* (1998). Naturalistic action impairment in closed head injury. *Neuropsychology*, **12**, 13–28.

Scoville, W. B. and Milner, B. (1957). Loss of recent memory after bilateral hippocampal lesions. *Journal of Neurology, Neurosurgery and Psychiatry*, **20**, 11–21.

Seale, G. S., Caroselli, J. S., High, W. M., Becker, C. L., Neese, L. E., and Scheibel, R. (2002). Use of the Community Integration Questionnaire (CIQ) to characterize changes in functioning for individuals with traumatic brain injury who participated in a post-acute brain injury rehabilitation programme. *Brain Injury*, **16**, 955–67.

Seidenberg, M. S. (1988). The cognitive neuropsychology of language – Coltheart, M., Sartori,G., Job, R. *Cognitive Neuropsychology*, **5**, 403–26.

Seidenberg, M. S. and McClelland, J. L. (1989). A distributed, developmental model of word recognition and naming. *Psychological Review*, **96**, 523–68.

Seron, T. and DeLoche, G. (1989). *Cognitive approaches in rehabilitation*. Hillsdale, NJ: Lawrence Erlbaum Associates.

Seron, X., van der Linden, M., and de Partz, M.-P. (1991). In defence of cognitive approaches in neuropsychological therapy. *Neuropsychological Rehabilitation*, **1**, 303–18.

Seyal, M., Ro, T. and Rafal, R. (1995). Increased sensitivity to ipsilateral cutaneous stimuli following transcranial magnetic stimulation of the parietal lobe. *Annals of Neurology*, **38**, 264–67.

Shallice, T. (2000) Cognitive neuropsychology and rehabilitation: is pessimism justified? *Neuropsychological Rehabilitation*, **10**, 209–17.

Shallice, T. (1988). *From Neuropsychology to Mental Structure*. Cambridge: Cambridge University Press.

Shallice, T. and Burgess, P. W. (1991a). Deficits in strategy application following frontal lobe damage in man. *Brain*, **114**, 727–41.

Shallice, T. and Burgess, P. W. (1991b). Higher-order cognitive impairments and frontal lobe lesions in man. In *Frontal Lobe Function and Dysfunction* H. S. Levin, (eds H. M. Eisenberg and A. L. Benton), pp. 125–38. New York: Oxford University Press.

Shallice, T. and Burgess, P. W. (1993). Supervisory control of action and thought selection. In *Attention: Selection, Awareness and Control* (eds A. D. Baddeley and L. Weiskrantz). Oxford: Oxford University Press.

Shallice, T. and Burgess, P. W. (1996). The domain of supervisory processes and the temporal organisation of behaviour. *Philosophical Transactions of the Royal Society of London B*, **351**, 1405–12. (Reprinted In *The Prefrontal Cortex: Executive and Cognitive Functions* (eds A. C. Roberts, T. W. Robbins and L. Weiskrantz), pp. 22–35. Oxford University Press, 1988.)

Shallice, T. and Burgess, P. (1996). The domain of the supervisory process and temporal organisation of behaviour. *Philosphical Transactions: Biological Sciences*, **351**, 1405–12.

Shallice, T. and Evans, M. E. (1978). The involvement of the frontal lobes in cognitive estimation. *Cortex*, **14**, 294–303.

Shallice, T., Burgess, P. W., Schon, F., and Baxter, D. M. (1989). The origins of utilisation behaviour. *Brain*, **112**, 1587–98.

Shapiro, A. M., Benedict, R. H. B., Schretlen, D., and Brandt, J. (1999). Construct and concurrent validity of the Hopkins Verbal Learning Test – Revised. *The Clinical Neuropsychologist*, **13**, 348–58.

Sheldrake, R. (1988). *The presence of the past.* New York: Times Books.

Shewan, C. M. and Kertesz, A. (1984). Effects of speech and language treatment in recovery from aphasia. *Brain and Language* **23**, 272–99.

Shiffrin, R. M. and Schneider, W. (1977). Controlled and automatic information processing: II. Perception, learning and automatic attending and a general theory. *Psychological Review*, **84**, 127–90.

Shores, E. A., Carstairs, J. R., and Crawford, J. R. (submitted). Crawford Excluded Letter Fluency Test (CELF): Norms and test-retest reliability data for healthy young adults.

Shores, E. A., Marosszeky, J. E., Sandanam, J., and Batchelor, J. (1986). Preliminary validation of a clinical scale for measuring the duration of post-traumatic amnesia. *The Medical Journal of Australia*, **144**, 569–73.

Sidman, M. and Stoddard, L. T. (1967). The effectiveness of fading in programming simultaneous form discrimination for retarded children. *Journal of Experimental Analysis of Behavior*, **10**, 3–15.

Silverman, W. A. (1998). *Where's the evidence? Debates in modern medicine.* New York: Oxford University Press.

Simmons-Mackie, N. (2001). Social approaches to aphasia intervention. In *Language intervention strategies in aphasia and related neurogenic communication disorders* (ed. R. Chapey). Baltimore, MD: Lippincott Williams and Wilkins.

Simmons-Mackie, N. and Damico, J. (2001). Intervention outcomes: a clinical application of qualitative methods. *Topics in Language Disorders*, **21**, 21–36.

Sivak, M., Hill, C. S., Henson, D. L., Butler, B. P., Silber, S. M., and Olson, P. L. (1984). Improved driving performance following perceptual training in persons with brain damage. *Archives of Physical Medicine and Rehabilitation*, **65**, 163–7.

Sixsmith, A., Stilwell, J., and Copeland, J. (1993). 'Rementia': challenging the limits of dementia care. *International Journal of Geriatric Psychiatry*, **8**, 993–1000.

Skeel, R. L. and Edwards, S. (2001). The assessment and rehabilitation of memory disorders. In *Rehabilitation of Neuropsychological Disorders: A Practical Guide for Rehabilitation Professionals* (eds B. Johnstone and H. Stonnington). Florence, KY: Psychology Press.

Skinner, C., Wirz, S., Thompson, I., and Davidson, J. (1984). *Edinburgh Functional Communication Profile.* Winslow: Winslow Press.

Small, S. (2002). Biological approaches to treatment of aphasia . In *Handbook of adult language disorders: integrating cognitive neuropsychology, neurology, and rehabilitation* (ed. A. E. Hillis), pp. 397–412. Philadelphia, PA: Psychology Press.

Small, G. W., Rabins, P. V., Barry, P. P., Buckholtz, N. S., DeKosky, S. T., Ferris, S. H., Finkel, S. I., Gwyther, L. P., Khachaturian, Z. S., Lebowitz, B. D., McRae, T. D., Morris, J. C., Oakley, F., Schneider, L. S., Streim, J. E., Sunderland, T., Teri, L. A., and Tune, L. E. (1997). Diagnosis and treatment of Alzheimer disease and related disorders: consensus statement of the American Association for Geriatric Psychiatry, the Alzheimer's Association and the American Geriatric Society. *Journal of the American Medical Association*, **278**, 1363–71.

Smith, J. L., Magill-Evans, J., and Brintnell, A. (1998). Life satisfaction following traumatic brain injury. *Canadian Journal of Rehabilitation*, **11**, 131–40.

Smith, G. V., Della Sala, S., Logie, R. H., and Maylor, E. A. M. (2000). Prospective and retrospective memory in normal ageing and dementia: A questionnaire study. *Memory*, **8**, 311–21.

Sohlberg, M. M. (2002). An overview of approaches for managing attention impairments. In *Perspectives on Neurophysiology and Neurogenic Speech and Language Disorders* (Issue ed. M. R. T. Kennedy), **12**(3), 4–8.

Sohlberg, M. M. and Mateer, C. A. (1987). Effectiveness of an attention training program. *Journal of Clinical and Experimental Neuropsychology*, **9**, 117–130.

Sohlberg, M. M. and Mateer, C. A. (1989). Training use of compensatory memory books: A three stage behavioral approach. *Journal of Clinical and Experimental Neuropsychology*, **11**, 871–91.

Sohlberg, M. M. and Mateer, C. A. (1989). *Introduction to cognitive rehabilitation. Theory and practice.* New York: Guilford Press.

Sohlberg, M. M. and Mateer, C. A. (2001). *Cognitive rehabilitation: An integrative neuropsychological approach.* New York: Guilford Press.

Sohlberg, M. M., Glang, A., Todis, B. (1998). Improvement during baseline: Three case studies encouraging collaborative research when evaluating caregiver training. *Brain Injury,* **12**(4), 333–46.

Sohlberg, M. M., Mateer, C. A., and Stuss, D. T. (1993). Contemporary approaches to the management of executive control dysfunction. *Journal of Head Trauma Rehabilitation,* **8**, 45–58

Sohlberg, M. M., McLaughlin, K. A., Todis, B., Larsen, J., and Glang, A. (2001). What does it take to collaborate with families affected by brain injury? A preliminary model. *Journal of Head Trauma Rehabilitation,* **16**, 498–511.

Sohlberg, M. M., Sprunk, H., and Metzelaar, K. (1988). Efficacy of an external cueing system in an individual with severe frontal lobe damage. *Cognitive Rehabilitation,* **6**, 36–41.

Sohlberg, M. M., Todis, B., and Glang, A. (1998). SCEMA: A team-based approach to serving secondary students with executive dysfunction following brain injury. *Aphasiology,* **12**(12), 1047–92.

Sohlberg, M. M., Avery, J., Kennedy, M., Yorkston, K., Coelho, C., Turkstra, L., and Ylvisaker, M. (2003). Practice guidelines for direct attention training. *Journal of Medical Speech-Language Pathology,* **11**(3), xix–xxxix.

Sohlberg, M. M., McLaughlin, K. A., Pavese, A., Heidrich, A., and Posner, M. (2000). Evaluation of attention process training and brain injury education in persons with acquired brain injury. *Journal of Clinical and Experimental Neuropsychology,* **22**(5), 656–76.

Solveri, P., Brown, R. G., Jahanashi, M., Caraceni, T., and Marsden, C. D. (1997). Learning manual pursuit tracking skills in patients with Parkinson's disease. *Brain,* **120**, 1325–37.

Sonde, L., Nordstrom, M., Nilsson, C. G., Lokk, J., and Viitanen, M. (2001). A double-blind placebo-controlled study of the effects of amphetamine and physiotherapy after stroke. *Cerebrovascular Diseases,* **12**, 253–7.

Spearman, C. (1927). *The Abilities of Man.* New York: Macmillan.

Spector, A., Orrell, M., Davies, S., and Woods, B. (2001). Can reality orientation be rehabilitated? Development and piloting of an evidence-based programme of cognition-based therapies for people with dementia. *Neuropsychological Rehabilitation,* **11**, 377–97.

Spector, A., Orrell, M., Davies, S., and Woods, R. T. (1998). *Reality orientation for dementia: a review of the evidence for its effectiveness* (Issue 4). Oxford: Update Software.

Spector, A., Thorgrimsen, L., Woods, B., Royan, L., Davies, S., Butterworth, M., and Orrell, M. (2003). Efficacy of an evidence-based cognitive stimulation therapy programme for people with dementia: randomised controlled trial. *British Journal of Psychiatry,* **183**, 248–54.

Spence, C. J. and Driver, J. (1996). Audiovisual links in covert spatial attention. *Journal of Experimental Psychology: Human Perception and Performance,* **22**, 1005–30.

Spikman, J. M. (2001). Attention, mental speed and executive control after closed head injury: deficits, recovery and outcome. Doctoral thesis, State University Groningen.

Spikman, J. M., Deelman, B. G., and van Zomeren, A. H. (2000). Executive functioning, attention and frontal lesions in patients with chronic CHI. *Journal of Clinical and Experimental Neuropsychology,* **22**, 325–38.

Spikman, J. M., Kiers, H. A. L., Deelman, B. G., and Van Zomeren, A. H. (2001). Construct validity of concepts of attention in healthy controls and closed head injured patients. *Brain and Cognition,* **47**, 446–70.

Spikman, J. M., van Zomeren, A. H., and Deelman, B. G. (1996). Deficits of attention after closed head injury: Slowness only? *Journal of Clinical and Experimental Neuropsychology,* **18**, 755–67.

Spreen, O. and Strauss, E. (1998). *A compendium of neuropsychological tests: Administration, norms and commentary.* New York: Oxford University Press.

Spreen, O. and Strauss, E. (1998). *A Compendium of Neuropsychological Tests,* 2nd edn. New York: Oxford University Press

Squire, L. R. (1992). Declarative and nondeclarative memory: Multiple brain systems supporting learning and memory. *Journal of Cognitive Neuroscience,* **4**, 232–43.

Squire, L. R. (1998). Memory systems. *C. R. Academy of Science, Paris, Life Sciences,* **321**, 153–6.

Squire, L. R. and Knowlton, B. J. (1995). Memory, hippocampus and brain systems. In *The Cognitive Neurosciences* (ed. M. Gazzaniga). Boston: MIT Press.

Squires, E. J., Hunkin, N. M., and Parkin, A. J. (1997). Errorless learning of novel associations in amnesia. *Neuropsychologia,* **35**, 1103–11.

Stablum, F., Umilta, C., Mogentale, C., Carlan, M., Guerrini, C. (2000). Rehabilitation of executive deficits in closed head injury and anterior communicating artery aneurysm patients. *Psychological Research*, **63**, 265–78.

State University of New York at Buffalo (1990). *Guide for the uniform data set for medical rehabilitation (FIM)*. Buffalo, NY: SUNY.

Sterzi, R., Bottini, G., Celani, M., Righetti, E., Lamassa, M., Ricci, M., and Vallar, G. (1993). Hemianopia, hemianaesthesia and hemiplegia after right and left hemisphere damage. A hemispheric difference. *Journal of Neurology, Neurosurgery and Psychiatry*, **56**, 308–10.

Stewart, F. M., Sunderland, A., Sluman, S. (1996). The nature and prevalence of memory disorder after stroke. *British Journal of Clinical Psychology*, **35**, 369–79.

Strich, S. J. (1956). Diffuse degeneration of the cerebral white matter in severe dementia following head injury. *Journal of Neurology, Neurosurgery and Psychiatry*, **19**, 163–85.

Sturm, W. and Willmes, K. (1991). Efficacy of a reaction training on various attentional and cognitive functions in stroke patients. *Neuropsychological Rehabilitation*, **1**, 259–80.

Sturm, W., Willmes, K., Orgass, B., and Hartje, W. (1997). Do specific attention deficits need specific training? *Neuropsychological Rehabilitation*, **7**, 81–103.

Stuss, D. T. and Alexander, M. P. (2000). Executive functions and the frontal lobes: A conceptual view. *Psychological Research*, **63**, 289–98.

Stuss, D. T. and Benson, D. F. (1984). Neuropsychological studies of the frontal lobes. *Psychological Bulletin*, **95**, 3–29.

Stuss, D. T. and Benson, D. F. (1986). *The Frontal Lobes*. New York: Raven Press.

Stuss, D. T., Alexander, M. P., Floden, D., Binns, M. A., Levine, B., McIntosh, A. R., Rajah, N., and Hevenor, S. J. (2002). Fractionation and localisation of distinct frontal lobe precesses: Evidence from focal lesions in humans. In *Principles of Frontal Lobe Function* (eds D. T. Stuss and R. K. Knight), pp. 392–407. New York: Oxford University Press.

Stuss, D. T., Eskes, G. A., and Foster, J. K. (1994). Experimental neuropsychological studies of frontal lobe functions. In *Handbook of Neuropsychology* (eds F. Boller and J. Grafman), Vol. 9. Amsterdam: Elsevier Science B. V.

Stuss, D. T., Levine, B., Alexander, M. P., Hong, J., Palumbo, C., Hamer, L., Murphy, K. J., and Izukawa, D. (2000). Wisconsin Card Sorting Test performance in patients with focal frontal and posterior brain damage: Effects of lesion location and test structure on separable cognitive processes. *Neuropsychologia*, **38**, 388–402.

Stuss, D. T., Shallice, T., Alexander, M. P., and Picton, T. W. (1995). A mulitidisclinary approach to anterior attentional functions. *Annals of the New York Academy of Sciences*, **769**, 191–211.

Stuss, D. T., Toth, J. P., Franchi, D., Alexander, M. P., Tipper, S., and Craik, F. I. M.(1999). Dissociation of attentional processes in patients with focal frontal and posterior lesions. *Neuropsychologia* **37**, 1005–27.

Stuss, D. T., Winocur, G., and Robertson, I. (1999). *Cognitive Neurorehabilitation*. Cambridge: Cambridge University Press.

Styles, E. A. (1997). *The psychology of attention*. Hove: Psychology Press.

Sunderland, A., Bowers, M. P., Sluman, S. M., Wilcock, D. J., and Ardron, M. E. (1999). Impaired dexterity in the ipsilateral hand after stroke and the relationship to cognitive deficit. *Stroke*, **30**, 949–55.

Sunderland, A., Harris, J. E., and Baddeley, A. D. (1988). Do laboratory tests predict everyday memory? A neuropsychological study. *Journal of Verbal Learning and Verbal Behaviour*, **22**, 341–57.

Tamamoto, F., Sumi, Y., Nakanishi, A., Okayasu, K., Maehara, T., and Katayama, H. (2000). Usefulness of cerebral blood flow (CBF) measurements to predict the functional outcome for rehabilitation in patients with cerebrovascular disease (CVD). *Annals of Nuclear Medicine*, **14**, 47–52.

Tatemichi, T. K., Desmond, D. W., Stern, Y., Paik, M., Sano, M., and Bagiella, E. (1994). Cognitive impairment after stroke: frequency, patterns and relationship to functional abilities. *Journal of Neurology, Neurosurgery and Psychiatry*, **57**, 202–7.

Taub, E. and Wolf, S. L. (1997). Constraint induced movement techniques to facilitate upper extremity use in stroke patients. *Topics in Stroke Rehabilitation*, **3**, 38–61.

Taub, E., Miller, N. E., Novack, T. A., Cook, E. W., Fleming, W. C., Nepomuceno, C. S., Connell, J. S., and Crago, J. E. (1993). Technique to improve chronic motor deficit after stroke. *Archives of Physical Medicine and Rehabilitation*, **74**, 347–54.

Taylor, L. B. (1979). Psychological assessment of neurosurgical patients. In *Functional Neurosurgery* (eds T. Rassmussen and R.Marino). New York: Raven Press.

Taylor, R. and O'Carroll, R. E. (1995). Cognitive estimation in neurological disorders. *British Journal of Clinical Psychology*, **34**, 223–8.

Temple, C. M. (1987). *Developmental cognitive neuropsychology*. Hove: Psychology Press.

Terrace, H. S. (1963). Discrimination learning with and without "errors". *Journal of Experimental Analysis of Behavior*, **6**, 1–27.

Thiel, A., Herholz, K., and Koyuncu, A. *et al.* (2001). Plasticity of language networks in patients with brain tumors: a positron emission tomography activation study. *Annals of Neurology*, **50**, 620–29.

Thoene, A. I. T. and Glisky, E. L. (1995). Learning of face-name associations in memory impaired patients: a comparison of different training procedures. *Journal of the International Neuropsychological Society*, **1**, 29–38.

Thomas-Stonell, N., Johnson, P., Schuller, R., Jutai, J. (1994). Evaluation of a computer-based program for remediation of cognitive-communication skills. *Journal of Head Trauma Rehabilitation*, **9**, 25–37.

Thompson, C. (1998). Treating sentence production in agrammatic aphasia. In *Approaches to the treatment of aphasia* (eds N. Helm-Estabrooks and A. Holland). San Diego: Singular Publishing Group.

Thompson, C. K., Fix, S. C., Gitelman, D. R., Parrish, T. B., Mesulam, M. M. (2000). FMRI studies of agrammatic sentence comprehension before and after treatment. *Brain and Language*, **74**, 387–91.

Thompson, J. B. and Kerns, K. A. (1999). Mild traumatic brain injury in children. In *Neuropsychological management of mild traumatic brain injury* (eds S. A. Raskin and C. A. Mateer), pp. 233–51. New York: Oxford University Press.

Thulborn, K. R., Carpenter, P. A., Just, M. A. (1999). Plasticity of language-related brain function during recovery from stroke. *Stroke*, **30**, 749–54.

Tinson, D. J. (1989). How stroke patients spend their days. An observational study of the treatment regime offered to stroke patients in hospital with movement disorders following stroke. *International Disability Studies*, **11**, 45–49.

Tinson, D. J. and Lincoln, N. B. (1987). Subjective memory impairment after stroke. *International Disability Studies*, **9**, 6–9.

Tipper, S. P., Howard, L. A., and Houghton, G. (1999). Action based mechanisms of attention. In *Attention space and action: Studies in cognitive neuroscience* (eds G. W. Humphreys, J. Duncan and A. Treisman), pp. 232–47. Oxford: Oxford University Press.

Togher, L. (2001). Discourse sampling in the 21st century. *Journal of Communication Disorders*, **34**, 131–50.

Togher, L., McDonald, S., Code, C., and Grant, S. (2004). Training communication partners of people with traumatic brain injury: a randomised controlled trial. *Aphasiology*, **18**, 313–35.

Toglia, J. R. (1993). *Contextual Memory Test*. San Antonio,Texas: Therapy Skill Builders (a division of the Psychological Corporation).

Tombaugh, T. N. (1996). *Test of Memory Malingering*. New York: Multi-Health Systems.

Tombaugh, T. N. (1997). The Test of Memory Malingering: Normative data from cognitively intact and cognitively impaired individuals. *Psychological Assessment*, **9**, 260–8.

Tonelli, M. R. (2001). The limits of evidence-based medicine. *Respiratory Care*, **46**(12), 1435–41.

Towle, D. and Lincoln, N. B. (1991). Development of a questionnaire for detecting everyday problems in stroke patients with unilateral visual neglect. *Clinical Rehabilitation*, **5**, 135–40.

Towle, D., Edmans, J. A., and Lincoln, N. B. (1990). An evaluation of a group treatment programme for stroke patients with perceptual deficits. *Int Jour Rehab Res*, **13**, 328–35.

Traversa, R., Cincinelli, P., Bassi, A., Rossini, P. M., and Bernardi, G. (1997). Mapping of motor cortical reorganisation after stroke: A brain stimulation study with focal magnetic pulses. *Stroke* **28**, 110–7.

Treisman, A. (1999). Feature binding, attention and object perception. In *Attention space and action: Studies in cognitive neuroscience* (eds G. W. Humphreys, J. Duncan and A. Treisman), pp. 91–111. Oxford: Oxford University Press.

Treisman, A. M. and Gelade, G. (1980). A feature integration theory of attention. *Cognitive Psychology*, **12**, 97–136.

Troyer, A. K. Moscovitch, M., Winucur, G., Alexander, M. P., and Stuss, D. T. (1998). Dissociation of attentional processes in patients with focal frontal and posterior lesions. *Neuropsychologia* **37**, 1005–27.

Tulving, E. (1972). Episodic and semantic memory. In *Organization of memory* (eds E. Tulving and W. Donaldson), pp. 381–403. New York: Academic Press.

Tulving, E. (1983). *Elements of episodic memory.* Cambridge: Cambridge University Press.

Tulving, E. (2002). Episodic memory from mind to brain. *Annual Review of Psychology*, **53**, 1–25.

Tulving, E. and Markowitsch, H. J. (1998). Hippocampus and episodic memory. *Hippocampus*, **8**, 198–204.

Tulving, E. and Markowitsch, H. J. (in prep.). Where is the uniqueness of human memory in the brain?

Tulving, E., Kapur S., Craik, F. I. M., Moscovitch, M., and Houle, S. (1994). Hemispheric encoding/Retrieval asymmetry in episodic memory: positron emission tomography findings. *Proceedings of the National Academy of Sciences of the USA*, **91**, 2016–20.

Tunis, S. R., Stryer, D. B., and Clancy, C. M. (2003). Practical clinical trials: Increasing the value of clinical research for decision making in clinical and health policy. *Journal of the American Medical Association*, **290**, 1624–32.

Turner, J. M., Green, G., and Braunling-McMorrow, D. (1990). Differential reinforcement of low rates of responding to reduce dysfunctional social behaviours of a head injured man. *Behaviour Residential Treatment*, **5**, 15–27.

Turner-Stokes, L., Nyein, K., Turner-Stokes, T., and Gatehouse, C. (1999). The UK FIM+FAM: development and evaluation. *Clinical Rehabilitation*, **13**, 277–88.

Twum, M. and Parente, R. (1994). Role of imagery and verbal labeling in the performance of paired associates tasks by persons with closed head injury. *Journal of Clinical and Experimental Neuropsychology*, **16**, 630–39.

Tyler, K. L. and Malessa, R. (2000). The Goltz-Ferrier debates and the triumph of cerebral localizationalist theory. *Neurology*, **55**, 1015–24.

Ulatowska, H. K., Olness, G. S., Wertz, R. T., Thompson, J. L., Keebler, M. W., Hill, C. L., and Auther, L. L. (2001). Comparison of language impairment, functional communication and discourse measures in African-American aphasic and normal adults. *Aphasiology*, **15**, 1007–16.

Ungerleider, L. G. and Mishkin, M. (1982). Two cortical visual systems. In *Analysis of visual behaviour* (eds D. Ingle, M. A. Goodale, R. J. W. Mansfield), pp. 459–86. Cambridge, MA: MIT Press.

Uttl, B., Graf, P., and Richter, L. K. (2002). Verbal paired-associate tests: limits on validity and reliability. *Archives of Clinical Neuropsychology*, **17**, 567–81.

Valenstein, E. S., Bowers, D., Verfaellie, M., Heilman, K. M., Day, A., and Watson, R. T. (1987). Retrosplenial amnesia. *Brain*, **110**, 1631–46.

van den Broek, M. D., Bradshaw, C. M., and Szabadi, E. (1993). Utility of the Modified Wisconsin Card Sorting Test in neuropsychological assessment. *British Journal of Clinical Psychology*, **32**, 333–43.

Van Reekum, R. Bayley, M., Garner, S. *et al.* (1995). N of 1 study: amantadine for the amotivational syndrome in a patient with traumatic brain injury. *Brain Injury*, **9**, 49–53.

Van Zomeren, A. H. and Spikman, J. M. (2003). Assessment of attention. In *Handbook of clinical neuropsychology* (eds P. W. Halligan, U. Kischka and J. C. Marshall). Oxford: Oxford University Press.

Van Zomeren, A. H., Brouwer, N. H., and Deelman, B. G. (1984). Attention deficits: The riddle of selectivity, speed and alertness. In *Closed head injury: Psychological, social and family consequences* (ed. N. Brooks), pp. 74–107. Oxford: Oxford University Press.

Van Zomeren, A. H. and Van Den Burg, W. (1985). Residual complaints of patients two years after severe head injury. *Journal of Neurology, Neurosurgery, and Psychiatry*, **48**, 21–8.

vanDellen, A., Blakemore, C., Deacon, R. *et al.* (2000). Delaying the onset of Huntington's in mice. *Nature*, **404**, 721–2.

Vandenberghe, R., Price, C., Wise, R., Josephs, O., and Frackowiak, R.S.J. (1996). Functional anatomy of a common semantic system for words and pictures. *Nature*, **383**, 254–6.

Vanier, M., Gauthier, L., and Lambert, J. (1990). Evaluation of left visuospatial neglect: norms and discrimination power of two tests. *Neuropsychology*, **4**, 87–96.

Vargha-Khadem, F., Gadian, D. G., Watkins, K. E., Connelly, A., Van Paesschen, W., and Mishkin, M. (1997). Differential effects of early hippocampal pathology on episodic and semantic memory. *Science*, **277**, 376–80.

Varney, N. R. and Menefee, L. (1993). Psychosocial and executive deficits following closed head injury: implications for orbital frontal cortex. *Journal of Head Trauma Rehabilitation*, **8**, 32–44.

Veltman, J. C., Brouwer, W. H., Zomeren, A. H. van, and Wolffelaar, P. C. van (1996). Central executive aspects of attention in subacute severe and very severe closed head injury patients: planning, inhibition, flexibility and divided attention. *Neuropsychology*, **10**, 1–11.

Vignolo, L. A. (1964). Evolution of aphasia and language rehabilitation: a retrospective exploratory study. *Cortex*, **1**, 344–67.

Vogel, W. B., Rittman, M., Bradshaw, P. *et al.* (2002). Outcomes from stroke rehabilitation in Veterans Affairs rehabilitation units: Detecting and correcting for selection bias. *Journal of Rehabilitation Research and Development*, **39**, 367–84.

Volpe, B. T., Ledoux, J. E., and Gazzaniga, M. S. (2000). Information processing of visual stimuli in an 'extinguished' field. In *Cognitive neuroscience: A reader* (ed. M. S. Gazzaniga). Oxford: Blackwell Publishing Ltd.

von Cramon, D. Y. and Matthes-von Cramon, G. (1990). Frontal lobe dysfunctions in patients – therapeutical approaches. In *Cognitive Rehabilitation in Perspective* (eds R. Ll. Wood and I. Fussey), pp. 164–179. London: Taylor and Francis.

von Cramon, D. Y. and Matthes-von Cramon, G. (1992). Reflections on the treatment of brain injured patients suffering from problem-solving disorders. *Neuropsychological Rehabilitation*, **2**, 207–30.

von Cramon, D. Y. and Matthes-von Cramon, G. (1994). Back to work with a chronic dysexecutive syndrome? (A case report). *Neuropsychological Rehabilitation*, **4**, 399–417.

von Cramon D. Y., Matthes-von Cramon, G., and Mai, N. (1991). Problem-solving deficits in brain injured patients: A therapeutic approach. *Neuropsychological Rehabilitation*, **1**, 45–64.

Waddell, G. (2002). *Models of disability, using low back pain as an example.* London: The Royal Society of Medicine Press Ltd.

Wade, D. T. (2000). Personal context as a focus for rehabilitation. *Clinical Rehabilitation*, **14**, 115–18.

Wade, D. T. (2001a). Disability, rehabilitation and spinal injury. In *Brain's textbook of neurology* (ed. M. Donaghy), 11th edn, pp. 185–209. Oxford: Oxford University Press.

Wade, D. T. (2001b). Social context as a focus for rehabilitation. *Clinical Rehabilitation*, **15**, 459–61.

Wade, D. T. (2002). Cognitive assessment and neurological rehabilitation. *Clinical Rehabilitation*, **16**, 117–18.

Wade, D. T. (2005). Applying the WHO ICF framework to the rehabilitation of patients with cognitive deficits. In *Effectiveness of rehabilitation for cognitive deficits* (eds P. W. Halligan and D. T. Wade). Oxford: Oxford University Press.

Wade D. T. and Collin, C. (1988). The Barthel ADL Index: a standard measure of physical disability? *International Disability Studies*, **10**, 64–6722.

Wade D. T. and Halligan, P. (2003). New wine in old bottles: the WHO ICF as an explanatory model of human behaviour. *Clinical Rehabilitation*, **18**, 349–54.

Wade, D. T., Hewer, R. L., David, R. M., and Enderby, P. M. (1986). Aphasia after stroke: natural history and associated deficits. *Journal of Neurology, Neurosurgery and Psychiatry*, **49**, 11–16.

Wahrborg, P., Borenstein, N., Linell, S., Hedberg-Borenstein, E., and Asking, M. (1997). Ten-year follow-up of young aphasic participants in a 34-week course at a Folk High School. *Aphasiology* **11**, 709–15.

Walker, S. (1992). Assessment of Language Dysfunction in Crawford JR, Parker DM and McKinlay WW *A Handbook of Neuropsychological Assessment* (eds). Hove: Lawrence Erlbaum Associates.

Walker, C. M., Sunderland, A., Sharma, J., and Walker, M. F. (2004). The impact of cognitive impairment on upper body dressing difficulties after stroke: A video analysis of patterns of recovery. *Journal of Neurology, Neurosurgery and Psychiatry*, **75**, 43–48.

Walker, C. M., Walker, M. F., and Sunderland, A. (2003). Dressing after a stroke: A survey of current occupational therapy practice. *British Journal of Occupational Therapy.* **66**, 263–68.

Walker-Batson, D. (2000). Use of pharmacotherapy in the treatment of aphasia. *Brain and Language*, **71**, 252–4.

Walker-Batson, D., Curtis, S., Natarajan, R., Ford, J., Dronkers, N., Salmeron, E., Lai J., and Unwin, D. H. (2001). A double-blind placebo-controlled use of amphetamine in the treatment of aphasia. *Stroke*, **32**, 2093–8.

Walker-Batson, D., Devous, M. D., Curtis, S., Unwin, D. H., and Greenlee, R. G. (1991). Response to amphetamine to facilitate recovery from aphasia subsequent to stroke. *Clinical Aphasiology*, **21**, 137–43.

Walker-Batson, D., Smith, P., Curtis, S., Unwin, H., and Greenlee, R. (1995). Amphetamine paired with physical therapy accelerates motor recovery after stroke. Further evidence. *Stroke*, **26**, 2254–9.

Walsh, B. F. and Lamberts, F. (1979). Errorless discrimination and fading as techniques for teaching sight words to TMR students. *American Journal of Mental Deficiency*, **83**, 473–9.

Warburton, E., Swinburn, K., Price, C. J. *et al.* (1999). Mechanisms of recovery from aphasia: evidence from positron emission tomographic studies. *Journal of Neurology, Neurosurgery and Psychiatry*, **66**, 155–61.

Ware, J. J. and Sherbourne, C. D. (1992). The MOS 36-item short-form survey (SF-36): I Conceptual framework and item selection. *Medical Care*, **30**, 473–83.

Warrington, E. K. and Weiskrantz, L. (1970). Amnesic syndrome: Consolidation or retrieval? *Nature*, **228**, 628–30.

Warrington, E. K. (1984). *Recognition Memory Test.* Windsor: NFER-Nelson.

Warrington, E. K. (1996). *The Camden Memory Tests.* Hove: Psychology Press.

Warrington, E. K. (2000). Homophone meaning generation: A new test of verbal switching for the detection of frontal lobe dysfunction. *Journal of the International Neuropsychological Society*, **6**, 643–8.

Watson, R. T., Fleet, S., Rothi, L. J. G., and Heilman, K. M. (1986). Apraxia and the supplementary motor area. *Archives of Neurology*, **43**, 787–92.

Watt, K. J. and O'Carroll, R. E. (1999). Evaluating methods for estimating premorbid intellectual ability in closed head injury. *Journal of Neurology, Neurosurgery and Psychiatry*, **66**, 474–9.

Webster, J. S. and Scott, R. R. (1983). The effects of self-instructional training on attentional deficits following head injury. *Clinical Neuropsychology*, **5**, 69–74.

Wechsler, D. (1998a). *Wechsler Memory Scale-III.* San Antonio, TX: The Psychological Corporation.

Wechsler, D. (1998b). *Wechsler Adult Intelligence Scale-III.* San Antonio, TX: The Psychological Corporation.

Weekes, B. and Coltheart, M. (1996). Surface dyslexia and surface dysgraphia: Treatment studies and their theoretical implications. *Cognitive Neuropsychology*, **13**, 277–315.

Weiller, C. (2000). Brain imaging in recovery from aphasia. *Brain and Language*, **74**, 385–7.

Weiller, C., Isensee, C., Rijntjes, M. *et al.* (1995). Recovery from Wernicke's aphasia: a positron emission tomographic study. *Annals of Neurology*, **37**, 723–32.

Weinstein, E. A. and Kahn, R. L. (1955). *Denial of illness. Symbolic and physiological aspects.* Springfield, IL: Charles C Thomas.

Weiskrantz, L. (1986). *Blindsight: A case study and implications.* Oxford: Oxford University Press.

Weniger, D. (1990). Diagnostic tests as tools of assessment and models of information processing: a gap to bridge. *Aphasiology*, **4**, 109–13.

Weniger, D. and Sarno, M. (1990). The future of aphasia therapy: More than just new wine in old bottles? *Aphasiology*, **4**, 301–6.

Wepman, J. M. (1951). *Recovery from aphasia.* New York: Ronald Press.

Wernicke, C. (1874). *Der aphasische Symptomenkomplex.* Breslau: Cohn and Weigert.

Wertz, R., Collins, M., Weiss, D., Kurtzke, J., Friden, T., Brookshire, R., Pierce, J., Holtzapple, P., Hubbard, D., Porch, B., West, J., Davis, L., Matovitch, V., Morley, G., and Resurreccion, E. (1981). Veterans administration cooperative study on aphasia: a comparison of individual and group treatment. *Journal of Speech and Hearing Research*, **24**, 580–94.

Wertz, R., Weiss, D., Aten, J., Brookshire, R., Garcia-Bunuel, L., Holland, A., Kurtzke, J., LaPointe, L., Milianti, F., Brannegan, R., Greenbaum, H., Marshall, R., Vogel, D., Carter, J., Barnes, N., and Goodman, R. (1986). Comparison of clinic, home and deferred language treatment for aphasia: a veterans administration cooperative study. *Archives of Neurology*, **43**, 653–8.

Whitworth, A., Perkins, L., and Lesser, R. (1997). *Conversation analysis profile for people with aphasia.* London: Whurr.

Whitworth, A. B., Webster, J., and Howard, D. (in press). *A cognitive neuropsychological approach to assessment and intervention in aphasia: A clinician's guide.* Hove: Psychology Press.

WHO (2001). *The international classification of functioning, disability and health (ICF).* Geneva: World Health Organisation.

Whurr, R. (1996). *The aphasia screening test,* 2nd edn San Diego, CA: Singular Publishing Group.

Whurr, R., Lorch, M. P., and Nye, C. (1992). A meta-analysis of studies carried out between 1946 and 1988 concerned with the efficacy of speech and language therapy treatment for aphasic patients. *European Journal of Disorders of Communication,* **27**, 1–17.

Whyte, J. (1997). Distinctive methodologic challenges. In *Assessing medical rehabilitation practices: the promise of outcome research* (ed. M. J. Fuhrer), pp. 43–59. London: Paul H. Brookes.

Whyte, J. (2002). Traumatic brain injury rehabilitation: are there alternatives to randomized clinical trials? *Archives of Physical Medicine and Rehabilitation,* **83**, 1320–2.

Whyte, J. and Hart, T. (2003). It's more than a black box; it's a Russian doll: Defining rehabilitation treatments. *American Journal of Physical Medicine and Rehabilitation,* **82**, 639–52.

Wickens, C. D. (1991). Processing resources and attention. In *Multiple-task performance* (ed. D. I. Damos). London: Taylor and Francis.

Wiggins, E. C. and Brandt, J. (1988). The detection of simulated amnesia. *Law and Human Behaviour,* **12**, 57–78.

Wilkinson, R., Bryan, K., Lock, S., Bayley, K., Maxim, J., Bruce, C., Edmundson, A., and Moir, D. (1998). Therapy using conversational analysis: Helping couples adapt to aphasia in conversation. *International Journal of Language and Communication Disorders,* **33**, 144–9.

Will, B. and Kelche, C. (1992). Environmental approaches to recovery of function from brain damage: A review of animal studies (1981 to 1991). In *Recovery from brain damage: Reflections and directions* (eds F. D. Rose and D. A. Johnson), pp. 79–103. New York: Plenum.

Williams, W. H., Evans, J. J., and Wilson, B. A. (2003). Neurological rehabilitation for two cases of post-traumatic stress disorder following traumatic brain injury. *Cognitive Neuropsychiatry.*

Williams, L., Weinberger, M., Harris, L., Clark, D., and Biller, J. (1999). Development of a stroke-specific quality of life scale. *Stroke,* **30**, 1362–9.

Willmes, K. and Poeck, K. (1984). Ergebnisse einer multizentrischen Untersuchung über die Spontanprognose von Aphasien vaskulärer Aetiologie. *Nervenartz,* **55**, 62–71.

Willmes, K. and Poeck, K. (1993). To what extent can aphasic syndromes be localized? *Brain,* **116**, 1527–40.

Wilshire, C. E. and Coslett, H. B. (2000). Disorders of word retrieval in aphasia: theories and potential applications. In *Aphasia and language: Theory to practice* (eds S. E. Nadeau, L. J. Gonzalez-Rothi and B. Crosson). New York: Guilford Press.

Wilson, B. A. (1987). *Rehabilitation of memory.* New York, London: The Guilford Press.

Wilson, B. A. (1995). Management and remediation of memory problems in brain-injured adults. In *Handbook of memory disorders* (eds A. D. Baddeley, B. A. Wilson and F. N. Watts), pp. 451–79. Chichester: John Wiley.

Wilson, B. A. (1997). Cognitive rehabilitation: How it is and might be. *Journal of the International Neuropsychological Society,* **3**, 487–96.

Wilson, B. A. (1999). *Case Studies in Neuropsychological Rehabilitation.* New York: Oxford University Press.

Wilson, B. A. (2002). Towards a comprehensive model of cognitive rehabilitation. *Neuropsychological Rehabilitation,* **12**(2), 97–110.

Wilson, B. A. and Evans, J. (1996). Therapy for the injured brain. *MRC News,* 36–40.

Wilson, B. A. and Evans, J. (2002). Does cognitive rehabilitation work? Clinical and economic considerations and outcomes. In *Clinical neuropsychology and cost-outcome research: An introduction* (ed. G. Prigatano), pp. 329–49. Hove: Psychology Press.

Wilson, B. A. and Patterson, K.E. (1990). Rehabilitation and cognitive neuropsychology. *Applied Cognitive Psychology,* **4**, 247–60.

Wilson, B. and Robertson, I. H. (1992). A home based intervention for attentional slips during reading following head injury: A single case study. *Neuropsychological Rehabilitation* **2**, 193–205.

Wilson, B. A., Alderman, N., Burgess, P. W., Emslie, H., and Evans, J. J. (1996). *BADS – Behavioural Assessment of the Dysexecutive Syndrome.* Bury St. Edmunds: Thames Valley Test Company.

Wilson, B. A., Baddeley, A. D., Evans E., and Shiel, A. (1994). Errorless learning in the rehabilitation of memory impaired people. *Neuropsychological Rehabilitation,* **4**, 307–26.

Wilson, B. A., Clare, L., Cockburn, J. M., Baddeley, A. D., Tate,R., and Watson, P. (1999). *The Rivermead Behavioural memory Test- Extended Version*. Bury St Edmunds: Thames Valley Test Company.

Wilson, B. A., Cockburn, J., and Baddeley, A. (1985). *The Rivermead Behavioural Memory Test*. Bury St Edmunds: Thames Valley Test Company.

Wilson, B. A., Cockburn, J., and Baddeley, A. (2003). *The Rivermead Behavioural Memory Test. Second Edition*. Bury St Edmunds: Thames Valley Test Company.

Wilson, B. A., Cockburn, J., and Halligan, P. (1987). *Behavioural Inattention Test*. Bury St Edmunds: Thames Valley Test Company.

Wilson, B. A., Emslie, H., Quirk, K., and Evans, J. (1999). George: Learning to live independently with NeuroPage®. *Rehabilitation Psychology*, **44**, 284–96.

Wilson, B. A., Emslie, H., Quirk K., and Evans J. J. (2001). Reducing everyday memory and planning problems by means of a paging system: a randomised control crossover study. *Journal of Neurosurgery, Neurology and Psychiatry*, **70**, 477–82.

Wilson, B. A., Evans, J. J., Emslic H., and Malinek, V. (1997). Evaluation of NeuroPage: A new memory aid. *Journal of Neurology Neurosurgery and Psychiatry* **63**, 113–15.

Wilson, F. A. W., Ó Scalaidhe, S. P., and Goldman-Rakic, P. S. (1993). Dissociation of object and spatial processing domains in prefrontal cortex. *Science* **260**, 1955–8.

Wilson, B. A., Watson, P. C., Baddeley, A. D., Emslie, H., and Evans, J. J. (2000). Improvement or simply practice? The effects of twenty repeated assessments on people with and without brain injury. *Journal of the International Neuropsychological Society*, **6**, 469–79.

Wise, R. J. S., Greene, J., Buchel, C., and Scott, S. K. (1999). Brain regions involved in articulation. *Lancet*, **353**, 1057–61.

Wood, R. L. and Fussey, I. (1987). Computer-based cognitive retraining: A controlled study. *International Disability Studies*, **9**, 149–53.

Wood, R. Ll. and Worthington, A. D. (1999). Outcome in community rehabilitation: measuring the social impact of disability. *Neuropsychological Rehabilitation*, **9**, 505–16.

Wood, R. Ll, McCrea, J. D., Wood, L. M., and Merriman, R. N. (1999). Clinical and cost-effectiveness of post-acute neurobehavioural rehabilitation. *Brain Injury*, **13**, 69–88.

Wood, R. Ll. and Worthington, A. D. (2001). Neurobehavioural rehabilitation: a conceptual paradigm. In *Neurobehavioural Disability and social handicap following traumatic brain injury*, (eds. R. Ll. Wood and T. M. McMillan), pp. 107–131. Hove: Psychology Press.

Woods, R. T. (1996). Psychological 'therapies' in dementia. In *Handbook of the Clinical Psychology of Ageing* (ed. R. T. Woods), pp. 575–600. Chichester: John Wiley and Sons Ltd.

Woods, R. T. (2002). Reality orientation: a welcome return? Editorial. *Age and Ageing*, **31**, 1–2.

Woolf, S. H. (1993). Practice guidelines: a new reality in medicine, III: impact on patient care. *Archives of Internal Medicine* **153**, 2646–55.

World Health Organisation (1980). *International Classification of Impairments, Disabilities and Handicaps: A Manual of Classification Relating to the Consequences of Disease*. Geneva: WHO.

World Health Organisation (1998). *International Classification of Impairments, Disabilities and Handicaps* (2). World Health Organisation. Available at: www.who.int/msa/mnh/ems/icidh/introduction.htm.

World Health Organisation (2001). *International classification of functioning, disability and health*. Geneva, Switzerland: WHO.

Worrall, L. E. (1992). *Everyday Communicative Needs Assessment*. Department of Speech and Hearing, University of Queensland, Australia.

Worrall, L. E. (1999). *Functional communication therapy planner*. Winslow: Winslow Press.

Worrall, L. E. (2000). A conceptual framework for a functional approach to acquired neurogenic disorders of communication and swallowing. In *Neurogenic communication disorders: A functional approach* (eds L. E. Worrall and C. M. Frattali). New York: Thieme.

Worrall, L. E. and Holland, A. L. (2003). Quality of life in aphasia. *Aphasiology*, **17**, 329–32.

Worrall, L. E., McCooey, R., Davidson, B., Larkins, B., and Hickson, L. (2002). The validity of functional assessments of communication and the activity/participation components of the ICIDH-2: do they reflect what really happens in life? *Journal of Communication Disorders*, **35**, 107–37.

Worthington, A. (1999). Dysexecutive paramnesia: Strategic retrieval deficits in retrospective and prospective remembering. *Neurocase*, **5**, 47–57.

Worthington, A. D., Williams, C., Young, K., and Pownall, J. (1997). Re-training gait components for walking in the context of abulia. *Physiotherapy Theory and Practice,* **13**, 247–56.

Wortman, P. M. (1994). Judging research quality. In *The handbook of research synthesis* (eds H. Cooper and L. V. Hedges), pp. 97–109. Sage: New York.

Wright, P., Rogers, N., Hall, C., Wilson, B., Evans, J., Emslie, H., and Bartram, C. (2001). Comparison of pocket-computer memory aids for people with brain injury. *Brain Injury,* **15**(9), 787–800.

Wykes, T. (1998). What are we changing with neurocognitive rehabilitation? Illustrations from two single cases in neuropsychological performacne and brain systems as measured by SPECT. *Schizophrenia Research,* **34**, 77–86.

Wykes, T., Brammer, M., Mellers, J. *et al.* (2002). Effects on the brain of a psychological treatment – cognitive remediation therapy: functional magnetic resonance imaging in schizophrenia. *British Journal of Psychiatry,* **181**, 144–52.

Wykes, T., Reeder, C., Williams, C., Corner, J., and Everitt, B. (1999). The effects of neurocognitive remediation on executive processing in patients with schizophrenia. *Schizophrenia Bulletin,* **25**, 291–307.

Xerri, C., Coq, J. O., Merzenich, M. M., and Jenkins, W. M. (1996). Experienced-induced plasticity of cutaneous maps in the primary somatosensory cortex of adult monkeys and rats. *Journal of Physiology, Paris,* **90**, 277–87.

Yates, M., Bowen, A., Mukhtar, N., Hill, E., and Tallis, R. C. (2000). Use of a novel contingency stimulator in unilateral spatial neglect. *Neurorehabilitation,* **15**, 79–85.

Ylvisaker, M. and Feeney, T. (1998). *Collaborative brain injury intervention: positive everyday routines.* San Diego, CA: Singular Publishing Group.

Ylvisaker, M., Coelho, C., Kennedy, M., Sohlberg, M. M., Turkstra, L., Avery, J., and Yorkston, K. (2002). Reflections on evidence-based practice and rational clinical decision making. *Journal of Medical Speech-Language Pathology,* **10**(2), xxv–xxxiii.

Yonelinas, A. P. (2002). The nature of recollection and familiarity: a review of 30 years of research. *Journal of Memory and Language,* **46**, 441–517.

Yonelinas, A. P., Kroll, N. E. A., Dobbins, I., Lazzara, M., and Knight, R. T. (1998). Recollection and familiarity deficits in amnesia: convergence of remember-know, process dissociation, and receiver operating characteristic data. *Neuropsychology,* **12**, 323–39.

Zangwill, O. L. (1947). Psychological aspects of rehabilitation in cases of brain injury. *British Journal of Psychology,* **37**, 60–9.

Zangwill, O. L. (1966). Psychological deficits associated with frontal lobe lesions. *International Journal of Neurology,* **5**, 395–402.

Zarit, S. H., Zarit, J. M., and Reever, K. E. (1982). Memory training for severe memory loss: effects on senile dementia patients and their families. *The Gerontologist,* **22**, 373–37.

Zencius, A., Wesolowski, M. D., and Burke, W. H. (1990). A comparison of four memory strategies with traumatically brain-injured clients. *Brain Injury* **4**, 33–8.

Zimmerman, P. and Fimm, B. (2002). A testbattery for attentional performance, TAP. In *Applied neuropsychology of attention* (eds M. Leclercq and P. Zimmerman). London: Psychology Press.

Zülch, K. J. (1976). A critical appraisal of 'Lokalisationslehre' in the brain. *Naturwissenschaften,* **63**, 255–65.

Index